Applying the Gender Perspective in Psychiatry and Psychotherapy

Mayte López-Atanes
Margarita Sáenz-Herrero
Editors

Applying the Gender Perspective in Psychiatry and Psychotherapy

Springer

Editors
Mayte López-Atanes
Department of Psychiatry
University Hospital Galdakao-Usansolo
Galdakao, Spain

Margarita Sáenz-Herrero
Cruces University Hospital
Basque University
Barakaldo, Spain

ISBN 978-3-032-17882-4 ISBN 978-3-032-17883-1 (eBook)
https://doi.org/10.1007/978-3-032-17883-1

This Springer imprint is published by the registered company Springer Nature Switzerland AG
The registered company address is: Gewerbestrasse 11, 6330 Cham, Switzerland

Foreword

The integration of a gender perspective in healthcare is an essential transformation in the way we approach global health, particularly women's health. The androcentric bias that permeates all societies, positioning men as the universal reference and rendering women invisible, has had a profound impact on research and medical practices. In this context, integrating a gender perspective across all areas of health ensures the equitable inclusion of women throughout the research and intervention processes. This gender perspective is not limited to recognizing the biological differences between men and women but also involves understanding and incorporating the specificities of women's health, while considering the influence of gender-based social constructs in the approach to health.

The gender perspective is especially relevant in the field of mental health. Gender influences all aspects related to mental health, from the stressful situations that may trigger the onset of mental disorders to how symptoms manifest, how individuals seek help, the treatment they receive within the healthcare system, the social support available, and the societal expectations that shape these processes. Gender also plays a fundamental role in defining what is considered "normal" and "pathological."

The lack of a gender perspective in mental health has led to numerous blind spots: the overdiagnosis of certain conditions in women and the underdiagnosis of others in men; the pathologization of behaviors that deviate from gender norms; and a widespread disregard for how systemic factors—such as gender-based violence, caregiving responsibilities, reproductive health, and socioeconomic inequality—affect mental well-being. Gender bias also permeates clinical research, where diagnostic criteria, assessment tools, and treatment protocols have historically been developed without adequately accounting for sex and gender differences.

Furthermore, in mental healthcare, women have experienced androcentrism both as patients and as professionals. Throughout the history of psychiatry and psychotherapy, women have been silenced, pathologized, and marginalized. Their experiences have often been interpreted through lenses of hysteria, fragility, or emotional excess, rather than acknowledged as legitimate responses to trauma, systemic oppression, and the burden of navigating a world structured by patriarchal norms.

As President of the International Association for Women's Mental Health, I am proud to present *Applying the Gender Perspective in Psychiatry and Psychotherapy*, edited by Margarita Sáenz-Herrero and Mayte López-Atanes, both widely recognized experts in the fields of gender and mental health. This book is the product of collaboration among experts from various disciplines and countries, united in the collective recognition that mental health must always account for gender.

The book is structured into six main sections, each addressing a key dimension of the intersection between gender and mental health. It begins with general principles, offering a solid theoretical foundation. These chapters define key terms such as sex, gender roles, socialization, and stereotypes, and explore the neurobiological foundations of gender, as well as the socioeconomic and structural factors—including violence and systemic discrimination—that shape mental health.

The historical section provides crucial context for understanding how women have been represented and treated within the mental health professions, both as professionals and as patients. From the early alienists to contemporary psychiatry, it reveals patterns of exclusion and bias that continue to inform current practices.

The third section delves into gender and psychopathology, examining how diagnostic criteria and clinical research have often failed to account for gender differences. It also challenges the medicalization of emotional suffering and highlights how gender norms influence the prevalence and expression of mental health disorders.

In the fourth and fifth sections, the focus shifts to therapeutic interventions, both general and diagnosis-specific. Here, the authors present innovative approaches to psychotherapy that incorporate a gender perspective—from cognitive-behavioral and systemic therapies to integrative, humanistic, and creative modalities. These sections also explore how gender intersects with conditions such as depression, bipolar disorder, anxiety, trauma, eating disorders, psychosis, personality disorders, addiction, and more.

Finally, the last section addresses special populations and contexts, including child and adolescent psychiatry, perinatal mental health, the mental health consequences of sex-based violence, transcultural inclusion of the gender perspective, the experiences of the LGTBI+ community, as well as the mental health consequences for women in prostitution.

This book is enriched by the voices of authors from diverse backgrounds and regions, bringing invaluable international perspectives. I am especially honored to highlight that two of the contributors have been past Presidents of the International Society for Women's Mental Health, a testament to the depth of experience and leadership that has shaped this work.

This volume is more than a textbook; it is a call to action—for clinicians, researchers, educators, and policymakers alike. Let it serve as both a guide and a challenge to improve the approach to mental health, avoiding androcentric biases and promoting well-being for all people.

Psychiatrist, Parc Sanitari Sant Joan de Deu
Barcelona, Spain
Judith Usall

President of International Association
of Women Mental Health
Potomac, MD, USA

Contents

Part I

General Principles

Theoretical Background: Definitions of Sex, Gender, Gender Roles, Gender Stereotypes, Gender Socialization

1

Marta Jimenez Carrillo

Current psychiatry and psychotherapy were developed under a predominantly male gaze. Until the end of the twentieth century, the description and study of mental illnesses was dominated by the androcentric model, in which the experiences of men were supposed to be generalizable. Based on this model, the results were extrapolated to the rest of individuals. For example, homosexuality and gender dysphoria were considered mental disorders and used as diagnoses. Similarly, the diagnosis of hysteria was not removed from the Diagnostic and Statistical Manual of Mental Disorders by the American Psychiatric Association until the 1950s.

In order to introduce the sex/gender perspective into clinical practice, it is necessary, first of all, to include it in research and to base the clinical practice on studies with good gender sensitivity. Sex/gender sensitivity in research begins with the correct use of both concepts. Sex is a biological quality or classification of sexually reproducing organisms, usually female, male, and/or intersex, according to functions that derive from chromosomal complement, reproductive organs, or specific hormones or environmental factors that affect the expression of phenotypic traits that are strongly associated with females or males within a given species. Gender refers to cultural expectations, behaviors, and beliefs about what constitutes being male or female. Although these concepts are often treated as a binary, they can also be viewed in a continuum or as interrelated [1, 2]. For example, Judith Butler rejects the dichotomous view and understands sex itself as a social construct, because of the ways cultural values and practices interrelate with "natural" biology, and so inherently effect the classification of bodies as either "male" or "female."

M. J. Carrillo (✉)
Institut Català de Salut (ICS), Barcelona, Spain

Research Group on Social Determinants of Health and Demographic Change (OPIK), Sociology Department, University of Basque Country (UPV/EHU), Leioa, Spain
e-mail: martajimenez.bcn.ics@gencat.cat

M. López-Atanes, M. Sáenz-Herrero (eds.), *Applying the Gender Perspective in Psychiatry and Psychotherapy*, https://doi.org/10.1007/978-3-032-17883-1_1

The introduction of sex and gender as fundamental pillars of research excellence is a relatively new phenomenon. The academic study of gender dates back to the late 1960s, with the second wave of feminism. Until then, the gender construct was not included in research as such, and differences in health were attributed to biological differences. In the particular case of psychotherapy, the Freudian model merely attributed the etiology of mental pathology to gender (specifically with regard to the relationship with parents). Nowadays, numerous international institutions, such as Canadian Institute of Health Research [3], the European Union [4, 5] or the European Association of Science Editors [6], have published recommendations on how to correctly introduce the variables of sex, gender, as well as their interaction with other sociodemographic variables such as race or migration background. The recognition that individuals are defined by multiple intersecting dimensions, such as gender, social class, ethnicity, (dis)ability, sexuality, age, etc., is called intersectionality, and some authors suggest the inclusion of power relations based on gender and social context [7].

A critical analysis of current praxis is needed to identify research gaps and promote more gender-inclusive clinical practice. This means considering how sex, gender, and associated factors may influence the approach to the patient, the efficacy of therapy, or the manifestation of psychopathology. It is also important to evaluate the current research that supports clinical practice and to assess whether or not the gender perspective was included. For example, it is necessary to assess whether the clinical trials underpinning our clinical practices also included non-binary or trans individuals and whether they took into account an intersectional approach.

In this book, we aim to offer a critical view of current psychiatry and psychotherapy, as well as to provide alternatives from a gender perspective based on existing evidence and gender theories. It is important to keep in mind that gender studies is not synonymous with women's studies and that our aim is also to assess how the masculine gender impacts the mental health of people who identify as men. At the same time, we intend to evaluate how other concepts such as gender identity, sexual orientation or race, intimately linked to gender, can modify mental health. Here, we offer a possible structure that may help to develop the various chapters. This does not imply that all chapters must follow the following structure, as some may not need to address all points.

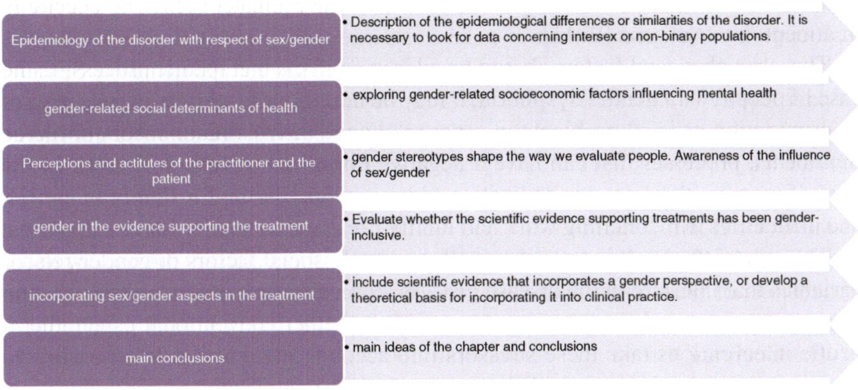

1.1 Epidemiology of the Disorder

Sex/gender differences in the epidemiology, symptomatology, and risk factors for mental illness have been described. In general, women tend to be overrepresented in anxious depressive or trauma-related disorders, whereas men constitute the majority of patients with substance abuse disorders and psychopathic behaviors. Other disorders, however, lack sex/gender differences, such as bipolar disorder type 1 [8]. In addition, the onset of presentation also varies; in the case of psychosis, women have a higher risk of late onset psychosis. With respect to non-binary or transgender individuals, research is scarce and they are often relegated in clinical guidelines or psychiatry textbooks. The main reason is the persistent idea that gender is a binary construct and, for this reason, these populations are neglected.

One of the aims of the book is to provide a brief description of sex/gender differences or similarities in mental illness. It would also be necessary to examine whether the course of illness differs or, on the contrary, is similar according to sex/gender. In addition, if there are published studies, information on the epidemiology of mental disorders in non-binary and transgender populations should be included.

1.2 Gender-Related Social Determinants of Health

The World Health Organization's Commission on Social Determinants of Health has defined SDH as "the conditions under which people are born, grow, live, work and age" and "the fundamental drivers of these conditions." The term "social determinants" often refers to factors which can influence health-related behaviors. In fact, they can account for between 30% and 55% of health outcomes.

Sex and gender interact with other sociodemographic variables, such as age, race, sexual orientation, caregiver strain, or experience of discrimination. Gender can also influence exposure to diseases or risk factors and access to health care. For example, older women with addiction problems have greater difficulty accessing treatment due to stigma [9–11].

These psychosocial factors should be addressed in the therapeutic process. In the case of people with gender dysphoria, it may be necessary to address experiences of discrimination or legal problems in order to change their name or access hormone treatments, processes that can have a negative impact on their mental state. In the case of women, their greater dedication to housework, caring for family members, and difficulties in reconciling work and family life can lead to depressive symptoms.

The aim of the book is to evaluate all the psychosocial factors or gender-related variables that interfere in the disease process, clinical course, symptomatology, and access to treatment. It is necessary to consider whether conventional psychotherapeutic interventions take these stressors into account and whether it is possible to improve them in order to provide better psychotherapeutic care.

1.3 Perceptions and Attitudes of the Practitioner and the Patient

Gender stereotypes are general expectations about certain members of social groups. Gender stereotypes reflect the primary importance we place on task performance when judging men and on social relationships when considering women. People often rely on these beliefs and convictions without realizing it. People behave differently toward women and men and have different attitudes and expectations toward them. More importantly, it has been shown that individuals who exhibit counter-stereotypical behaviors or behaviors that do not conform to our stereotypical idea are often undervalued by the observer. Although individuals may be reluctant to admit that they hold these beliefs, the truth is that most of us rely on these ideas and demonstrate it in our behavior, choices, and evaluation of others [12, 13].

Language also represents a fundamental part of human communication. Do professionals use different language depending on the gender of a patient with a given mental disorder? What language do they use when confronted with a woman with substance abuse disorders? Do they engage in more judgmental terminology and are they aware of it? With respect to the patient, gender influences health-seeking behaviors, illness perception, and healthcare utilization. How the patient acts and reacts is of utmost importance, as many diseases include diagnostic criteria based on patient behavior. For example, histrionic personality disorder includes excessive seductive behavior. However, this is assessed according to the practitioner's perception of what it means to be seductive. It is also possible that a given patient may show different responses or reveal different life experiences depending on the gender and attitude of the practitioner. All these factors should be evaluated (if research exists to address them) or theorized if possible.

The aim of the book is to explain how gender influences the attitudes, perceptions, evaluations, or behaviors of both therapists and patients. For example, in women with substance abuse disorders, professionals may show a critical attitude unconsciously, due to the stigma that weighs on this population. The same is true for males with eating disorders: being a pathology mainly associated with women, professionals take longer to diagnose them due to gender stereotypes. There may be no research or recommendations on how the therapist should address his or her own attitudes or stereotypes regarding gender. in that case, it would be reasonable to develop a new theoretical construct or provide recommendations on how to address these aspects in the psychotherapeutic process.

1.4 Gender in the Evidence Supporting Treatment Decisions

The aim of the book is to explore the current evidence and assess the extent to which sex/gender has been included. Both clinical practice guidelines and the main studies behind the clinical recommendations can be explored. Some of the points to assess are:

- The representativeness of the sample: Have men, women, and non-binary individuals been included in the sample under study?
- the inclusion of gender-related variables, such as sexual orientation, age, race, or domestic work.
- Disaggregation of data: Have sex/gender disaggregated data been provided or have they been generalized?

In addition, it is pertinent to look for studies with good gender sensitivity and compare whether their results are similar or different from those that do not include it. In general, the guidelines do not differentiate between women, men, or intersex individuals. The SAGER guidelines can serve as a guideline for assessing the gender sensitivity of studies [6].

1.5 Incorporating the Gender Perspective in Treatment

The last point, and probably the most important, is to provide advice on how to introduce the gender perspective in the therapy and evaluation of patients. Although there are recommendations on how to work with specific populations in which gender is fundamental (victims of gender violence or gender diverse people), it is necessary to include this perspective in all therapeutic processes, since gender is a fundamental element of the human experience. The experience of a disease cannot be separated from the experience of gender. In interpersonal relationships, including the psychotherapeutic environment, the experience of gender is also present and influences how we behave.

Psychosocial aspects must be included. For example, female victims of gender-based violence may present with depressive symptoms but, in this case, treatment would involve gender empowerment interventions and psychosocial support to help the patient emerge from her situation of violence. Transgender people are victims of ongoing discrimination, difficulties to access the job market and social isolation. In this context, often present with depressive symptoms, substance abuse, and suicidal ideation, symptoms that cannot be separated from the social context in which they take place. Studies have shown that men present attitudinal barriers to accessing mental health treatment, concluding that service delivery must adapt to better respond to dominant masculine ideals while also improving men's ease of access.

How to effectively make effective gendered interventions in all of these situations is yet to be determined and in many other therapeutic contexts will probably have to be developed from scratch. Each chapter of the book should adapt this perspective to the given topic, first by reviewing the literature but also by putting forward a new model of psychotherapy and psychiatric approach that works with these aspects.

References

1. Clayton JA, Tannenbaum C. Reporting sex, gender, or both in clinical research? JAMA. 2016;316(18):1863–4.
2. Krieger N. Genders, sexes, and health: what are the connections—and why does it matter? Int J Epidemiol [Internet]. 2003;32(4):652–7. Available from: https://doi.org/10.1093/ije/dyg156.
3. Government of Canada CI of HR. How to integrate sex and gender into research – CIHR [Internet]. 2018. Available from: https://cihr-irsc.gc.ca/e/50836.html.
4. European Commission, Directorate-General for Research and Innovation. Approaches to inclusive gender equality in research and innovation (R&I). Publications Office of the European Union; 2022.
5. European Commission, Directorate-General for Research and Innovation. Gender in EU-funded research: toolkit. Publications Office; 2014.
6. Heidari S, Babor TF, De Castro P, Tort S, Curno M. Sex and gender equity in research: rationale for the SAGER guidelines and recommended use. Res Integr Peer Rev. 2016;1:2.
7. Hammarström A, Johansson K, Annandale E, Ahlgren C, Aléx L, Christianson M, et al. Central gender theoretical concepts in health research: the state of the art. J Epidemiol Community Health (1978). 2014;68(2):185–90.
8. Riecher-Rössler A. Sex and gender differences in mental disorders. Lancet Psychiatry. 2017;4(1):8–9.
9. Blow FC, Barry KL. Use and misuse of alcohol among older women. Alcohol Res Health. 2002;26(4):308–15.
10. Koenig TL, Crisp C. Ethical issues in practice with older women who misuse substances. Subst Use Misuse [Internet]. 2008;43(8–9):1045–61. Available from: https://doi.org/10.1080/10826080801914246.
11. Brennan PL, Moos RH, et al. Gender differences in the individual characteristics and life contexts of late-middle-aged and older problem drinkers. Addiction [Internet]. 2021;88(2):127–38. Available from: https://doi.org/10.1080/08952841.2019.1684176.
12. Ellemers N. Gender stereotypes. Annu Rev Psychol [Internet]. 2018;69(1):275–98. Available from: https://doi.org/10.1146/annurev-psych-122216-011719.
13. Nadal KL. Gender stereotypes. In: The SAGE encyclopedia of psychology and gender. Thousand Oaks: SAGE; 2017. p. 1–24.

Sex, Gender, and Neurobiology of the Brain

2

Rafael Segarra Echevarria, María Santaolalla Sánchez, and Beatriz Isabel Molina Cañas

2.1 A Brief Introduction to the Concept of "Healthy" Sexuality

Human sexuality is a multifaceted construct shaped by biological, psychological, and socio-cultural factors. As inherently social beings, humans rely on relational networks for emotional and physical development. Neuroscientists like Damasio [1] emphasize that interpersonal interactions form the basis of selfhood and consciousness, with feelings playing a critical role in cultural and psychological processes.

Three pillars underpin human sexuality:

1. Biological Factors: hormonal, genetic, and neurodevelopmental mechanisms drive sexual differentiation. More recent studies have founded new hypothesis such that immune system derives mast cells which are a primary target for the masculinizing hormone estradiol and that mast cells are in turn the primary mediators of brain sexual differentiation. These findings identify a novel non-neuronal origin of brain sex differences and resulting motivated behaviors [2]. A study published more recently [3] highlights the role of estradiol-responsive mast cells in brain masculinization, cerebral cortical copy number variations

R. S. Echevarria (✉)
Basque Country University, Leioa, Biscay, Spain

Psychiatry Department, Cruces University Hospital, Bilbao, Spain
e-mail: RAFAEL.SEGARRAECHEVARRIA@osakidetza.eus

M. S. Sánchez
Department of Psychiatry, Reina Sofía University Hospital, Córdoba, Spain

B. I. M. Cañas
Cruces University Hospital, Bilbao, Spain

M. López-Atanes, M. Sáenz-Herrero (eds.), *Applying the Gender Perspective in Psychiatry and Psychotherapy*, https://doi.org/10.1007/978-3-032-17883-1_2

(CNVs) contributing to neural diversity and evolving genetic/genomic insights into brain structure and behavior.
2. Individual Psychosexuality: encompasses sexual identity, emotional bonds, and personal life experiences.
3. Socio-cultural Environment: Shapes, Norms, and Expressions of Sexuality.

John Money's "relay race" model [4] illustrates how genetic, hormonal, environmental, and psychosocial factors sequentially influence sexual development, with all interacting to achieve mature, healthy sexuality. This integrative framework underscores the dynamic interplay of nature and nurture in human sexual identity.

2.2 Psychosexual Development

The sex of the embryo is usually determined at the moment of fertilization, depending on the chromosome of the spermatozoid, either X or Y. However, during human embryogenesis, some weeks go by without noticeable differences, even under an electronic microscope, between a female and a male fetus [5]. This is known as the sexually undifferentiated period in the sexual development [6].

Recent studies have shown that male rates had greater numbers and more activated mast cells in the cortical preoptic area (POA), a brain region essential for male copulatory behavior, than female littermates during the critical period for sexual differentiation. Inhibiting mast cells with a stabilizing agent blunted the masculinization of both POA neuronal and microglial morphology and adult sex behavior, whereas activating mast cells in females, even though fewer in number, induced masculinization. Treatment of newborn females with a masculinizing dose of estradiol increased mast cell number and induced mast cells to release histamine, which stimulated the microglia to release prostaglandins and thereby induced male typical synaptic patterning. These findings identify a novel non-neuronal but immunity an inflammatory origin of brain sex differences and resulting motivated behaviors [2].

Or even it almost demonstrated the existence of myriad CNVs which genomically diversify neural cells before incorporation into the mature organization of the brain [3].

During the undifferentiated period, the gonadal crests, outlines of the future gonads, are bipotential, and will evolve into testicles or ovaries depending on the genetic make-up. In parallel, in the same mesoderm, we find Wolff's mesonephric duct and Müller's paramesonephric duct, both outlines of the internal genitalia as well, but unipotentials in this case.

With regard to the external genitalia, they result from the cloaca and the cloacal membrane, the urorectal septum being in charge of the urogenital division of the rectum. All the genital outlines are bipotential, with a differentiation dependent on the presence or absence of testicular hormones.

Sexual differentiation comes to establish, in normal conditions, around the seventh week of the embryonic development, considered since the last menstruation date [6].

Thus, in the XY individuals, the gonadal crests are differentiated forming the fetal testicles, the germinal cells of which, differentiated into spermatogonial cells, will divide through mitosis, not entering meiosis until puberty. These cells are accompanied, forming the seminiferous tubules, by the Sertoli cells, of somatic origin, and the Leydig cells, at an interstitial level, in charge of the expression of proteins that are key in the consequent sexual differentiation, among which we can find the Anti-Müllerian Hormone (AMH).

In the case of fetuses XX, the gonads stay with an undifferentiated appearance for a longer period of time. Moreover, and also unlike the XY fetus, the germinal cells, differentiated into oogonial cells, proliferate through mitosis until the fourth month, when they initiate the meiosis stage until the diplotene stage, which stops shortly before birth, restarting at puberty with each ovaric cycle.

The presence of the functional Y chromosome becomes the determining factor of the sexual development of the fetal gonad. Concretely, in its short arm, we find the SRY gene (Sex-determining Region Y-chromosome). Although the cell mechanisms through which it works aren't precisely known yet, the gene SRY is deemed to perform the migration function and that of differentiating all the three main cell structures [6]:

- We find the germinal cells differentiation into spermatogenic cells.
- The Sertoli cells start to show a specific pattern of expression characterized by an increase of SOX9 (protein of the SRY family) and of AMH, together with a reduction of DAX1 levels, its gene being located in the X chromosome.
- There is experimental evidence that SRY and DAX1 interact in early stages of the gonadal crests. Thus:

  In XY individuals, there is only one allele of the SRY gene, and just one allele of the DAX1 gene. In such conditions, SRY seems to be dominant and allows the testicular differentiation with the resulting expression of genes typically testicular, such as SOX9 and AMH. Nevertheless, not only the SRY levels but also their chronology of expression will be determining, given that a delay in the expression of SRY would allow an anti-testicular action of DAX1.

  In XX individuals, the absence of SRY results in an increase of DAX1 levels in the gonad that is differentiated in an ovaric sense. In spite of that, DAX1 does not appear to be essential for the development of the ovary, for mice DAX1 Knock-out do present, a fact that has classically led to conclude that the mere absence of SRY results in the ovary development. However, although the absence of SRY is imperative, it seems logical to imagine that some kind of pro-ovaric genes must exist, unknown to date.
- Finally, from week eighth of pregnancy, the Leydig cells will be in charge of the androgen production.

On the basis of such provisions, we can sum up the sexual differentiation process as follows.

- Internal genitalia. Under the action of the testicular androgens, the Wolffian mesonephric ducts give rise in the male fetus to the epididymis, vasa deferentia and seminal vesicles. In the female sex, given the absence of anti-Müllerian hormone (AMH), the Müllerian paramesonephric ducts form the uterine tubes, the uterus, and the upper third of the vagina. Therefore, the Wollfian ducts degenerate in the XX fetus due to the lack of androgens, whereas the Müllerian ducts return in the XY fetus by action of the AMH. It should be noted that the action time frame of the AMH is short: the testicular secretion starts by the end of the seventh week, and the Müllerian ducts become refractory to its action from the tenth week.
- External genitalia: the undifferentiated outlines evolve into male structures under the action of the dihydrotestosterone, a powerful androgen derived from the action of the 5-α-reductase enzyme on the testosterone. Thus, the genital tubercle originates the penis, whereas the labioscrotal folds enlarge and fuse in the ante-posterior sense to form the scrotal bags. In the female fetus, the lack of androgens allows the genital tubercle to originate the clitoris, and the urogenital folds to remain separate forming the labia majora. However, the mere presence of testosterone and AMH is not enough, for the final action will depend on the binding of each molecule to its specific receptor, and on the proper functioning of the subsequent molecular cascade.

Well then, that same sexual differentiation phenomenon proves to be more complex and determinant, given that under the influence of the sexual hormones circulating in the fetus, the dimorphic development of certain brain areas is produced as well. Furthermore, the brain like the internal genitalia is monotypic and in it also prevails the feminization principle, unless there is an adequate level of circulating androgens [7].

Sexual differentiation of the human brain takes place approximately between weeks 16 and 28 of the embryonic development, and the specific hypothalamic and hypophyseal functions (cyclic in women and no cyclic in men) are determined in that moment.

The hypothalamus is considered to be the main regulating center of sexual behavior in humans. The preoptic nucleus is produced by the hormone that releases gonadotropins (GnRH), which stimulates the anterior pituitary so it can in turn produce the luteinizing hormone (LH) and the follicle-stimulating hormone (FSH). Both control the steroid hormone secretion by the gonads (estradiol, progesterone, and testosterone).

This complex system of hypothalamus-hypophysis-gonads presents a secretory self-regulation by means of positive and negative feedback mechanisms [7]. Moreover, the GnRH modulates the catecholaminergic neurotransmission, direct and indirect arbiter of the sexual output of the individual (while dopamine stimulates the sexual function, and serotonin and prolactin inhibit it, becoming crucial in this field the balance between dopamine and serotonin). Other substances implicated in the complex world of the neurochemical interactions that modulate human sexuality are GABA, ACTH, cortisol-releasing peptide, endogenous opioids, and acetylcholine [8].

A gender approach should be taken into consideration regarding neurotransmitter systems and their clinical differences. Altered glutamatergic transmission is linked to schizophrenia (SCZ), with sex-specific differences observed. Women with SCZ show unique genetic risks (e.g., GRIA3 polymorphisms on the X chromosome) [9, 10], elevated glutamine synthetase (regulating glutamate) [10], and higher NMDA receptor density, which may mitigate symptoms by countering NMDA hypofunction [11]. These findings suggest protective mechanisms in women and underscore the need for gender-tailored therapies [12].

Secondary sexual characteristics, regulated by the Central Nervous System (CNS) and hormonal surges (androgens/estrogens), emerge during puberty, though the exact CNS trigger remains unclear, potentially linked to reduced hypothalamic sensitivity to feedback [13]. Hormonal imbalances can alter physical traits, but psychosocial factors dominate sexual desire and behavior post-puberty. McConaghy suggests that psychosocial influences are stronger in females, though research gaps persist [14].

Sexual identity forms through early social interactions and affective bonds, with healthy sexuality rooted in intimacy, empathy, and trust, transcending mere reproduction. While Freud emphasized libidinal pleasure, post-Freudians like Fairbairn prioritize relational dynamics [15].

Psychoanalytic theories highlight early relationships in shaping gender identity and orientation. Kernberg links object–relation dyads (self-object-affect) to internal psychological structures [13, 14], while Stoller notes gender identity forms in infancy [16–19]. The Oedipal Complex is now deemphasized as a cultural myth, with critiques of psychoanalysis' androcentrism and the marginalization of paternal roles [20].

Sexual arousal, tied to the limbic system, integrates cognitive-affective states, driving both physiological responses (e.g., genital arousal) and psychological excitement [1]. Because the sexual activation also includes the implementation of the limbic system under the influence of a particular cognitive-affective state, which stimulates the peripheral and central nervous systems that determine the congestion, lubrication, and increases focused sensitivity of the genital organs, providing a central feedback "self-realization" of that genital activation and the subsequent psychological excitement.

In that regard, Kernberg [13, 14, 21, 22] adds that the sexual arousal is a specific affection that shows all the features of the affective structures and constitutes the central building block of the so-called sexual or libidinal drive as general motivational system. Sexual arousal is the basic affection that constrains the appearance of a more complex psychological phenomenon, erotic desire, in which the sexual arousal appears bound with the emotional relationship with a specific subject.

The source of desire is not an anatomic body, but a body that is built through the array of discourses and intersubjective practices. Both girls and boys organize themselves through their relationship with other subjects (for instance, the mother) who are not just objects for the child, because both the girl and the boy are able to recognize that subject as different from them and, at the same time, as akin. That way the intersubjectivity plays a role in the structuring of the psychological world. It may be noted that uneven consequences arise from a double sexual standard, the fact that admiring women or giving them recognition only for their physical attributes poses a difficulty to their mental balance, as well as the extra-work to which the female psyche is set out if it intends to reconcile the multiplicity of demands of its motivational systems [23].

To conclude this brief thought, we will attempt to define in a simple and operational way what there is a general agreement to consider an "abnormal or deviant" sexual behavior, that is:

That is destructive or damaging to the subject who displays it and to those who get involved in it.
That is not oriented to the other in a strict sense.
That excludes the stimulation of the own genital organs and those of the partner.
That is inappropriately associated to feelings of guilt and/or anxiety.
And that shows a repetitive nature of a compulsive kind.

We share with many authors a preoccupation arisen from the manifest neglect in the clinical practice to document the medical/sexual history and its psychopathological manifestations in the individuals who visit the doctor. More frequently than would be desirable, it is the health professional themselves (unlike the patients) who perceive this issue as a complicated area to explore, and thus subject to be avoided. It is essential to explore the patient's love life, including sexual patterns as well as the fantasies and the nature of the object–relations that are established in the context of their sexual behavior [24].

References

1. Damasio A. The strange order of things: life, feeling and the making of cultures. Toronto: Penguin Random House Canada Limited; 2018.
2. Lenz KM, Pickett LA, Wright CL, Davis KT, Joshi A, McCarthy MM. Mast cells in the developing brain determine adult sexual behavior. J Neurosci. 2018;38(37):8044–59.
3. Rohrback S, April C, Kaper F, Rivera RR, Liu CS, Siddoway B, Chun J. Submegabase copy number variations arise during cerebral cortical neurogenesis as revealed by single-cell whole-genome sequencing. PNAS. 2018;115(42):10804–9.
4. Money J. Handbook of sexology. New York: Elsevier/North Holland; 1978.
5. McCarthy MM. A new view of sexual differentiation of mammalian brain. J Comp Physiol A Neuroethol Sens Neural Behav Physiol. 2020;206:369–78.
6. Rey RA. Fetal sex differentiation: from molecules to anatomy. Rev Chil Anat. 2001;19(1):75–82.
7. Young S, Cocallis K. A systematic review of relationship between neurodiversity and psychosexual functioning in individuals with Autism Spectrum Disorder (ASD) or Attention-Deficit/Hyperactivity Disorder (ADHD). Neuropsychiatr Dis Treat. 2023;19:1379–95.
8. Rey RA, Grinspon RP. Normal male sexual differentiation and aetiology of disorders of sex development. Best Pract Res Clin Endocrinol Metab. 2011;25(2):221–38.
9. Wickens MM, Bangasser DA, Briand LA. Sex differences in psychiatry disease: a focus on the glutamate system. Front Mol Neurosci. 2018;11:197.
10. Magri C, Gardella R, Valsecchi P, Barlati SD, Guizzetti L, Imperadori L. Study on GRIA2, GRIA3 and GRIA4 genes highlights a positive association between schizophrenia and GRIA3 in female patients. Am J Med Genet B Neuropsychiatr Genet. 2008;147B:745–53.

11. Martins-de-Souza D, Maccarrone G, Wobrock T, Zerr I, Gormanns P, Reckow S. Proteome analysis of the thalamus and cerebrospinal fluid reveals glycolysis dysfunction and potential biomarkers candidates for schizophrenia. J Psychiatr Res. 2010;44:1176–89.
12. Nudmamud-Thanoi S, Reynolds GP. The NR1 subunit of the glutamate/NMDA receptor in the superior temporal cortex in schizophrenia and affective disorders. Neurosci Lett. 2004;372:173–7.
13. Lotter LD, Sabieri A, Hansen JY, Misic B, Paquola C, Barker GJ, Arun L, Bodke W, Desrivieres S, Flor H, Grigis A, et al. Relating patterns of human cortex development correlate with underlying neurobiology. Nat Commun. 2024;15:7987.
14. Kernberg O. Love relations. Normality and pathology. New Haven: Yale University Press; 1998.
15. Kernberg O. The sexual couple. A psychoanalytic exploration. Psychoanal Rev. 2011;98:217–45.
16. Fairbairn WRD. Psychoanalytic studies of personality. London: Taylor & Francis Ltd.; 1969.
17. Stoller RJ. The transsexual experiment. London: Karnac Books; 1975.
18. Stoller RJ. Sex and gender. London: Karnac Books; 1984.
19. Stoller RJ. Presentations of gender. New Haven: Yale Univ Press; 1985.
20. Stoller RJ. Perversion, the erotic form of hatred. London: Karnac Books; 1986.
21. Dio Bleichmar E. Female sexuality. Barcelona: Paidós; 1997.
22. Kernberg O. Limitations to the capacity to love. In: Kernberg O, editor. The inseparable nature of love and aggression. Washington, DC: American Psychiatric Publishing; 2012.
23. Kernberg O. Sexual pathology in borderline patients. In: Kernberg O, editor. The inseparable nature of love and aggression. Washington, DC: American Psychiatric Publishing; 2012.
24. Irigaray L. This sex which is not one. New York: Cornell University Press; 1985.

Gender-Related Determinants and Socioeconomic Aspects of Mental Health

3

Tilman Brand and Daniela Fuhr

3.1 Introduction

Mental health disorders represent a major global health challenge, contributing significantly to the overall burden of disease. Epidemiological studies have consistently demonstrated gender disparities in the prevalence of mental health conditions. For instance, the Global Burden of Disease Study 2019 reported that women experience higher disability-adjusted life-year (DALY) rates due to major depressive disorder compared to men—564 versus 354 per 100,000 individuals, respectively. This disparity persists across various age groups and regions worldwide [40].

While numerous studies have highlighted gender differences in mental health, it is essential to acknowledge that measurement and reporting biases may influence observed patterns. Research indicates that women are more likely to report symptoms and seek help, which could contribute to higher diagnosed prevalence rates. However, studies have found no significant gender differences in the severity of reported symptoms or the likelihood of disclosing them, suggesting that such biases do not fully explain the observed disparities [52, 75].

In this chapter, we examine gender differences in mental health within the broader framework of the social determinants of health by:

- Describing the general association between socioeconomic inequality and mental health;
- Elaborating on the intersection of gender, other indicators of socioeconomic position, and mental health; and

T. Brand (✉) · D. Fuhr
Leibniz Institute for Prevention Research and Epidemiology – BIPS, Bremen, Germany
e-mail: brand@leibniz-bips.de; fuhr@leibniz-bips.de

M. López-Atanes, M. Sáenz-Herrero (eds.), *Applying the Gender Perspective in Psychiatry and Psychotherapy*, https://doi.org/10.1007/978-3-032-17883-1_3

- Analyzing exposures that are either differentially distributed across genders or have gender-specific effects on mental health.

Finally, we illustrate the impact of social and gender-related determinants on mental health using the example of the Covid-19 pandemic.

3.2 Socioeconomic Inequality and Mental Health

The World Health Organization's framework on the social determinants of health posits that health inequities—unjust differences in health outcomes between social groups—are driven by structural factors and mediated by more proximal influences such as health-related behaviors [64]. Structural factors encompass the socioeconomic and political conditions that shape the social hierarchy and define individuals' socioeconomic positions (SEPs).

SEP is primarily determined by education level, occupation, and income (plus wealth). These dimensions are interrelated: education influences access to certain occupations, which in turn affects potential income [25]. In essence, SEP determines access to scarce societal resources—such as knowledge, money, political power, and social networks—that individuals can leverage to protect and promote their health [51]. Each component of SEP has distinct health implications: education enhances cognitive skills necessary to navigate complex health systems [68]; occupation defines levels of workplace stress as a result of job-related demand and control [65], and income provides individuals with the means to improve their living conditions—such as residing in safe, green neighborhoods—and access healthcare services [9, 79, 83, 85].

SEP is a well-established determinant of mental health. Individuals with lower SEP face an increased risk of various mental disorders, including depression, anxiety, and substance use disorders [3, 34, 42]. For example, a study conducted in the Basque Country, Spain, found that individuals aged 1–30 years from lower-income households exhibited higher prevalence rates of mental disorders and were at greater risk of psychiatric hospitalization and mortality [43].

The WHO framework outlines two primary models to explain the relationship between socioeconomic status (SES) and mental health:

- Social Causation Model: This model suggests that stressors associated with low SEP—such as financial strain, limited access to resources, and unsafe living environments—increase the risk of developing mental health problems.
- Social Selection Model: This model posits that individuals with mental health disorders may experience downward social mobility due to difficulties in maintaining employment or achieving educational goals.

These models are not mutually exclusive and may interact, contributing to a cyclical relationship between socioeconomic inequality and mental health.

3.3 Intersection of Gender, Socioeconomic Inequality, and Mental Health

The intersection of gender and SEP further compounds mental health disparities. As demonstrated by the Gender Inequality Index, women around the world often occupy a lower socioeconomic position than men, characterized by reduced access to secondary education and lower labor market participation [78]. In addition to lower participation, labor markets tend to be gender-segregated both horizontally (with more women working in lower paid economic sectors) and vertically (with fewer women in top positions within occupations), contributing to lower overall earnings among women [23]. While gender inequality is more pronounced in low- and middle-income countries, it remains a significant issue in high-income countries as well. For example, the Gender Overall Earnings Gap 2024 index shows that the average monthly income of women in Germany was 37% lower than that of men—largely due to lower labor market participation and a higher prevalence of part-time employment among women. Even after excluding these factors, the unadjusted Gender Pay Gap in Germany shows a wage difference of 16% per hour worked between women and men, while the adjusted Gender Pay Gap, which controls for both horizontal and vertical labor market segregation, still indicates a difference of 6% [17]. Additionally, approximately 80% of all single-parent households in the EU are headed by women. Single parenthood is a major risk factor for poverty and is associated with a higher mental health burden [38, 56]. Taken together, these underlying processes of social stratification place women at greater risk for socioeconomic hardship—and, consequently, for poorer mental health outcomes.

3.4 Differential Exposures and Consequences

Beyond structural inequalities, gender norms shape differential exposures to stressors and influence how certain life events affect the mental health of women and men.

- Multiple Burden and "Women in the Middle": Despite increasing labor market participation, women still disproportionately bear the burden of domestic responsibilities and unpaid caregiving [22, 28]. Many women balance paid employment with caregiving duties, especially middle-aged women who care for both their children and elderly parents or in-laws—often referred to as "women in the middle" or "sandwich carers" [60]. Women tend to provide unpaid care not only more frequently but also more intensively, exposing them to chronic stress [21]. While caregiving and fulfilling multiple roles can be rewarding, research consistently shows that informal caregiving—especially sandwich caregiving—negatively impacts mental health for both women and men [54, 88]. Studies focusing on gender differences have found that the negative effects of caregiving are more pronounced in women than in men [8, 14, 81].
- Exposure to Intimate Partner and Sexual Violence: Gender inequalities in society are often mirrored by power imbalances in the domestic sphere. While men are

more frequently exposed to physical interpersonal violence, women are significantly more likely to experience intimate partner and sexual violence [29, 48]. These experiences contribute to increased rates of post-traumatic stress disorder (PTSD), depression, and anxiety among women [50]. Furthermore, a recent population-wide survey from Sweden highlighted the intersection of gender and sexual orientation, finding that non-heterosexual women and men are at the highest risk for recurrent sexual victimization [16].

- Marital and Employment Instability: Earlier research suggested that men benefit more from marriage than women in terms of mental well-being and mortality in heterosexual couples [76]. However, more recent findings from international surveys and longitudinal studies show that marriage is associated with better mental health for both women and men. Specifically, married women are at lower risk of substance abuse, while married men show reduced risks of depression and panic disorders [27, 61]. The dissolution of marriages or cohabiting relationships has become increasingly common in Western societies, and negative mental health effects—such as increased antidepressant use—have been observed in both genders [33]. Some studies indicate that women report the highest mental health burden in the period before separation, while men report the greatest burden after the breakup [58]. Additionally, men tend to re-partner sooner, while women often experience longer term economic disadvantages, increasing their risk of poverty [39]. Besides family status, job loss and job insecurity have been identified as important mental health stressors in working-age adults [13, 36]. Due to gender-segregated labor markets, women are more likely to experience job insecurity [44]. However, research suggests that job loss and job insecurity have a greater negative impact on men's mental health, potentially due to underlying gender norms and societal expectations [69].

In summary, gendered patterns of exposure to life events and adversities significantly influence mental health outcomes. In some cases, men and women experience and respond to these stressors in different ways. Overall, differential exposure to stressors helps explain, at least in part, why women tend to report a higher mental health burden.

3.5 Example: Mental Health During the Covid-19 Pandemic

It was in the first quarter of 2020 when the WHO declared Covid-19 to be a global pandemic [11]. Early advice included to halt the spread of the disease by social distancing measures which was at the height of the outbreak enforced by governments through national lockdowns, closure of borders, and compulsory quarantine of infected persons [10]. This was recommended to not only contain local and national outbreaks but to also protect vulnerable population groups such as the chronically ill and the elderly from negative health consequences. The shutdown of economies drastically affected work arrangements and income for entire populations, but also social life as direct contact with friends and next of kin had to be avoided [1]. Multiple stress factors accumulated and led to high psycho-social distress among many. Stressors included indirect threats to poor mental health such as economic instability, the worry of loss of income, lack of social support and social isolation, and at times increased conflict within the family [87]. Psychological distress was also incurred by more direct threats, and this included the fear of risk of exposure to Covid-19 and the anxiety of infecting loved ones and vulnerable family members. Symptoms of depression surged by 27% during the first year of the pandemic, and similar increments were seen for anxiety disorders (25%, respectively) [5]. Harmful use of alcohol increased too and was often used as a coping mechanism to deal with uncertainties and worries surrounding the pandemic, particularly by men [72]. Not everyone's mental health deteriorated though. Mental health trends with regard to prevalence and mental health trajectories were not linear, and a substantive proportion of the population remained resilient or did improve their mental health from the first to the later waves [53, 71].

It did not take long before it became apparent that the pandemic exacerbated the influence of social determinants of mental health and widened health inequalities for specific groups [63]. For example, female gender, people with socio-economic difficulties (i.e., living in deprivation), and those with pre-existing health conditions were named as risk factors of poor mental health during the pandemic, although evidence is mixed for people who already had a mental health condition at the onset of the pandemic [1, 5, 66]. Due to its synergistic effect on health outcomes, Covid-19 was characterized as syndemic [31] as the virus did intersect with those broader social and economic determinants of mental health and created distinct challenges for these particular groups.

Women seem to have been greatly affected during the Covid-19 pandemic [5] and gender discrepancy in prevalence of depression during the pandemic may be due to a variety of factors including gender norms, inequality in household responsibilities [20, 41], but also hormonal and biological mechanisms [2] reflecting the etiology of the disease. A double burden was experienced and often articulated by women who were juggling paid work, children as well as family life simultaneously which resulted in a high mental load [15]. Consequently, higher symptoms of depression, anxiety, and post-traumatic stress disorder (PTSD) were reported by women compared to men [20]. Help-seeking may be greater among women than men [49] and women may be generally more likely to report symptoms of common mental health problems, contributing to the higher prevalence that we see [73]. Still, evidence also suggests that women who underwent paid regular work were more likely to lose their jobs during the pandemic, exposing them to precarious social and financial circumstances; this was due to the fact that women are usually to a greater extend employed informally [32, 77]. This is why some studies reported that a reduction in income was associated with higher psycho-social distress among women, but not men [20]. Contributing factors to poorer mental health among women may have also been conflicts within the family and gender-based violence which spiraled during enforced stay-at-home orders [55]. Interpersonal violence included not only physical harm but encompassed psychological, sexual, and economic harms with one in three women experiencing gender-based violence during the pandemic contributing to poor mental health [35]. A high mental health burden was also discovered among front healthcare workers who were drastically exposed to Covid-19-related adversities. Most healthcare workers are women, and this did not change during the pandemic as females make up the majority of the nursing workforce in the European Region [84]. Evidence shows that they disproportionally suffered from burnout and trauma leading to post-traumatic stress symptoms or disorders among some [86].

Low-income women and women from minority groups including migrants and refugees were severely impacted as the intersectionality of gender and socio-economic hardship had a compounding effect on their mental health [19, 74]. Interpersonal violence may transcend socio-economic income levels, however, negative health outcomes may be felt hardest among the socio-economically deprived [4]. Access to mental health care has been hampered for both men and women, but was especially difficult for those who endured economic hardship and lived in poorly resourced areas, even before Covid-19 [67]. While access to face-to-face health services decreased, mobile technologies for mental health expanded [24]; however, certain population groups were left out as digital technologies for mental health required personal monies to afford certain devices, and a level of digital health literacy to navigate support and care [18]. Moreover, most technologies for mental health support did not tailor the intervention to the specific cultural need of ethnic or minority populations, leaving people from certain backgrounds behind [18].

Compounding effects on mental health could be detected among men too. Indeed, more men than women were hospitalized during Covid-19 due to severe infections, and this was also associated with a higher death rate [7, 47]. Those who were hospitalized often faced heightened psychological stress, particularly those who experienced severe illness or required intensive care [82]. Evidence shows that patients who were admitted to intensive care units, faced not only the physical challenges of recovery but also significant mental health distress [70]. These symptoms have shown to persist up to 1 year after in-patient care, with similar levels of post-traumatic stress disorder and depression found in both men and women [80]. Looking closely at the prevalence of psychological distress and the prevalence of mental health symptoms among men, there seems to have been an inverse relationship between age and the severity of mental health problems in men with mental health issues being more pronounced in younger men than in their older counterparts [26, 45]. As the pandemic unfolded, there was a notable increase in alcohol consumption too which was used as coping mechanism for the heightened emotional and psychological pressures people faced. Research conducted during the pandemic revealed a rise in alcohol consumption among men, although the evidence is mixed across studies and heterogenous [6, 46, 57]. While evidence indicates that men generally consumed more alcohol than women on average, they may have also experienced a more significant decrease in both the quantity and intensity of their alcohol consumption during lockdowns [6, 59]. Drinking motives seem to have been largely responsible for this with women being more likely than men to consume alcohol in order to cope with stress, and men's drinking being more related to financial worries and employment loss, thereby magnifying socio-economic disparities in alcohol consumption [46, 59]. Also, men of middle-age have historically had higher suicide rates than women, with the number of deaths for men being more than twice than those for women [12]. However, a recent meta-analyses indicates that during the pandemic, rates of completed suicide did not change significantly compared to the years before the pandemic [89], although an upward trend of suicidal ideation and suicide attempts was observed, particularly among men. Factors that were protective against suicide ideation and attempts among men were being in a relationship/being married, being in paid work and social supports from friends [62].

In recent years, there was more and more research that called for the impact of social determinants of mental health to be made more explicit in intervention and programmed development as Covid-19 magnified this effect [37]. Intersectoral programs addressing the root causes of mental health problems were designed and evaluated that especially served disadvantaged population groups [30]. To alleviate poor mental health, it is important to implement these programs, especially in times of adversity, ensuring that tailored support is provided to the most vulnerable communities as outlined in this chapter.

3.6 Conclusion

This chapter has examined the complex and multifaceted relationship between gender, socioeconomic position, and mental health, framed through the lens of the social determinants of health. While mental health disorders are a global concern affecting all populations, the burden is not evenly distributed. Women, in particular, face a disproportionately high mental health burden—a disparity shaped by structural inequalities, gender norms, and differential exposures to stressors.

Socioeconomic inequalities, gendered labor market disparities, and unequal caregiving responsibilities compound women's vulnerability to poor mental health. These challenges are further exacerbated during periods of crisis, as clearly demonstrated during the Covid-19 pandemic. The pandemic not only increased psychological distress across populations but also revealed how deeply entrenched social and gender inequalities amplify mental health risks for certain groups—particularly low-income women, single mothers, minority populations, and frontline healthcare workers.

Importantly, while men also experienced significant mental health challenges during the pandemic—including increased hospitalization rates, alcohol misuse, and suicidal ideation—these manifested differently and were often linked to socioeconomic stressors and shifting gender role expectations. These findings underscore that gendered experiences of mental health are dynamic and intersectional, shaped by both societal structures and individual circumstances.

To reduce mental health disparities and promote psychological well-being, interventions must go beyond individual-level treatment and address the broader social and economic contexts in which people live. This includes developing and implementing intersectoral policies that target the root causes of inequality, improving access to culturally appropriate mental health care and ensuring support systems are inclusive and responsive to the diverse needs of different gender and socioeconomic groups. As the Covid-19 pandemic has made clear, a more equitable approach to mental health is not only necessary—it is urgent.

References

1. Ahmed N, Barnett P, Greenburgh A, et al. Mental health in Europe during the COVID-19 pandemic: a systematic review. Lancet Psychiatry. 2023;10:537–56.
2. Albert PR. Why is depression more prevalent in women? J Psychiatry Neurosci. 2015;40:219–21.
3. Allen J, Reuben B, Ruth B, et al. Social determinants of mental health. Int Rev Psychiatry. 2014;26:392–407.
4. American Psychological Association. Violence and socio-economic status. Washington, DC: APA; 2022.
5. Anonymous. Global prevalence and burden of depressive and anxiety disorders in 204 countries and territories in 2020 due to the COVID-19 pandemic. Lancet. 2021;398:1700–12.
6. Anonymous. Alcohol during the pandemic: steady for women, down for men. Alcohol Drug Abuse Wkly. 2022;34:8–8.
7. Appunni S, Rubens M, Ramamoorthy V, et al. Gender differences in hospital outcomes among COVID-19 hospitalizations. South Med J. 2024;117:75–9.
8. Bom J, Bakx P, Schut F, et al. The impact of informal caregiving for older adults on the health of various types of caregivers: a systematic review. The Gerontologist. 2019;59:e629–42.
9. Carnazza G, Liberati P, Resce G. Income-related unmet needs in the European countries. Socio Econ Plan Sci. 2023;87:101542.
10. Chen F, Liu Y, Ya B, et al. Latest effective measures to combat COVID-19: a review. Iran J Public Health. 2021;50:640–8.
11. Cucinotta D, Vanelli M. WHO declares COVID-19 a pandemic. Acta Biomed. 2020;91:157–60.
12. Davis Weaver N, Bertolacci GJ, Rosenblad E, et al. Global, regional, and national burden of suicide, 1990–2021: a systematic analysis for the Global Burden of Disease Study 2021. Lancet Public Health. 2025;10:e189–202.
13. De Witte H, Pienaar J, De Cuyper N. Review of 30 years of longitudinal studies on the association between job insecurity and health and well-being: is there causal evidence? Aust Psychol. 2016;51:18–31.
14. De Zwart PL, Bakx P, Van Doorslaer EKA. Will you still need me, will you still feed me when I'm 64? The health impact of caregiving to one's spouse. Health Econ. 2017;26(Suppl 2):127–38.
15. Delaney C, Bobek A, Clavero S. "It was too much for me": mental load, mothers, and working from home during the COVID-19 pandemic. Front Psychol. 2023;14:1208099.
16. Deogan C, Bergström J, Heimer G, et al. Socioeconomic inequalities in sexual victimisation in a nationally representative sample of the Swedish population. Scand J Public Health. 2023;51:552–60.
17. Destatis. Gender pay gap. 2025.
18. Duden GS, Gersdorf S, Stengler K. Global impact of the COVID-19 pandemic on mental health services: a systematic review. J Psychiatr Res. 2022;154:354–77.
19. El Tatary G, Gill N. The impact of the COVID-19 pandemic on the mental health and wellbeing of refugees and asylum seekers-a narrative review of the literature. Australas Psychiatry. 2022;30:728–31.
20. Eugene D, Nöthling J, Tarsitani L, et al. Mental health during the Covid-19 pandemic: an international comparison of gender-related home and work-related responsibilities, and social support. Arch Womens Ment Health. 2025;28:359–74.

21. Eurofond. European quality of life survey 2017: quality of life, quality of public services, and quality of society. Luxembourg: European Commission; 2016.
22. European Commission. Informal care in Europe. Brussels: European Commission; 2018.
23. European Commission's Expert Group on Gender and Employment (Egge). Gender segregation in the labour market. Root causes, implications and policy responses in the EU. Luxembourg: Publications Office of the European Union; 2009.
24. Fuhr DC, Wolf-Ostermann K, Hoel V, et al. Digitale Technologien zur Verbesserung der psychischen Gesundheit. Bundesgesundheitsbl Gesundheitsforsch Gesundheitsschutz. 2024;67:332–8.
25. Ganzeboom HBG, De Graaf PM, Treiman DJ. A standard international socio-economic index of occupational status. Soc Sci Res. 1992;21:1–56.
26. Gottert A, Shattuck D, Pulerwitz J, et al. Meeting men's mental health needs during COVID-19 and beyond: a global health imperative. BMJ Glob Health. 2022;7(4):e008297.
27. Grundström J, Konttinen H, Berg N, et al. Associations between relationship status and mental well-being in different life phases from young to middle adulthood. SSM Popul Health. 2021;14:100774.
28. Harryson L, Strandh M, Hammarström A. Domestic work and psychological distress–what is the importance of relative socioeconomic position and gender inequality in the couple relationship? PLoS One. 2012;7:e38484.
29. Hashemi L, Fadeeva A, Khan N, et al. Intimate partner violence and physical health in England: gender stratified analyses of a probability sample survey. Womens Health (Lond). 2025;21:17455057251326419.
30. Hinrichsen C, Nielsen L, Tamminen N, et al. Intersectoral mental health promotion—a practice-oriented taxonomy of roles and a study of intersectoral dynamics. SSM Mental Health. 2022;2:100136.
31. Horton R. Offline: COVID-19 is not a pandemic. Lancet. 2020;396:874.
32. Hossain M. COVID-19 and gender differences in mental health in low- and middle-income countries: young working women are more vulnerable. SSM Mental Health. 2021;1:100039.
33. Hu Y, Metsä-Simola N, Malmberg S, et al. Trajectories of antidepressant use before and after union dissolution and re-partnering in later life: a prospective total population register-based cohort study. J Epidemiol Community Health. 2024;78:277–83.
34. Jacobi F, Höfler M, Strehle J, et al. Mental disorders in the general population: study on the health of adults in Germany and the additional module mental health (DEGS1-MH). Nervenarzt. 2014;85:77–87.
35. Kifle ME, Aychiluhm SB, Anbesu EW. Global prevalence of intimate partner violence during the COVID-19 pandemic among women: systematic review and meta-analysis. BMC Womens Health. 2024;24:127.
36. Kim TJ, Von Dem Knesebeck O. Perceived job insecurity, unemployment and depressive symptoms: a systematic review and meta-analysis of prospective observational studies. Int Arch Occup Environ Health. 2016;89:561–73.
37. Kirkbride JB, Anglin DM, Colman I, et al. The social determinants of mental health and disorder: evidence, prevention and recommendations. World Psychiatry. 2024;23:58–90.
38. Lanza-León P, Cantarero-Prieto D. The loud silent side of single parenthood in Europe: health and socio-economic circumstances from a gender perspective. J Fam Econ Issues. 2024;46(2):479–91.
39. Leopold T. Gender differences in the consequences of divorce: a study of multiple outcomes. Demography. 2018;55:769–97.
40. Li S, Xu Y, Zheng L, et al. Sex difference in global burden of major depressive disorder: findings from the global burden of disease study 2019. Front Psych. 2022;13:789305.
41. Li G, Li Y, Lam AIF, et al. Understanding the protective effect of social support on depression symptomatology from a longitudinal network perspective. BMJ Ment Health. 2023;26(1):e300802.
42. Lorant V, Deliège D, Eaton W, et al. Socioeconomic inequalities in depression: a meta-analysis. Am J Epidemiol. 2003;157:98–112.

43. Mar J, Larrañaga I, Ibarrondo O, et al. Socioeconomic and gender inequalities in mental disorders among adolescents and young adults. Span J Psychiatry Ment Health. 2024;17:95–102.
44. Menéndez-Espina S, Llosa JA, Agulló-Tomás E, et al. The influence of gender inequality in the development of job insecurity: differences between women and men. Front Public Health. 2020;8:526162.
45. Mental Health Commission of Canada. Mental health and substance use during COVID-19: spotlight on youth, older adults & stigma. Ottawa: Mental Health Commission of Canada; 2021.
46. Monk RL, Qureshi AW, Richardson GB, et al. UK alcohol consumption during the COVID-19 pandemic: the role of drinking motives, employment and subjective mental health. PLoS One. 2023;18:e0283233.
47. Nguyen NT, Chinn J, De Ferrante M, et al. Male gender is a predictor of higher mortality in hospitalized adults with COVID-19. PLoS One. 2021;16:e0254066.
48. Öberg M, Heimer G, Lucas S. Lifetime experiences of violence against women and men in Sweden. Scand J Public Health. 2021;49:301–8.
49. Oliver MI, Pearson N, Coe N, et al. Help-seeking behaviour in men and women with common mental health problems: cross-sectional study. Br J Psychiatry. 2005;186:297–301.
50. Oram S, Khalifeh H, Howard LM. Violence against women and mental health. Lancet Psychiatry. 2017;4:159–70.
51. Phelan JC, Link BG, Tehranifar P. Social conditions as fundamental causes of health inequalities: theory, evidence, and policy implications. J Health Soc Behav. 2010;51(Suppl):S28–40.
52. Piccinelli M, Wilkinson G. Gender differences in depression. Crit Rev Br J Psychiatry. 2000;177:486–92.
53. Pierce M, Mcmanus S, Hope H, et al. Mental health responses to the COVID-19 pandemic: a latent class trajectory analysis using longitudinal UK data. Lancet Psychiatry. 2021;8:610–9.
54. Pinquart M, Sörensen S. Differences between caregivers and noncaregivers in psychological health and physical health: a meta-analysis. Psychol Aging. 2003;18:250–67.
55. Piquero AR, Jennings WG, Jemison E, et al. Domestic violence during the COVID-19 pandemic – evidence from a systematic review and meta-analysis. J Crim Justice. 2021;74:101806.
56. Rattay P, Von Der Lippe E, Borgmann LS, et al. The health of single mothers and fathers in Germany. J Health Monit. 2017;2:23–41.
57. Rehm J, Kilian C, Ferreira-Borges C, et al. Alcohol use in times of the COVID 19: implications for monitoring and policy. Drug Alcohol Rev. 2020;39:301–4.
58. Rober Koch-Institut. Gesundheitliche Lage der Männer in Deutschland [Men's Health in Germany]. Berlin: Robert Koch-Institut; 2014.
59. Sallie SN, Ritou V, Bowden-Jones H, et al. Assessing international alcohol consumption patterns during isolation from the COVID-19 pandemic using an online survey: highlighting negative emotionality mechanisms. BMJ Open. 2020;10:e044276.
60. Schlesinger B, Raphael D. The woman in the middle: the sandwich generation revisited. Int J Sociol Fam. 1993;23:77–87.
61. Scott KM, Wells JE, Angermeyer M, et al. Gender and the relationship between marital status and first onset of mood, anxiety and substance use disorders. Psychol Med. 2010;40:1495–505.
62. Seidler ZE, Wilson MJ, Oliffe JL, et al. Suicidal ideation in men during COVID-19: an examination of protective factors. BMC Psychiatry. 2023;23:46.
63. Shim RS. Mental health inequities in the context of COVID-19. JAMA Netw Open. 2020;3:e2020104.
64. Solar O, Irwin A. Conceptual framework for action on the social determinants of health. In: Social determinants of health discussion paper 2 (policy and practice). Geneva: World Health Organization; 2010.
65. Stansfeld S, Candy B. Psychosocial work environment and mental health—a meta-analytic review. Scand J Work Environ Health. 2006;32(6):443–62.
66. Stein J, Pabst A, Berger K, et al. Mental health of individuals with pre-existing mental illnesses at the beginning of the COVID-19 pandemic: results of the German National Cohort (NAKO). Front Public Health. 2024;12:1451631.

67. Stepanova E, Thompson A, Yu G, et al. Changes in mental health services in response to the COVID-19 pandemic in high-income countries: a rapid review. BMC Psychiatry. 2024;24:103.
68. Stormacq C, Van Den Broucke S, Wosinski J. Does health literacy mediate the relationship between socioeconomic status and health disparities? Integrative review. Health Promot Int. 2019;34:e1–e17.
69. Strandh M, Hammarström A, Nilsson K, et al. Unemployment, gender and mental health: the role of the gender regime. Sociol Health Illn. 2013;35:649–65.
70. T'ng K, Kenardy J, Hartanto A. Evaluating mental health outcomes in COVID-19 ICU survivors: a scoping review of measurement tools. J Clin Med. 2024;13(11):3191.
71. Tarsitani L, Pinucci I, Tedeschi F, et al. Resilience of people with chronic medical conditions during the COVID-19 pandemic: a 1-year longitudinal prospective survey. BMC Psychiatry. 2022;22:633.
72. Taylor S, Paluszek MM, Rachor GS, et al. Substance use and abuse, COVID-19-related distress, and disregard for social distancing: a network analysis. Addict Behav. 2021;114:106754.
73. Tedstone Doherty D, Kartalova-O'doherty Y. Gender and self-reported mental health problems: predictors of help seeking from a general practitioner. Br J Health Psychol. 2010;15:213–28.
74. Thibaut F, ELNahas G. Women's mental health and lessons learnt from the COVID-19 pandemic. Psychiatr Clin N Am. 2023;46:415–26.
75. Tousignant M, Brosseau R, Tremblay L. Sex biases in mental health scales: do women tend to report less serious symptoms and confide more than men? Psychol Med. 1987;17:203–15.
76. Umberson D, Thomeer MB, Williams K. Family status and mental health: recent advances and future directions. In: Aneshensel CS, Phelan JC, Bierman A, editors. Handbook of the sociology of mental health. Dordrecht: Springer Netherlands; 2013. p. 405–31.
77. UN. Women in the informal economy. New York: UN Women; 2023.
78. United Nations Development Program. Gender Inequality Index (GII). 2025.
79. Urbanos-Garrido RM. Income-related inequalities in unmet dental care needs in Spain: traces left by the great recession. Int J Equity Health. 2020;19:207.
80. Van Houwelingen F, Van Dellen E, Visser-Meily JMA, et al. Mental, cognitive and physical outcomes after intensive care unit treatment during the COVID-19 pandemic: a comparison between COVID-19 and non-COVID-19 patients. Sci Rep. 2023;13:14414.
81. Verbakel E, Tamlagsrønning S, Winstone L, et al. Informal care in Europe: findings from the European Social Survey (2014) special module on the social determinants of health. Eur J Pub Health. 2017;27:90–5.
82. Waite AA, Cherry MG, Brown SL, et al. Psychological impact of an intensive care admission for COVID-19 on patients in the United Kingdom. J Intensive Care Soc. 2025;26:17511437241312113.
83. Wen M, Zhang X, Harris CD, et al. Spatial disparities in the distribution of parks and green spaces in the USA. Ann Behav Med. 2013;45(Suppl 1):S18–27.
84. WHO. Health workforce. Copenhagen: WHO; 2023.
85. Williams TG, Logan TM, Zuo CT, et al. Parks and safety: a comparative study of green space access and inequity in five US cities. Landsc Urban Plan. 2020;201:103841.
86. Wojnar-Gruszka K, Miernik M, Cichoń J, et al. Prevalence of the symptoms of post-traumatic stress disorder (PTSD) and burnout syndrome (BOS) among intensive care unit (ICU) healthcare workers during the COVID-19 pandemic. Psychol Health Med. 2025;30:1–12.
87. Wright L, Steptoe A, Fancourt D. Are we all in this together? Longitudinal assessment of cumulative adversities by socioeconomic position in the first 3 weeks of lockdown in the UK. J Epidemiol Community Health. 2020;74:683–8.
88. Xue B, Lacey RE, Di Gessa G, et al. Do mental and physical health trajectories change around transitions into sandwich care? Results from the UK household longitudinal study. Public Health. 2025;239:224–9.
89. Yan Y, Hou J, Li Q, et al. Suicide before and during the COVID-19 pandemic: a systematic review with meta-analysis. Int J Environ Res Public Health. 2023;20(4):3346.

4 Violence Against Women: Systemic Violence and Medical Violence

Marina Carretero-Gómez

4.1 Systemic Violence

Systemic violence against women refers to power structures and social norms that perpetuate gender inequality, discriminating against and subjugating women in different spheres, such as work, education, politics, and family. This type of violence is characterized by its structural nature, that is, it is embedded in institutions and everyday practices and it is reflected in the lack of access to resources, unequal pay, discriminatory laws, and traditional social expectations that limit women's freedom [1].

This violence is not only manifested in individual actions, but is deeply linked to norms, policies, and practices that perpetuate gender inequality.

Violence against women has existed throughout history in various forms and under different contexts, but systemic violence is distinguished by the fact that it is institutionalized, accepted, or even promoted by power structures and dominant cultural norms. Throughout history, women have been treated as second-class citizens in many countries [2], and patriarchal structures have perpetuated various forms of violence, such as

- *Limited political and social rights*: for centuries, women were excluded from political, social, and economic life. In many parts of the world, women did not have the right to vote, could not access education or paid work, and their rights were considered secondary to those of men. This constituted a form of systemic violence, as power structures not only ignored women, but actively maintained their subordinate position. Even today, there are still countries where women are excluded from political, social, and economic life; where they lack their own

M. Carretero-Gómez (✉)
Infanta Sofia Hospital, Madrid, Spain

M. López-Atanes, M. Sáenz-Herrero (eds.), *Applying the Gender Perspective in Psychiatry and Psychotherapy*, https://doi.org/10.1007/978-3-032-17883-1_4

rights and are subjected to men, to whom they are inferior and on whom they must depend for survival. There are still places [3] such as Afghanistan, where women cannot attend school or university (exclusion from education), work (exclusion from the labor market and impossibility of economic independence), dress as they wish, leave the house without the company of a close male relative, play sports, ride a bus with men (segregation of transportation), choose who they marry, how many children they want to have and when to have sex, be seen, protest (denial of freedom of expression).

- *Sexist legislation*: In many countries, laws have been designed to protect the interests of men, while women were treated unequally. For example, in some places, well into the twentieth century, women could not own property or have access to their inheritance or were forced to follow the will of their husbands. These laws contributed to maintaining women's economic and social dependence [1–3].
- *Patriarchal culture and gender-based violence*: At a cultural level, patriarchal societies have normalized the subordination of women, devaluing their contributions to the economy and social life. Sexual violence, harassment, and physical abuse were long considered "men's stuff," often minimized or ignored by institutions [1].
- *Domestic violence*: Domestic violence is a clear example of systemic violence. For many years, the laws of many countries did not adequately protect women from domestic violence, and in some cases, husbands were considered "entitled" to their wives [2]. Although laws have changed in many parts of the world, domestic violence remains a manifestation of how social and cultural structures allow or minimize women's suffering. There are still countries in the world where domestic violence is not only underreported or ignored but legitimized [3].
- *Sexual harassment in the workplace*: In many cultures, sexual harassment was tolerated or even ignored for years. Women who reported harassment were often blamed and feared that they would be accused of being "troublemakers." The lack of clear policies and an efficient legal system to protect women in the workplace contributed to the perpetuation of this violence.
- *Job discrimination and wage inequality*: The wage gap between men and women is another example of systemic violence. Although women perform the same amount of work, they often receive lower wages than men for the same job [1, 2]. This wage inequality is supported by a series of labor norms and structures that devalue women's work, perpetuating their economic disadvantage.
- *Femicides and gender-based violence*: Extreme violence against women, such as femicides (gender-based killings of women), is another manifestation of systemic violence. In many countries, femicide is seen as an isolated problem or as a "private" matter, rather than being addressed as a consequence of structural violence against women.
- *Patriarchal justice system*: Women who suffer sexual or physical violence often face a justice system that blames them or minimizes their suffering. In many places, women victims of violence are questioned for their behavior, their dress,

or their decisions prior to the incident, which allow aggressors to go unpunished and them to be revictimized by an unjust system.

- *Cultural practices, such as female genital mutilation (FGM)*: In some cultures, practices such as female genital mutilation (FGM) are encouraged and tolerated by social structures. This form of violence is institutionalized in certain contexts and is perpetuated by cultural norms that view control over female sexuality as a means to ensure women's honor or purity.

As Lerner explains [1], patriarchy—a social system based on male domination—is not natural, but a historical construct that developed in diverse cultures over time. Patriarchy emerged gradually throughout history, particularly in the transition from matrilineal to patriarchal societies. According to the author, early human societies were more egalitarian, with women playing a central role in the economy, religion, and social organization. However, with the development of agriculture, private property, and the consolidation of hierarchical structures, power shifted to men.

Patriarchy was not only consolidated in political institutions but was also legitimized through religion, philosophy, and law, establishing ideologies that justified the subordination of women. Women were systematically excluded from power, property decisions, and civil rights, which led them to a position of dependence and subordination in society.

This system of ideas has been the basis from which historical, medical, and animal kingdom findings have been interpreted. Margarita Sánchez Herrero [4] explains in her book, *Prehistory of women*, how prehistoric findings have been explained from a patriarchal point of view: females have been relegated to a passive and submissive role, while men performed activities such as hunting or fighting, something that does not correspond to the actual findings. From this patriarchal bias, the erroneous message of male supremacy over women has been transmitted as something natural.

Similarly, for centuries, findings of the animal kingdom have been explained under a patriarchal light [5] , where observation and interpretation have been guided by a patriarchal system of thought, relegating females to a position of docility and submission. Being biologically "female" defined and restricted what it meant to be a woman [5–7]. For a long time, even scientific fundamentals—questioned and reinterpreted from a feminist perspective—have served to justify gender inequality [8]. For example, during the nineteenth and twentieth centuries, scientists such as Paul Broca, one of the founders of neuroscience, argued that the female brain was smaller and less developed than the male brain, which was interpreted as a sign of "inferiority." These studies were used to justify women's inadequacy in holding positions of power, studying scientific fields, or participating fully in public life.

Many studies of the time presented differences in abilities between men and women as innate and biological, when in reality the observed differences were often due to social, cultural, and economic factors. For example, the notion that women were less competitive and less rational was argued, justifying their exclusion from the public sphere or politics.

Another key issue in gender differences was the study of testosterone, where flawed research led to an overinterpretation of biological differences. Testosterone has been associated with aggression and male superiority, while the impact of hormones on women has been dismissed, reinforcing stereotypes that women are less aggressive and therefore less suitable for leadership roles.

Scientific studies have played a crucial role in constructing and perpetuating gender inequality, often unintentionally but equally damaging.

Systemic violence against women is a complex phenomenon involving a combination of cultural, social, economic, and political factors. The historical oppression of women highlights the need to transform patriarchal structures and create a more equal society. The fight against systemic violence requires not only of individual actions but also a profound change in the social, political, and cultural structures that allow and perpetuate inequality and violence. To eradicate it, it is essential that women's rights are preserved, that discriminatory laws be eliminated, and that changes in the way societies perceive the role of women be promoted.

4.2 Medical Violence

Women have historically been ignored, excluded, or underestimated in the development of science and technology. Patriarchal structures within the scientific world have relegated women to the background, both in terms of visibility and access to resources and opportunities [6].

Medical violence against women happens when women are mistreated, misinformed, or negligently treated in the healthcare setting specifically because of their gender. This violence can manifest itself in many ways: from the overmedicalization of women's lives to explicit discrimination or denial of treatment. Medical violence against women includes abusive, negligent, or derogatory practices within the healthcare system, especially in areas such as childbirth, reproductive management and health, mental health, and sexuality.

Throughout history, medical violence has been a systematic form of control over women's bodies, and it persists in many forms today. Historically, women have been subjected to medical interventions without their consent [9], erroneous or derogatory diagnoses (such as the pathologization of menstruation or female sexuality) and even forced sterilizations, especially in contexts of colonization, racism, and poverty.

According to Carme Valls [9], there is an unconscious bias among medical professionals, which leads them to under-diagnose women's pathologies and to medicalize natural and physiological processes such as childbirth, pregnancy, and menopause. Women's symptoms have remained masked as psychosomatic complaints or as psychological problems [10], that is, invisible to medicine, which has continued to prescribe psychotropic drugs at the first visit of any female patient even before any examination.

Cultural, social, and psychological stereotypes can affect how women's health issues are identified and treated. These factors may lead to incorrect diagnoses, ineffective examinations, and treatments that do not address the intended conditions or may worsen them.

As Pastor states [11], the three rules of patriarchy write on female bodies the structures of its power: the *naturalization* of sexual differences according to its stereotypes, the *fragmentation* of experience and the body, and the *conversion* into an object constitute the pillars on which this symbol of patriarchal power rests.

4.3 History of Medical Violence Against Women

Throughout history, and more particularly, since the establishment of medicine as a scientific field, women have suffered different types of violence. These are more easily recognized when in relation to exclusive women's health issues surrounding the reproductive cycle and childbirth. The fact that women were removed from medicine studies has resulted in various well-spread forms of medical violence against women. Such as

- *Gender-based misdiagnosis and treatment*: for centuries, women have been subject to misdiagnosis due to gender bias. The medical establishment, especially in the nineteenth and early twentieth centuries, often viewed women as "hypersensitive" or "emotional," which led to women being disproportionately diagnosed with psychosomatic illnesses [6, 9, 10, 12]. Women with mental health issues were often labeled as "hysterical" [7] and subjected to treatments such as isolation or "hysterectomy," often without medical justification.
- *Obstetric and gynecological abuse*: abuse during childbirth, also known as "obstetric abuse," is a form of medical violence against women that has been documented worldwide. This term can include everything from performing procedures without the woman's consent, to humiliating comments, excessive use of force, and denial of adequate pain treatment. For centuries, women were treated as passive objects in childbirth, without considering their wishes or needs. Obstetric and gynecological abuse includes medicalization of pregnancy and childbirth and control over female reproduction, eugenics, and forced sterilization:

  Medicalization of pregnancy and childbirth: Throughout history, women have been denied the right to decide over their own bodies regarding childbearing. Throughout the twentieth century, childbirth went from being a natural process largely controlled by women and their communities to being medicalized and controlled by medical staff. Control over childbirth and the decision on how it is carried out (cesarean section, induction of labor, etc.) has historically been a form of medical violence; especially when women have no say in decisions or are pressured to opt for invasive procedures without medical necessity. Cesarean section, for example, has been used in some contexts without proper medical justification, simply for convenience or because of external pressures.

Control over female reproduction, eugenics, and forced sterilization: Throughout the twentieth century, in many countries, women, particularly those belonging to marginalized or minority groups (such as indigenous women, women of African descent, or women with disabilities), were subjected to forced sterilization under "eugenics" programs. These programs sought to reduce the "procreation" of certain groups considered "undesirable" or "inferior," and women were sterilized without their knowledge or consent. In the United States, for example, it is estimated that between the 1930s and 1970s, thousands of women were sterilized without their consent under these policies. For many years, medicine has exerted control over women's reproductive capacity. Women's reproductive health was managed by physicians without their consent: from imposed sterilization to performing abortions without anesthesia.

- *Control over female sexuality*: Throughout history, women have been subjected to medical violence related to their sexuality. The practice of "hymenoplasty" or hymen reconstruction (surgical procedure to reconstruct the hymen of women) remains an example of how social control over women's bodies is perpetuated. In addition, medicine has used practices such as female genital mutilation (FGM) in some cultures, which represents one of the most serious forms of medical violence.
- *Misinformation, lack of informed consent, paternalistic treatment, and dehumanization*: Women have historically been treated in the medical field in a paternalistic manner, which meant that they were deprived of autonomy over their own bodies. Doctors often did not listen to their experiences or symptoms and made decisions without their informed consent. This approach dehumanizes women and places them in a position of subjugation to the physician, who assumes that he or she knows what is best for the patient. In situations such as surgical interventions or medical treatments, women often do not have all the necessary information about risks, benefits, and available alternatives, which can lead to decisions that do not reflect their wishes and interests.
- *Medical malpractice and discrimination in care*: Women, especially black, indigenous, and women from marginalized communities, often receive unequal treatment in hospitals and health centers. In some cases, their pain and symptoms have been dismissed, which can lead to misdiagnosis or even death [6, 10]. A well-known case is the dismissal of black women's pain in prenatal care, a practice that has been linked to structural racism within health systems.
- *Pathologization of women*: Women have been misdiagnosed with mental illness or anxiety and depressive disorders in the belief that their emotions were pathological due to their "feminine nature." In addition, symptoms of menstrual or menopausal pain were often minimized or ignored.

During the nineteenth and twentieth centuries, in both Europe and North America, men had the legal right to confine their wives or daughters to a psychiatric hospital, even if they presented no mental illnesses. Within psychotherapy, patriarchal dominance prevailed and women, labeled as hysterical, were routinely beaten, deprived of sleep, food, exercise, sunlight, and all contact with the outside world. Some were even murdered. Therapeutic bias also came from psychiatric associations, where almost all of the members were men, while two-thirds of the patients were women.

Inequality, discrimination, and stereotypes undermine self-esteem and restrict women's opportunities [7]. Oppression causes trauma, especially when those who suffer from it are blamed for their own misfortune and diagnosed as a pathology. Under psychiatric imperialism, women have been further mistreated: labeled and punished, over-sedated, sexually abused during treatment, hospitalized against their will, subjected to shock therapy, lobotomies, described as aggressive, promiscuous, depressed, ugly, old, angry, fat, or incurable.

How is it possible that a world that believes itself to be scientific has been able to forget the problems of half the population and, on the contrary, has medicalized almost all the natural stages of women's lives? [9] In few clinical issues—such as menstruation and clinical gynecology—there is such a marked imbalance between the number of people who suffer and how marginal it is for medical and scientific research. The proportion of women who suffer from some kind of reproductive or gynecological pathology during their lifetime is one in three, but in most cases the problem ends when the contraconceptive pills are prescribed. Hormonal treatment is precisely one of the keys to the lack of progress in research on the menstrual cycle [13]. This is also the case, for example, with the treatment of hot flashes in menopause; one of the most important longitudinal studies on menopause, the Study of Women's Health Across the Nation (SWAN), has as one of its main conclusions the correlation between the frequency of hot flashes and the risk of suffering from cardiovascular disease [14]. Hot flashes are the symptoms that are first suppressed and hidden, by hormonal medicalization of women, and therefore more difficult to assess.

Science has historically ignored women's testimony about menstruation and the problems associated with it [13]. For example, during the COVID-19 pandemic, many women reported alterations in the menstrual cycle after vaccination. Most of the adverse effects of the vaccine were suffered by women [15]. We now know [9] that if the vaccine is administered early in the menstrual cycle it is altered, while if the vaccination occurs after ovulation, it does not alter the cycle. Research suggests that also the seasonal vaccine against the common flu can alter the menstrual cycle. It is more advisable for women to receive any vaccination 20 days after they have had their previous menses. And yet this has not led to any changes in any clinical guidelines. Questions regarding the phase of the menstrual cycle have not been incorporated into medical interviews when scheduling vaccinations to female patients.

The practices and rituals during menstruation [16] (e.g., menstrual isolation) hide a submission of the female gender with respect to men, demanding from them practices to become fit again before society that they do not have to go through.

Women experience more pain-related diseases, representing 70% of chronic conditions. Most of autoimmune diseases that cause pain are predominantly female, in a ratio of 9 to 1 [9, 10]. Comen [6] discusses how women who suffer from chronic pain conditions, such as endometriosis or chronic fatigue syndrome, are often dismissed by physicians. Research indicates that women are more likely to be misdiagnosed, and their symptoms are often minimized. For example, endometriosis, a painful condition that affects millions of women, was historically ignored or misunderstood. Endometriosis takes an average of 8–10 years to be diagnosed by physicians [17]. Women suffering from this condition receive misdiagnoses, such as depression or anxiety, instead of proper treatment for their condition. Comen highlights how the lack of research on women-specific conditions has been a reflection of medicine's neglect of their needs [6].

Cardiovascular diseases, traditionally viewed as a male health problem, have also been diagnosed and treated differently in women [6, 9]. For decades, research on heart diseases focused primarily on men, ignoring gender differences in the symptoms and manifestations of these diseases in women. A relevant fact is that women [12] often do not experience the male-typical symptoms of a heart attack, such as chest pain; but rather more vague symptoms, such as fatigue or neck pain, which makes early diagnosis difficult. However, due to gender bias in medicine, women's symptoms were downplayed, contributing to a lower rate of detection and proper treatment.

For a long time, women were excluded from clinical trials, especially in areas of medical research that directly affect them, such as heart disease or osteoporosis. This meant that medical interventions and treatments were based on male models, leading to inappropriate or even harmful treatment for women. Until relatively, recently [6], most clinical trials were conducted exclusively with men, resulting in medical responses to diseases and treatments that were inadequate for women. As a measure of political and economic control, women's bodies have been invisible to science and a weapon of power.

4.4 Conclusion

Medical violence against women is a serious human rights violation that has historically been systematic and structural. Although important advances have been made in women's health care, forms of discrimination and abuse persist in many health systems. The struggle for respect of reproductive rights and women's right to make informed decisions about their bodies and health remain essential to eradicate these forms of medical violence. Raising awareness of these issues, as well as strengthening legislation and training of health professionals, are crucial steps toward the elimination of this violence.

References

1. Lerner G. The creation of Patriarchy, 1986, en su traducción española: La creación del patriarcado. Katakrak Luburuak; 2017.
2. Beauvoir S. El segundo sexo. Ediciones Cátedra; 2017.
3. https://www.es.amnesty.org/.

4. Sánchez Romero M. Prehistorias de mujeres. Ediciones destino; 2022.
5. Cooke LH. Una guía revolucionaria sobre el sexo, la evolución y la fémina animal. Argumentos, Anagrama; 2025.
6. Comen E. No seas exagerada. Historia de cómo la medicina olvidó a las mujeres y por qué es importante arreglarlo. Ed Temas de Hoy; 2025.
7. Chesler P. Mujeres y locura. Continta me tienes; 2019.
8. Saini A. Inferior. Cómo la ciencia infravalora a la mujer y cómo las investigaciones reescriben la historia. Círculo de tiza; 2017.
9. Valls C. Mujeres invisibles para la medicina. Desvelando nuestra salud. Capitán Swing; 2021.
10. Cleghorn E. Enfermas. Una historia sobre las mujeres, la medicina y sus mitos en un mundo de hombres. Paidós; 2022.
11. Pastor R. Cuerpo y género: representación e imagen corporal. In: Barberá Heredia E, Martínez Benlloch I, Bonilla Campos A, editors. Psicología y género. Madrid: Pearson Educación; 2004. p. 223.
12. Muntane I, Coll B. Eres una exagerada. Sesgo de género y sexo en salud. Rayo Verde Editorial, S.L; 2025.
13. Zuil Navarro M, Villarreal A. La mitad que sangra. Cómo y por qué hemos ignorado históricamente la menstruación. Libros del K.O; 2024.
14. https://www.swanstudy.org.
15. Wong KK, Heilig CM, Hause A, Myers TR, Olson CK, Gee J, Marquez P, Strid P, Shay DK. Menstrual irregularities and vaginal bleeding after COVID-19 vaccination reported to v-safe active surveillance, USA in December, 2020-January, 2022: an observational cohort study. Lancet Digit Health. 2022;4(9):e667–75.
16. Stein E, Kim S. Flow: the cultura story of menstruation. St. Martin's Griffin; 2009.
17. Fernández Parra, J.; Dolores, M.; Ruiz, L.; Rodríguez Olivares, M.A., Diagnóstico y clasificación de la endometriosis, 2008.

The Gender Perspective and Gender Analysis

5

Mayte López-Atanes, Iratxe Escajadillo, and Leire Erkoreka

5.1 Introduction

Gender is probably one of the most important variables when it comes to determining our experiences as human beings. In fact, gender is a primary characteristic in the perception of people. Children and adults immediately and implicitly group unfamiliar people according to their gender, even if this is not relevant for the social interaction taking place [1]. From a very early age, children are implicitly taught about gender stereotypes and reproduce them in their own beliefs and behaviors. For example, as early as the age of 6, girls begin to associate the masculine stereotype with a high level of intellectual ability and begin to avoid activities that are for "smart children" [2, 3]. Gender, understood as the socially constructed roles, behaviors, expressions and identities of girls, women, boys, men, and gender diverse people [4], influences our thinking, our choices, our interactions with others and how we are perceived.

Obviously, in the same way that gender influences other aspects of life, it also interferes with the manifestation of mental illness and the therapeutic process.

M. López-Atanes (✉)
Department of Psychiatry, University Hospital Galdakao-Usansolo, Galdakao, Biscay, Spain

Center of Interdisciplinary Addiction Research University of Hamburg, Hamburg, Germany
e-mail: M.lopezatanes@centra.hamburg

I. Escajadillo
University Hospital Galdakao-Usansolo, Galdakao, Biscay, Spain

L. Erkoreka
University Hospital Galdakao-Usansolo, Galdakao, Biscay, Spain

University of the Basque Country, Leioa, Biscay, Spain

M. López-Atanes, M. Sáenz-Herrero (eds.), *Applying the Gender Perspective in Psychiatry and Psychotherapy*, https://doi.org/10.1007/978-3-032-17883-1_5

Already in the early days of contemporary Western psychotherapy, Freud emphasized that the majority of the patients affected by hysteria were women, and that a large number of them referred to childhood episodes of sexual abuse, which he explained in the framework of the Oedipus complex. In his human development theory, for example, he also spoke of different developmental processes in boys and girls [5]. However, he is nowadays criticized for taking the inferior psychological development of the latter for granted and describing women as the products of an incomplete and frustrated male development. Edipous complex is currently not supported by empirical research [6], and under a feminist lens, it can even be considered a normalization of children abuse and a negative influence on culture [7, 8].

Therefore, simply considering gender differences does not imply the inclusion of a gender perspective, neither does it solely influence the study of women. To do so goes beyond conceptualizing the man–woman dichotomy. This chapter aims to develop the definition of the gender perspective and clarify how to perform a gender analysis, exploring their implications for mental health and psychotherapy.

5.2 What Is the Gender Perspective?

Although there is not one universal definition of the gender perspective, according to the European institute of gender equality, it consists of the focus on gender-based differences in status and power, and the consideration on how such discrimination shapes the immediate needs, as well as the long-term interests, of women and men. In a policy context, taking a gender perspective is a strategy for making women's as well as men's concerns and experiences an integral dimension of the design, implementation, monitoring, and evaluation of policies and programs in all political, economic, and societal spheres, so that inequality is not perpetuated [9].

Nevertheless, there are some debates about the current tendencies to incorporate the gender perspective [10–12]. Some argue that the focus on the woman–man dualism can lead to an overemphasis on differences [13], whereas in many cases similarities between men and women have been found to be the norm. For example, men and women show equal increases in oxytocin levels 6 months after the birth of their first child [14], and there are also more similarities than differences in cognitive performance [15]. Another aspect is the shift from the use of "women's studies" to gender studies [10]. Although there is a need to study the particularities of women, the gender perspective is not a synonymous of women studies, and aims to include both women and men in scientific work [16]. Instead of focusing on women as an underprivileged group, the emphasis is now on the social construction of gender identities and on the nature of the relationships between them. This means to also include in research and interventions the non-binary population, which is usually neglected in clinical research [11]. In general, the LGBTQ collective is studied as a unit, and less often each group is studied separately. Studies that have compared each group separately show that certain minorities have specific needs. For example, bisexual women are at even greater risk than other subgroups for alcohol use disorders [17, 18] and trans people consume less alcohol than cis people, although the risk of the use of other substances remains higher [19]. It is therefore important that future studies also assess the specificities within this group.

5.3 What Is Gender Analysis?

The European Institute for gender equality defines gender analysis as the provision of the necessary data and information to integrate a gender perspective into policies, programs, and projects. As a starting point for gender mainstreaming, gender analysis identifies the differences between and among women and men in terms of their relative position in society and the distribution of resources, opportunities, constraints, and power in a given context. In this way, conducting a gender analysis allows for the development of interventions that address gender inequalities and meet the different needs of women, men, and non-binary individuals [20]. Gender analysis refers to the inclusion of the gender perspective in all research steps, from project design to data interpretation and discussion [21]. When a research project or intervention includes a gender perspective and uses gender analysis in its methodology, it can be considered gender sensitive, in contrast to what is usually referred to as gender blind research [22].

In psychiatry, one of the main methodological problems has been to relate differences between men and women to biological factors, rather than to include the gender dimension. Although gender may not have a major impact in other disciplines, it does in mental health [23]. Mental health is all about how a person thinks and feels. This reflects their biological health, but also their sense of self, how they think others perceive and treat them, and how they see their role in society. The role of sex and gender clearly needs to be acknowledged, and researchers also need to be aware of their own preconceptions and how these may affect both the scientific questions they have and their interpretation of the data [24].

Furthermore, both biology and the social context interplay, and it remains difficult to separate what is caused by biological differences and which fraction of distress is caused by social stressors. For example, in the study of the higher depression prevalence among women, only a minor effect could be related to biology and much came from life adversities, especially during childhood [25]. When facing trauma, especially interpersonal trauma, it has been shown that the cortisol axis dysregulates and is hypo or hyperactive, giving rise to a hormonal imbalance [26, 27]. As women are more frequently exposed to this kind of trauma, it makes sense that their hormonal dysregulation could also influence the higher proportion of depression [28].

Gender-sensitive research considers the differences between men and women in all aspects of the investigation, from an initial idea, formulating research questions, objectives, and methodologies to the outcomes and presentation of results. Sex and Gender-based analysis (SGBA) systematically inquiries about biological (sex-based) and socio-cultural (gender-based) differences between women and men, and boys and girls, without presuming that there are disparities. Apart from integrating gender into the content, the gender-sensitive approach strives to provide equal participation of both women and men in scientific work. The gender-sensitive method also considers the transgender population and should not understand gender as a binary category [15].

5.4 Gender Analysis: What Does it Entail?

Although a growing body of evidence supports the inclusion of gender analysis in research to achieve scientific excellence [11, 23, 29–33], researchers still struggle to properly separate sex and gender [34–37]. Moreover, there is no single consensus on how to include gender analysis in research, but rather different documents and recommendations from different agencies across countries. The World Health Organization (WHO) provided an overview of various gender tools, policies, and guidelines designed to help measure the impact of gender on human health. This document identifies different levels of gender analysis, considering personal and community-level impacts of gender, and identifies questions to ask when examining the interactions between sex and gender and their dual impact on health [38].

In the case of the European Union, it has advocated for gender equality in research and academia. For these reasons, the EU has developed a gender toolkit to help researchers integrate gender sensitivity [16]. They also published a gender equality strategy in 2020 in which they require that all EU-funded research proposals include gender as a variable to analyze in their program [39]. The European Association of Science Editors (EASE) established a Gender Policy Committee in 2012 and tasked it with developing a set of guidelines for reporting on Sex and Gender Equity in Research (SAGER), with the aim of promoting more transparent research and reporting practices that bridge the gender evidence gap. The guidelines provide a comprehensive set of recommendations for incorporating gender analysis at various stages of the research process [21]. Several high-impact journals, as well as the World Health Organization (WHO), have endorsed SAGER and the use of the checklist [40–42]. By doing this, they ensure that authors address the sex or gender dimensions of their research in all manuscripts and avoid ambiguity or conflation of terms.

The Cochrane Group also demonstrated its commitment to equity by establishing the Equity Methods Group in 2012 [43]. The main objectives of the group were to provide policy advice, training, and support on how to incorporate equity into systematic reviews and meta-analyses, although their main target is those reviews that address health equity to define social stratifying factors by which disadvantage can be measured: Place of residence; religion; occupation; gender or sex; race/ethnicity/language/culture; education; socioeconomic status; social capital; and additional characteristics such as age, sexual orientation and disability, as well as relationship characteristics and time-dependent circumstances [44].

5.5 Inclusion of Sex/Gender

Most authors and recommendations have a common point: They emphasize the importance of using the terms sex and gender correctly in health research, avoiding their interchange or use without a specific definition [12, 20, 21, 32, 41, 45, 46]. Sex refers to the biologically determined characteristics of men and women in terms of reproductive organs and functions, and it is based on chromosomal complement and physiology. Sex is globally understood as the classification of living things as male or female. Conceptually, it relies on the female/male binary, although there are many variations on the genetic chromosomal dichotomy [11, 12, 32]. Sex can also be conceptualized in interaction with gender, instead of as a static difference between females and males [47]. Gender refers to the social construction of femininity and masculinity, which varies in time and place and between cultures. As a static concept, it is defined as a person's self-representation as women or men, but relational theory describes it as a multidimensional concept [11].

However, it is common for authors to misuse both concepts and report gender (i.e., the identity referred to by the participants) and categorize it as sex [34, 46]. For this reason, it is recommended that authors should report how sex and gender were taken into account in the design of the study, ensure adequate representation of males and females, and justify reasons for the exclusion of males or females. The SAGER guidelines also recommend that, if only one sex/or gender was included in the study, this should be specified in the title or abstract of the paper [21].

5.6 Gender in Research Methods

The methodological aspects of gender analysis are of vital importance in order to produce quality scientific work. For this very reason, it remains a subject of discussion and constant development. The most fundamental issue, recognized by the European Union as one of the key steps in gender analysis, is the disaggregation of data by sex and gender [16]. To date, data outcomes have tended to be presented in a combined form, which has resulted in an inability to see the particularities of men and women [34, 37, 46, 48, 49]. This is even true in fields such as cardiology, where gender bias has long been cited as a source of poor data and the origin of delayed diagnoses and access to care in women [50].

The European Commission also underlines that data collection tools (such as questionnaires and interview checklists) must be gender-sensitive, use gender-neutral language and allow for the identification of the different realities of men and women. This will help to avoid gender bias. For example, answers to be provided by the "head of household" may not apply to all household members [16]. Dermody et al. reviewed the gender inclusivity of harmful drinking measures and although most included gender-neutral language (e.g., no gendered pronouns or terminology), there were still some that included gendered language and would not be appropriate for use with non-binary populations [51]. This highlights the need for researchers to make an effort to select psychometric tests that are gender inclusive.

Authors should also think about how to deal with gender in statistics. The concept of intersectionality should be incorporated [12, 52, 53]. Intersectionality is a methodology that systematically examines how gender and other social factors, such as age, disability, ethnicity, and migration status, interact with each other and create differences in needs, capacities, and inequalities among individuals and groups [53]. To examine this, an intersectional analysis should be performed. Typically, researchers perform a regression analysis where gender is usually included as a cofactor and therefore "controlled" for, forcing the relationship between the predictor and the outcome of interest to be the same across sex (i.e., male, female, and intersex) or gender (i.e., male, female, and gender minorities). Rather than controlling for sex and gender—whether statistically or in the application of an intervention—it is advisable to consider sex and gender as important variables that can explain, rather than confound, their research [52]. The intersectional analysis deals with the dynamics between sex/gender with other demographic factors, evaluating if these variables (e.g., race or migration status) have a different effect depending on the sex or gender of the individuals.

To identify these variables, authors should first make a list of sex-related variables relevant to the outcomes. A gender-related variable is a nonbiological variable that differs in magnitude, prevalence, and/or impact between people of different genders. For example, if the study is examining the psychological distress experienced by women, including the number of hours devoted to housing care in the study would serve as a gender-related variable, as it has been previously described that women experience difficulties with work–life balance that increase their depressive symptoms [54].

Finally, when interpreting the results obtained in a study, authors should evaluate the implications respecting sex or gender. This means to use a gendered theoretical framework or the gender perspective to explain the results, instead of the classic attribution of the results to biological factors. For example, if a study finds higher rates of depression in women than in men, a gendered interpretation of data should explore gender inequalities that could explain this difference, so just reporting a gender difference or attributing it to biological factors without further investigation would not be enough. Authors should also be aware of their own preconceptions and gender stereotypes, which may be used to explain results even without evidence to support it, as happened in studies on the mental health during COVID [34]. Additionally, according to the SAGER guidelines, the extent to which the findings can be generalized should also be evaluated. For example, if the study sample is overrepresented by men (e.g., 80%), the generalization of results to women should be cautious, as it could include a systematic gender bias [21].

5.7 Gender Perspective in the Clinical Practice

The final question is how to incorporate a gender perspective not only into the research process but also into clinical practice. Previous research has consistently shown that men are more likely to present with externalizing disorders, such as substance abuse, aggression, and risk-taking behavior, while women are more likely to present with internalizing disorders, such as depression or anxiety [55]. Although these sex and gender differences in mental health cannot be attributed solely to social factors [56], and biology also plays a role, a gender perspective can help practitioners intervene in the social aspects of illness.

First, gender roles and stereotypes profoundly influence behavior [1]. According to this, the masculine role promotes aggression, power, and dominance in men, while the feminine stereotype reinforces vulnerability, sensitivity, and powerlessness in women. Women are expected to be passive and are negatively evaluated when they display counter-stereotypical behaviors. When suffering from emotional distress (whether it be stress, depression, anxiety, or any kind of emotional suffering), men are more likely to exhibit aggressive behaviors, something that even led some authors to speak of "masculine depression" [57]. Women, on the other hand, are not encouraged to be independent and responsible, so they are more likely to present with internalizing disorders with feelings of hopelessness or depression [25]. These differences (men expected to be in control and women as submissive) create different barriers to accessing mental health care: men usually face cognitive barriers (feelings of failure when asking for help), while women face structural ones [58].

Second, being a woman, a man, or a non-binary person comes with different life experiences. Women experience more interpersonal trauma, such as gender-based violence and childhood abuse, factors associated with the development of anxiety and depression disorders, personality disorders, eating disorders, and trauma-related disorders [28]. Furthermore, they have lower wages, expend more time doing household chores and in childcare. In fact, in a nationwide study of the who on the prevalence of mental disorders, the narrowing of depression between genders was explained by changes in the traditional gender roles [55].

These factors should be recognized in clinical practice in order to address them appropriately. For example, in substance use disorders in men, the possible comorbidity of a depressive episode should be recognized, and in women, we should be aware of the additional stressor of social stigma, which may reduce access to health care. Respecting the psychosocial stressors related to sex and gender, we should try to address them as part of a multidisciplinary approach. For example, if a female victim of gender-based violence presents with depressive symptoms, a pharmacological approach alone may have little effect. Rather, we should organize safety planning and inform the patient about existing social and legal support. In the case of gender minorities, given the widespread discrimination that results in reduced access to the labor market, violence and even the risk of death or imprisonment in many countries, addressing these issues could help to dignify and validate the client.

5.8 Conclusions

Gender shapes the way we experience multiple aspects of human life, from relationships to decision making to emotion regulation. Because of its pervasive influence, gender shapes the manifestations of disease, and several studies have already shown that gender-biased science produces biased results and therefore low-quality data. Including gender in research is not just about studying women or focusing on the differences between women and men. Men, women, and non-binary patients are all gendered individuals, and gender may (or may not) lead to particularities in their disease expression, response to treatment, or access to health care. When applying gender analysis, it is important to correctly include sex and gender as a variable. Although not always necessary, sex/gender disaggregation of clinical data should be done, as studies have typically focused on males and extrapolated data to females and non-binary populations. Other variables, such as race, sexual orientation, or income, usually interact with gender, and the effect of this interaction can be measured using intersectional analysis. Besides that, current treatment services and recommendations should be evaluated from a gender perspective to identify potential shortcomings and improve care for men, women, and gender minorities.

References

1. Ellemers N. Gender stereotypes. 2017. Available from: https://doi.org/10.1146/annurev-psych-122216.
2. Bian L, Leslie SJ, Cimpian A. Gender stereotypes about intellectual ability emerge early and influence children's interests. Science (1979) [Internet]. 2017;355(6323):389–91. Available from: https://doi.org/10.1126/science.aah6524.
3. Steffens MC, Jelenec P, Noack P. On the leaky math pipeline: comparing implicit math-gender stereotypes and math withdrawal in female and male children and adolescents. J Educ Psychol. 2010;102(4):947–63.
4. Canadian Institutes of Health Research. Institute of Gender and Health Online Training Modules. What is gender? What is sex?
5. Morss JR. The concept of developmental stage: Hall, Freud, and Piaget [Internet]. Oxford University Press; 2020. Available from: https://oxfordre.com/psychology/view/10.1093/acrefore/9780190236557.001.0001/acrefore-9780190236557-e-531.
6. Spencer R. Freud's oedipus complex in the #metoo era: A discussion of the validity of psychoanalysis in light of contemporary research. Philosophies. 2020;5(4):27.
7. Joel P. The oedipus complex: a critical re-examination. Can Psychiatr Assoc J [Internet]. 1976;21(3):173–9. Available from: https://doi.org/10.1177/070674377602100308.
8. Olafson E, Corwin DL, Summit RC. Modern history of child sexual abuse awareness: cycles of discovery and suppression. Child Abuse Negl [Internet]. 1993;17(1):7–24. Available from: https://www.sciencedirect.com/science/article/pii/014521349390004O.
9. European Institute for Gender Equality. Gender perspective [Internet]. [cited 2025 Mar 21]. Available from: https://eige.europa.eu/publications-resources/thesaurus/terms/1257?language_content_entity=en.
10. Doyal L. Gender equity in health: debates and dilemmas. Soc Sci Med [Internet]. 2000;51(6):931–9. Available from: https://www.sciencedirect.com/science/article/pii/S0277953600000721.
11. Bauer GR. Sex and gender multidimensionality in epidemiologic research. Am J Epidemiol. 2023;192(1):122–32.
12. Hammarström A, Johansson K, Annandale E, Ahlgren C, Aléx L, Christianson M, et al. Central gender theoretical concepts in health research: the state of the art. J Epidemiol Community Health (1978). 2014;68(2):185–90.

13. Hammarström A. A tool for developing Gender research in medicine: examples from the medical literature on work life. Gend Med [Internet]. 2007;4:S123–32. Available from: https://www.sciencedirect.com/science/article/pii/S1550857907800532.
14. Gordon I, Zagoory-Sharon O, Leckman JF, Feldman R. Oxytocin and the development of parenting in humans. Biol Psychiatry [Internet]. 2010;68(4):377–82. Available from: https://doi.org/10.1016/j.biopsych.2010.02.005.
15. Hyde JS. Gender similarities and differences. Ann Rev Psychol. Annual Reviews Inc. 2014;65:373–98.
16. Trbovc JM, Hofman A. Toolkit for integrating gender-sensitive approach into research and teaching [Internet]. Available from: www.garciaproject.eu.
17. Schuler MS, Collins RL. Sexual minority substance use disparities: bisexual women at elevated risk relative to other sexual minority groups. Drug Alcohol Depend [Internet]. 2020;206:107755. Available from: https://www.sciencedirect.com/science/article/pii/S0376871619305320.
18. Schuler MS, Rice CE, Evans-Polce RJ, Collins RL. Disparities in substance use behaviors and disorders among adult sexual minorities by age, gender, and sexual identity. Drug Alcohol Depend [Internet]. 2018;189:139–46. Available from: https://www.sciencedirect.com/science/article/pii/S0376871618303235.
19. Cotaina M, Peraire M, Boscá M, Echeverria I, Benito A, Haro G. Substance use in the transgender population: a meta-analysis. Brain Sci. 2022;12(3):366.
20. European Comission for Gender Equality. Gender analysis [Internet]. [cited 2025 Mar 23]. Available from: https://eige.europa.eu/gender-mainstreaming/tools-methods/gender-analysis?language_content_entity=en.
21. Heidari S, Babor TF, De Castro P, Tort S, Curno M. Sex and gender equity in research: rationale for the SAGER guidelines and recommended use. Res Integr Peer Rev [Internet]. 2016;1(1):2. Available from: https://doi.org/10.1186/s41073-016-0007-6.
22. Howard LM, Ehrlich AM, Gamlen F, Oram S. Gender-neutral mental health research is sex and gender biased. Lancet Psychiatry [Internet]. 2017;4(1):9–11. Available from: https://doi.org/10.1016/S2215-0366(16)30209-7.
23. Lenz B, Derntl B. Sex-sensitive and gender-sensitive care for patients with mental disorders. Lancet Psychiatry [Internet]. 2025;12(4):244–6. Available from: https://doi.org/10.1016/S2215-0366(24)00330-4.
24. The Lancet Psychiatry. Sex and gender in psychiatry. Lancet Psychiatry [Internet]. 2016;3(11):999. Available from: https://doi.org/10.1016/S2215-0366(16)30310-8.
25. Kuehner C. Why is depression more common among women than among men? Lancet Psychiatry [Internet]. 2017;4(2):146–58. Available from: https://doi.org/10.1016/S2215-0366(16)30263-2.
26. von Majewski K, Kraus O, Rhein C, Lieb M, Erim Y, Rohleder N. Acute stress responses of autonomous nervous system, HPA axis, and inflammatory system in posttraumatic stress disorder. Transl Psychiatry [Internet]. 2023;13(1):36. Available from: https://doi.org/10.1038/s41398-023-02331-7.
27. Lawrence S, Scofield RH. Post traumatic stress disorder associated hypothalamic-pituitary-adrenal axis dysregulation and physical illness. Brain Behav Immun Health [Internet]. 2024;41:100849. Available from: https://www.sciencedirect.com/science/article/pii/S2666354624001273.
28. Copeland WE, Shanahan L, Hinesley J, Chan RF, Aberg KA, Fairbank JA, et al. Association of childhood trauma exposure with adult psychiatric disorders and functional outcomes. JAMA Netw Open [Internet]. 2018;1(7):e184493. Available from: https://doi.org/10.1001/jamanetworkopen.2018.4493.
29. Krieger N. Genders, sexes, and health: what are the connections—and why does it matter? Int J Epidemiol [Internet]. 2003;32(4):652–7. Available from: https://doi.org/10.1093/ije/dyg156.

30. Khan NA, Daskalopoulou SS, Karp I, Eisenberg MJ, Pelletier R, Tsadok MA, et al. Sex differences in acute coronary syndrome symptom presentation in young patients. JAMA Intern Med [Internet]. 2013;173(20):1863–71. Available from: https://doi.org/10.1001/jamainternmed.2013.10149.
31. Canadian Institutes of Health Research (CIHR), Institute of Gender and Health. Science is better with sex and gender: strategic plan 2018–2023. Canadian Institutes of Health Research (CIHR), Institute of Gender and Health; 2018. 35 p.
32. Clayton JA, Tannenbaum C. Reporting sex, gender, or both in clinical research? JAMA [Internet]. 2016;316(18):1863–4. Available from: https://doi.org/10.1001/jama.2016.16405.
33. Peters SAE, Woodward M. A roadmap for sex- and gender-disaggregated health research. BMC Med [Internet]. 2023;21(1):354. Available from: https://doi.org/10.1186/s12916-023-03060-w.
34. López-Atanes M, Sáenz-Herrero M, Zach N, Lakeberg M, Ugedo A, Fraile-García E, et al. Gender sensitivity of the COVID-19 mental health research in Europe: a scoping review. Int J Equity Health [Internet]. 2024;23(1):207. Available from: https://doi.org/10.1186/s12939-024-02286-1.
35. Jahn I, Börnhorst C, Günther F, Brand T. Examples of sex/gender sensitivity in epidemiological research: results of an evaluation of original articles published in JECH 2006–2014. Health Res Policy Syst [Internet]. 2017;15(1):11. Available from: https://doi.org/10.1186/s12961-017-0174-z.
36. Carcel C, Woodward M, Balicki G, Koroneos GL, de Sousa DA, Cordonnier C, et al. Trends in recruitment of women and reporting of sex differences in large-scale published randomized controlled trials in stroke. Int J Stroke [Internet]. 2019;14(9):931–8. Available from: https://doi.org/10.1177/1747493019851292.
37. Heidari S, Palmer-Ross A, Goodman T. A systematic review of the sex and gender reporting in covid-19 clinical trials. Vaccines. 2021;9(11):1322.
38. World Health Organization. Gender analysis in health. A review of selected tools [Internet]. WHO; 2002. Available from: www.inis.ie.
39. Debusscher P. Chapter 5: The EU gender equality strategy 2020–2025: the beginning of a new season? In: Social policy in the European Union: state of play 2022. ETUI and OSE.
40. Heidari S, Fernandez DGE, Coates A, Hosseinpoor AR, Asma S, Farrar J, et al. WHO's adoption of SAGER guidelines and GATHER: setting standards for better science with sex and gender in mind. The Lancet [Internet]. 2024;403(10423):226–8. Available from: https://doi.org/10.1016/S0140-6736(23)02807-6.
41. Raising the bar on sex and gender reporting in research. Nat Med [Internet]. 2022;28(6):1099. Available from: https://doi.org/10.1038/s41591-022-01860-w.
42. The Lancet Haematology. Sex and gender reporting advances in medicine. Lancet Haematol [Internet]. 2024;11(4):e241. Available from: https://doi.org/10.1016/S2352-3026(24)00074-7.
43. Petticrew M, Welch V, Tugwell P. 'It is surely a great criticism of our profession…' The next 20 years of equity-focused systematic reviews. J Epidemiol Community Health (1978) [Internet]. 2014;68(4):291. Available from: http://jech.bmj.com/content/68/4/291.abstract.
44. Parker R, Petkovic J, Pardo Pardo J, Darzi A, Dewidar O, Khabsa J, et al. The equity group: supporting Cochrane's social responsibility of improving health equity. Cochrane Evid Synth Methods [Internet]. 2023;1(3):e12012. Available from: https://doi.org/10.1002/cesm.12012.
45. Schiebinger L, Leopold SS, Miller VM. Editorial policies for sex and gender analysis. The Lancet [Internet]. 2016;388(10062):2841–2. Available from: https://doi.org/10.1016/S0140-6736(16)32392-3.
46. Johnson JL, Greaves L, Repta R. Better science with sex and gender: facilitating the use of a sex and gender-based analysis in health research. Int J Equity Health [Internet]. 2009;8(1):14. Available from: https://doi.org/10.1186/1475-9276-8-14.
47. Fausto-Sterling A, Books B. Sexing the body: gender politics and the construction of sexuality [Internet]. Basic Books; 2000. Available from: https://books.google.es/books?id=c3lhYfZzIXkC.

48. Hockham C, Thompson K, Carcel C, Pinho-Gomes AC, Woodward M, Peters SAE. What sex-disaggregated metrics are needed to explain sex differences in COVID-19? Front Glob Womens Health. 2020;1:2.
49. Carcel C, Harris K, Peters SAE, Sandset EC, Balicki G, Bushnell CD, et al. Representation of women in stroke clinical trials. Neurol Int. 2021;97(18):e1768–74. Available from: https://doi.org/10.1212/WNL.0000000000012767.
50. Bastian-Pétrel K, Rohmann JL, Oertelt-Prigione S, Piccininni M, Gayraud K, Kelly-Irving M, et al. Sex and gender bias in chronic coronary syndromes research: analysis of studies used to inform the 2019 European Society of Cardiology guidelines. Lancet Reg Health—Europe [Internet]. 2024;45:101041. Available from: https://doi.org/10.1016/j.lanepe.2024.101041.
51. Dermody SS, Uhrig A, Moore A, Raessi T, Abramovich A. A narrative systematic review of the gender inclusivity of measures of harmful drinking and their psychometric properties among transgender adults. Addiction. John Wiley & Sons Inc. 2023;118:1649–60.
52. Shapiro JR, Klein SL, Morgan R. Stop controlling for sex and gender in global health research. BMJ Glob Health. BMJ Publishing Group. 2021;6:e005714.
53. Geneva I. IOM intersectional gender analysis toolkit: summary [Internet]. 2024. Available from: www.iom.int.
54. Seedat S, Rondon M. Women's wellbeing and the burden of unpaid work. BMJ [Internet]. 2021;374:n1972. Available from: https://www.bmj.com/content/374/bmj.n1972.abstract.
55. Seedat S, Scott KM, Angermeyer MC, Berglund P, Bromet EJ, Brugha TS, et al. Cross-National Associations between gender and mental disorders in the World Health Organization World Mental Health Surveys. Arch Gen Psychiatry [Internet]. 2009;66(7):785–95. Available from: https://doi.org/10.1001/archgenpsychiatry.2009.36.
56. Li SH, Graham BM. Why are women so vulnerable to anxiety, trauma-related and stress-related disorders? The potential role of sex hormones. Lancet Psychiatry [Internet]. 2017;4(1):73–82. Available from: https://doi.org/10.1016/S2215-0366(16)30358-3.
57. von Zimmermann C, Hübner M, Mühle C, Müller CP, Weinland C, Kornhuber J, et al. Masculine depression and its problem behaviors: use alcohol and drugs, work hard, and avoid psychiatry! Eur Arch Psychiatry Clin Neurosci. 2024;274(2):321–33.
58. Harris MG, Baxter AJ, Reavley N, Diminic S, Pirkis J, Whiteford HA. Gender-related patterns and determinants of recent help-seeking for past-year affective, anxiety and substance use disorders: findings from a national epidemiological survey. Epidemiol Psychiatr Sci. 2016;25(6):548–61.

Part II

History

The Role of Women in the History of Psychiatry and Psychotherapy

6

Margarita Sáenz-Herrero

In the history of psychiatry, the pathological condition of the female body is a constant. For Greeks, hysteria is a word that means uterus. Plato [1] in his text *Timaeus* (which was later integrated into Western medical tradition through Galen and the Hippocratic writers) asserted that:

> The matrix or womb in women, which is a living creature within them, longs to bear children. If it is left unfertilized long beyond the normal time, it causes mayhem in the body, it blocks the breathing channels and causes, in consequence, acute distress and disorders of all kinds. If it is not "appeased by passion and love," the womb moved from its natural position within the body and, attaching itself to soft internal tissues, giving rise to a wide variety of symptomatic disturbances [1].

Through the history of psychiatry, the woman's body has been catalogued as being more prone to illness. Women suffer from nervous disease, neurasthenia, sickness, and gloom more frequently, while chlorotic women are often described in nineteenth- century Gothic literature. Galen, reproducing Greek's medicine model, thought women to be more likely to suffer mental illnesses and to be weaker and cripple. He also believed they were predisposed to be compliant and servile. The conception that female organs were inverted and under-developed within the body was held by Galen and subsequently by medieval philosophers. Albertus Magnus reckoned that women were not in their nature human beings but a failed birth. This conception of the female sex was maintained until the sixteenth century. Over history, the male sex is the only one that has been truly constructed, while the female has been constructed in opposition to him [2].

From a historical viewpoint, male domination was highlighted from the end of the Medieval period through the change of inheritance laws, the ban of women from

M. Sáenz-Herrero (✉)
Acute Unit, Cruces University Hospital, Barakaldo, Spain

M. López-Atanes, M. Sáenz-Herrero (eds.), *Applying the Gender Perspective in Psychiatry and Psychotherapy*, https://doi.org/10.1007/978-3-032-17883-1_6

universities, and the Church's debates on women's duties. Accordingly, the Church had a negative view, with the Dominicans and the Inquisition removing women from other professions (such as doctors or translators, which weren't infrequent in the Roman Era). On account of the influence exerted by the Church, women were confined within the domestic environment, the indissoluble matrimony making them disappear from public life [3].

Mithu Sanyal [2] has reviewed the invisibility of the female sex throughout the history of the Western world. In the first texts, the vulva was seen as principally a wound and then a crack by a world that rejected its existence through denial. Female genitals are the point where the interior meets the exterior. Psychoanalyst Harriet Lerner wrote in the 1970s about the difficulties experienced by many women in naming their own genitals and their inability to explore their own body. What they touched lacked a name. The absence of an explicit recognition and nomenclature for the girl's genitals had to have pathogenic consequences. At the end of the nineteenth century, the terms vulva, clitoris, and labia did not appear in the dictionary; just as the only word for female genitals in the dictionary today is vagina.

Freud deprived women of a self-determined sexuality. To challenge this is to fight a monster, a myth that has taken on life of its own through two words: penis envy. Sanyal asserts that psychoanalysis has committed matricide by killing the mother and placing the father at the heart of culture. It is odd that Lacan, who created the concept of the "Law of the Father," displayed reluctance to exhibit in his own home "The Origin of the World," Gustav Courbet's famous painting featuring a close-up of female genitalia. The painting, which may be seen nowadays at the *Museum d'Orsay* in Paris, was kept hidden behind a sliding door created by Surrealist painter, André Masson. With Freud, there is just one libido, the masculine one, from the moment it is identified with the forms of domination. Simone de Beauvoir in *The Second Sex* [4] criticizes psychoanalysis by stating that the concept of penis envy is symbolic of envy of power, symbolizing the privileges allowed to boys, the place the father holds in the family, and the universal predominance of boys, reinforcing masculine superiority. The descriptions of the female libido are poor, stemming their study from the male libido and not from itself.

If de Beauvoir's assertion [4] that "one is not born a woman but rather becomes one" is correct, woman is in itself a term in process, a becoming, a constructing that cannot rightfully be said to begin or end. As an ongoing discursive practice, it is open to intervention and resignification. This is the notion of body not as an available surface that awaits signification but as a set of individual and social limits that remain and acquire meaning politically. Referring to an original or authentic femininity is against the present need to analyze gender as a complex cultural construct [5].

Sexuality, violence, appropriated bodies, and medicated bodies are often related to women, as Michel Foucault [6] expressed in "*Histoire de la Folie à l'Âge Classique*," in which he questioned the medical view from the classical hysteria diagnosed by Charcot.

The twentieth century is considered revolutionary for women in Western culture. Society was deeply transformed in the manner in which male and female conception was perceived. Women could join the workforce and take up further education. In the 1950s, the arrival of the contraceptive pill brought a revolution in reproductive control changing the life of many Western women.

Unfortunately, at this point, we shall acknowledge that the revolution has not meant that women have entered the workforce and social life in the same way as men. The shift from private to public life has not guaranteed an actual transformation in real life for women throughout the world. Modern conceptions remain traditional. In today's world, media and the market, including the pharmaceutical one, are at the core of women's bodies. And the same can relate to the female sexual organs, for which a large market has grown, in contrast with men, such as creams to protect women from their own malodorousness.

The Madwoman in the Attic (by Sandra Gilbert and Susan Gubar) [7] explores how women have been represented in literature, particularly in the Gothic genre. In novels like those by the Brontë sisters, women are often depicted as mad, confined, and threatening. One prominent example is *Jane Eyre* by Charlotte Brontë, where Bertha Mason, the "madwoman" locked in the attic, becomes a symbol of female rage and repression.

This trope of the "madwoman" reflects the way society at the time viewed women's emotional and mental states as a threat when they stepped outside the confines of prescribed gender roles. Bertha, who ultimately sets the house on fire, embodies the consequences of this repression. In *The Madwoman in the Attic*, the authors argue that these women, though portrayed as insane, actually represent the suppressed desires and struggles of women in a patriarchal world.

The Brontë sisters' novels often depict women trapped by societal expectations, with the Gothic setting enhancing the atmosphere of entrapment and danger.

The portrayals of madness in the late nineteenth and early twentieth centuries were predominantly focused on women, as depicted in the book *The Madwoman in the Attic*, where writing is used as a way to express oppression and isolation. Let's not forget the lifelong confinement of Emily Dickinson, who was considered mentally ill for life, and it was only after her death that all her poems were discovered—works of great artistic quality created by a brilliant mind, not a person with a serious mental disorder. But for women at the time, sewing was the only acceptable activity. If they published, it was under a pseudonym, and Emily Dickinson used the metaphor of the artist spider weaving a place to hide and live. In her poem "The Paradise Tapestry" (J. 278), she expresses that in this paradise, she would not be a subversive spider, disguising herself and her meaning in webs of darkness, but a bare and shining figure. Here, she would not be forced to sew in the solitude of "North"; she would live loudly. Male poets have always inhabited that golden realm, but she, as a woman, lived camouflaged, from the beginning of her career as a poet to her quiet end. The poet Mary Elizabeth Coleridge also expresses this metaphor in "The Other Side of the Mirror," where she sees an enraged prisoner (herself) (Gilbert, 1998).

The figure of Nellie Bly [8], most recognized within the feminist advocacy sphere and an extremely popular character in American culture, joins the tradition of "fake mental patients" who, between the nineteenth and twentieth centuries, managed to bring the internal reality of psychiatric institutions to the general public.

Beyond the necessary social awareness, these cases caused a transformation in public opinion and a renewed reformist interest on the part of administrations that resulted in an improvement in patient treatment and a review of the state of psychiatric facilities.

Certainly, in many American states, it was necessary to have the requirement of two doctors to admit a patient to a mental asylum, since—as was the case in Europe— patients often refused to voluntarily go to them. To a large extent, this refusal was due to the bad reputation of these institutions, abusive treatments, or uncertainty about the length of confinement. Even so, not all those who ended up in such centers were precisely "crazy," as they were rarely evaluated by competent staff. Misunderstood or simply ignored, it was common for many patients to be transferred to asylums out of convenience, punishment, or misunderstood charity.

Nellie Bly, during her stay, was able to get a complete idea of how the asylum functioned. In fact, there seemed to be some sort of gradation in treatment, ranging from the moderately reasonable treatment received by less problematic patients to the absolutely degrading treatment provided to the most demented, violent, or supposedly dangerous inmates. Of the nearly 1600 inmates of the Asylum, the most unruly were confined in a special and independent module known as "The Lodge," a dark, dirty, and humiliating place that the more experienced inmates of the center advised her not to see. The patients interned there walked as part of the "gang rope": "A long rope was wound around leather belts, and these belts were closed around the waists of the fifty-two women. At the end of the rope was a heavy iron cart, and in it, two nurses […]. The women of 'the rope,' as the other patients called them, were completely occupied with their own disorders. Some shouted all the time."

Even though suspecting that Nellie was not actually ill and should not be there, Dr. Ingram did not discharge her, but only eased her confinement, from which she would only be freed by Peter A. Hendricks, one of the lawyers from The New York World. Because of this, Nellie would conclude: "The asylum on Blackwell's Island is a human trap. It is easy to enter, but once inside, it is impossible to leave."

De Beauvoir [4] asserts that the female body must be the situation and instrument of women's freedom and not a defining and limiting essence. This conversion process, which cannot be said to have a beginning or an end, is open to resignification. Hence, the body seems to be a set of individual and social limits. We women are fragments, pieces, and incompleteness; thus in this lack, we find the origin of distress and associated psychopathology. Alluding to an original or authentic femininity is a nostalgic ideal, as philosopher Judith Butler asserts. Following de Beauvoir's theory of "one is not born a woman but one becomes one," she proposes that the current need to analyze gender is a complex cultural construction. Hegelian tradition entwines desire with recognition; the desire is always a desire for recognition and anyone of us constitutes a viable social being only through the experience of recognition. Insofar as desire is involved in social standards, this is linked to the issue of power and the person who meets the requisites of what is recognized as human versus the person who does not [5]. Female human bodies are very often disdained by others and, as a consequence of this disdain, they are subject to abuse, ill-treatment, abasement, and murder. Female desire represents a dangerous energy for the established order, and the female body finds itself between disdain and exaltation. Many examples can be found in literature, cinema, and history: the femme fatale, vamps with come-to-bed eyes, with a dark gaze, provocative clothing, the cult of romantic love, and fatal destiny. The diva of this era is Marlene Dietrich in The Blue Angel. The dream of the First World War was the devil as a woman, the woman as desire, exotic, and sophisticated. The Second World War saw the appearance of pin-ups, girls with big cheeks. In the 1940s and 1950s, the most representative pin-up was Rita Hayworth, who was famously slapped in a scene showing the abuse of power [9]. By dint of this type of social determinism, servitude became voluntary and ended up finding pleasure in the renunciation of itself, as in the famous case of the triumphantly beautiful but ill-starred Marilyn Monroe, whose femininity was caricaturized until she took her own life; her sensuality laid in being tragic [9]. To censure the body is to censure, at the same time, the breath, the word. The subject is subordinated through language, and an individual prefers to exist in subordination than not to exist at all [5]. The pathologization of the female body has been a reality in the history of psychology, just as women do not appear in history until the nineteenth century. For practically, the whole of history "anonymous was a woman," as the writer Virginia Woolf [10] reminds us. In The Portrait of a Lady, Henry James explains:

> "There is no such thing as an isolated man or woman; we are each of us made up of a cluster of appurtenances. What do you call one's self? Where does it begin? Where does it end? It overflows into everything that belongs to us and then flows back again." A kind of collage, with the hope that things endure, however divided and fragmented they may be, like any mind [3]. The body seems to offer, in these conditions, the final anchorage point to cling onto. It is the anchorage point to be grasped as a being, to be organized, manipulated, transformed, exceeded as a person or individual in the eyes of others. This post-human perspective raises questions about certainty over identity and reassurance about oneself, which are also altered by the discovery of other experiences and other constructions of the body through the work of feminist artists (Nancy Spero, Judy Chicago, Cindy Sherman, Barbara Kruger), homosexual artists, and queer culture. Queer culture, according to Paul B. Preciado [11], goes much further by suggesting that this dichotomy does not exist, without even a difference between a true femininity/masculinity and another, impostured one. All gender identity is a performance, a masquerade.

The author and medical historian Edward Shorter says that each society has its own "symptom repertoire," the set of symptoms that we unconsciously trace when we start feeling unwell.

For example, a Victorian woman in distress would say she feels like fainting, while her modern equivalent in the United Kingdom would feel anxious or depressed, and a woman in China would have stomach pain. They all may have had identical experiences, perhaps all felt weak, nervous, or suffered physical pains, but the symptoms they paid more attention to were different, depending on what is considered normal in their society.

In Britain, "hysteria" was a disease believed to affect women and cause fainting, emotional outbursts, and nervousness. Today, the same mental phenomenon has other diagnoses, such as depression.

This fits with another increasingly popular concept, "expressions of distress," which suggests that each culture has certain acceptable and established ways of expressing emotional distress at any given time.

But then, are culture-related illnesses only a result of differences in how we label them? Another possibility is that the society we live in can actually changes how we get sick.

It was historically easy to have a woman committed to a psychiatric institution, both in England, as Charles Dickens attempted with his first wife (though unsuccessfully), and in Mussolini's Italy (where he confined his first wife and child for their entire lives). In France, Camille Claudel wrote letters begging her brother, a career diplomat, to help free her from the asylum, but without success. During Franco's regime in Spain, as reflected in Letters from the Asylum by Olga Villasante [12], similar abuses occurred. For instance, the book recounts the case of a woman suffering from endometriosis and addiction to pain medication, who was separated from her three children. This system essentially psychiatrized the lives of many women, women who could have been living their lives at home, instead of being institutionalized under dubious pretenses.

This reflects a pattern where psychiatric institutions were used as a means of control over women, often under the guise of medical necessity, but in reality, many of these women were simply suffering from issues that could have been better addressed outside of a psychiatric setting.

The imbalance of power between men and women becomes an increasingly accentuated process. In the era of Descartes, rationality was masculine and women moved to the private space. There were new urban strata in which the arrival of the bourgeoisie meant that the woman was spouse, mother, and housekeeper.

The French Revolution did not bring about a change for women. It was respectful with institutions and bourgeois values. The fifteenth century outstood Olympe de Gouges' contributions. The author of the famous Declaration of the Rights of Women (1791), which began with the following words: "Man, are you capable of being just? It is a woman who poses the question," was subsequently executed by guillotine. Mary Wollstonecraft, the author of the famous *Vindication of the Rights of Woman* (1792) as well as the feminist John Stuart Mill, who issued the first call in the British Parliament in favor of female suffrage (1867), were also key figures in the women's rights history. Finally, the voting right was granted in the United Kingdom and Germany in 1918, in Spain in 1931, and in France in 1944 (4 years ahead of de Beauvoir's book was published). In Switzerland, women were not allowed to vote until 1971, while some countries such as Saudi Arabia have just recently approved women's voting rights.

Sylvia Plath's work [13] is inseparable from her existence and the feminist view, as her contemporary, Anne Sexton, expressed in her poems. Both were women, poets, and committed suicide. Both were diagnosed with depression and were in psychiatric treatment. To fully understand her novels in depth, it is necessary to look at what a woman was supposed to be at that time. The following is part of the testimony of her friend and writer, Jillian Becker [14], on the final days of Sylvia Plath:

> I had met her in September 1962, shortly after her marriage to Ted Hughes had broken up. I felt sorry for her. I admired and envied her talent... On a freezing afternoon in February 1963, Sylvia arrived with her children... Her doctor spoke to me on the phone. He told me not to do everything for the children, that Sylvia must look after them, she must feel that they needed her. So, I asked her to come with me, when I took them to the bathroom, when I prepared their meals, when Nick needed feeding and changing. But she didn't pick up soap or a towel, or a spoon, or a safety pin. I'd leave the room, but she'd wait for me to return. My choice was to let them go unwashed, unfed, unchanged, or do the job myself. Mostly I did it...Sylvia suddenly said: "I must get back. I have to sort the laundry... My husband asked her if she was sure she wanted to go. She said she was. So, he drove her home. Only when he stopped at a red light did he hear the sound of weeping. He parked the car and went to sit on a jump seat opposite Sylvia. He implored her to let him bring them back to our house. She refused. He came back and told me that he wished she had stayed on with us, that he didn't think she could cope on her own. On the Monday morning at about eight o'clock the phone rang. I answered, and Dr Horder told me Sylvia had put her head in the gas oven and was dead.

As a confessional poet, Anne Sexton exploited the intimate details of her life for her poetry. "Poetry milks the unconscious," she said. Sexton lamented and celebrated female identity, sexuality, and power by revealing painful and shocking personal details about her life. Although she always insisted that her poetry was not autobiographical, her exploration of difficult and taboo female subjects, such as abortion, menstruation, menopause, masturbation, or desires, was made with such frankness that most readers and critics felt that the line between Anne the woman and Sexton the poet was often blurred.

Female subjectivity is constructed in relation to the body, taking care of others, and love as nuclear. Responsibility for others (children, husband, parents) occupies an important part of female identity. Values such as sacrifice, effort, caregiving responsibilities, and the ability to withstand hardship are part of most religions and culture and are a breeding ground for expressing psychic disturbances in women much more frequently than in men. Elfriede Jelinek (2004 Nobel Prize winner) [15] said in her novel Die Liebhaberinnen (Women as Lovers) that, in female lives, love is working. Art, literature, and history provide us with many examples of it.

Virginia Woolf, in her essay A Room of One's Own, published in 1929, expressed the real position of women at that time which still remains: "For most of history, Anonymous was a woman." "Imagine that men were only represented in literature as women's lovers, and were never friends, soldiers, thinkers, dreams; how few parts in the plays of Shakespeare could be allotted to them; how would the literature suffer." If this were the case, literature would be dramatically impoverished, and so, she argues, has happened by closing the doors on women's writing. Satirically, she describes her perplexity about why are there so many books written by men about women but none the other way round.

> A woman must have money and a room of her own if she is to write fiction." "It is fatal to be a man or woman pure and simple: one must be a manly woman, or a womanly man. [10]

References

1. Plato. Timaeus dialogue. Stanford Encyclopedia of Philosophy; 2005.
2. Sanyal MM. Vulva La revelación del sexo invisible. Anagrama; 2009.
3. Saenz-Herrero. Gender, corporality, and body image in psychopathology in women. A gender perspective. Springer; 2018.
4. Beauvoir S. The second sex. New York: Vintage Books; 1952.
5. Butler J. Gender trouble. Feminism and the subversion of identity. New York: Routledge; 1999.
6. Foucault M. Histoire de la folie á lâge classique. Paris: Gallimard; 1972.
7. Gilbert S, Gubar S. The madwoman in the attic. Madrid: Catedra; 1998. ISBN 10: 8437616689 ISBN 13: 9788437616681.
8. Blye N. Ten days in a Madhouse. Bucks Eds; 2009. ISBN-10. 8493747912.
9. El BA. cuerpo en el cine en Historia del cuerpo, vol. III. Madrid: Taurus; 2006.
10. Woolf V. A room of one's own; 1929.
11. Preciado PB. Manifiesto contrasexual. Barcelona: Opera Prima; 2002.
12. Viillasante O. Cartas desde el manicomio. Madrid: Catarata eds; 2018.
13. Plath S. Diarios completos. Barcelona: Alba Proyectos; 2016.
14. BBC. Sylvia Plath: Jillian Becker on the poet's last days. Feb 2013 [quoted in Oct 2018]. Available in https://www.bbc.com/news/magazine-21336933.
15. Jelinek E. Die Liebhaberinnen (women as lovers). Reinbek bei Hamburg: Rowohlt; 1975. ISBN 3-499-25064-0.

Alienated and Alienists

7

Margarita Sáenz-Herrero

The health problems faced by women share many common traits worldwide, but there are also significant differences determined by various living conditions. The health of girls and women is influenced by social and economic factors, such as access to education, family wealth, and place of residence. These differences are not only observed in developing countries but also within so-called developed nations. When we talk about poverty, we are talking about women. Therefore, poverty has the face of a woman. This also affects the health and mental health of girls and women. Traditionally, poverty has been defined purely in economic terms by the World Bank, but in 1997, a United Nations Human Development Report defined it in a much more accurate way, in my opinion, as "the denial of opportunities, such as the opportunity to lead a long, healthy, and creative life, and to enjoy a decent standard of living in freedom, dignity, and with the respect of all" [1].

Women suffer more than men from various forms of poverty, as they are victims of blatant inequalities: unequal access to education, health, means of production, property, and political responsibility positions. All these inequalities contribute to the feminization of poverty [1].

However, women play an important productive and social role in the community: agricultural and livestock work, commerce and financial income, social relationships, education, and the care of children and dependent people, etc. Women's poverty directly affects society as a whole [1].

In the seventeenth century, in France's first psychiatric hospital, La Salpêtrière, separate wings were reserved for prostitutes, poor women, young women, and those marginalized by society, as noted by Phyllis Chesler explained in her book [2] *Impoverished and prostituted women must have been victims of chronic violence, both sexual and physical, excessive in nature.*

M. Sáenz-Herrero (✉)
Acute Unit, Cruces University Hospital, Barakaldo, Spain

M. López-Atanes, M. Sáenz-Herrero (eds.), *Applying the Gender Perspective in Psychiatry and Psychotherapy*, https://doi.org/10.1007/978-3-032-17883-1_7

At the end of the nineteenth century, the crises these women experienced were not understood. They were not seen as responses to trauma. Charcot rediscovered hysteria and named it. He isolated it as a pure nosological object, separating it from epilepsy and other mental disorders. But this does not mean that he fully understood it or that he provided a therapeutic approach for these women. In fact, the author Didi Huberman questions the treatment given to this illness in his book "*The Invention of Hysteria*." In no case was attention given to the social and economic circumstances in which these women lived.

The pose was essential—it was necessary to take time to look, the framing, and the setting up of the body for the photographs. It gave the impression that the doctors (all men at that time) observed the "hysterics" as "in vivo" autopsies of patients.

In fact, many of the women hypnotized by Breuer and diagnosed with hysteria were prostitutes who had lived through traumatic events.

It is no coincidence that the pioneer of German feminism, founder of social services, and whose image was used on stamps for letters when she founded the first institution for marginalized women and their children, was simultaneously the first case of Breuer and Freud. This is how highly recognized but mostly ignored alienists were also patients and suffered from mental health problems (Anna O).

Berta Pappenheim (1859–1936), a Jewish feminist in the twentieth century who found fame as the first woman to found an orphanage in Germany, fought for women's rights and translated Wollstonecraft's Vindication of the Rights of Woman. Wollstonecraft was the mother of Mary Shelley (author of Frankenstein) but died in childbirth, leaving the baby to be raised by her father, a political anarchist. Mary was cast out by her father when she began a relationship with poet Shelley, with whom she had to flee the country in order to marry. Some articles show that perhaps the Frankenstein monster, who was able to think and feel emotions but was not human, recalls the situation of women in the late nineteenth century, when they were unable to study, had no access to family inheritance, lacked the vote, and were judged on whether they would form a good marriage. Berta Pappenheim was also famous in the history of psychiatry for being the subject of Breuer and Freud's famous case "Anna O." She suffered a "hysterical collapse" when she had to care for her infirm father [3]. Twenty-one at the time, Berta stopped eating and displayed multiple physical symptoms including mood swings and absences. She also had rage outbursts, during which she broke objects and suffered from headaches and morphine dependency. According to today's classifications, she might have been diagnosed with emotional instability disorder or borderline personality disorder. However, as mentioned above, her life took a different course. Such was her role in the social reintegration of women that her image was used for West Germany's first set of stamps, which were devoted to the benefactors of humanity. Many people are unaware of how Breuer and Freud's famous clinical case developed.

Another prominent case was that of *Blanche Wittman* [4], a Parisian nick-named "the Queen of Hysterics." She was admitted very young to the Salpêtriére Hospital where she got famous for her hysterical crises, which were recorded in paintings of the time. This took place in the context of what was called "moral therapy" imported by Pinel and implemented in asylums such as Salpêtriére. The aim of this "therapy" was to temper passions and destroy deliria through kindness, persuasion, and respect for the doctor's authority. Therapy sessions looked almost like authentic performances, as seen in the famous painting *A Lesson at the Salpêtriére* where one of Charcot's famous classes can be seen, in which Blanche, a Salpêtriére resident for many years, is held in Babinski's arms in a show to which members of Parisian high society were invited.

The large amounts of photographs from that time are well known. At the start of the century, very long exposure times and proper lighting were needed in order to create the right conditions for the photographs; the hysterical women were capable of warning of a possible "crisis" to allow the time for them to get ready [4]. The hysterical women of the Salpêtriére question the role of the doctor, who was none other than the great Charcot. However, few people know that following Charcot's death, Blanche left the Salpêtriére to return some years later as an employee, initially in the photographic laboratory and from 1900 on in the Radiology Service. She proved herself to be commanding, hardworking, and a good organizer in her work.

7.1 Sabina Spielrein (1885–1941)

She was born in Rostov on November 7, 1885. The eldest daughter of a wealthy Jewish couple, with three younger brothers. A younger sister died at the age of 6 from typhoid fever.

The relationship between the parents and their four children is described in Sabina's history as tumultuous and sadomasochistic. At 16, she displayed continuous mood swings, impulsive behavior, aimless escapes, and parasuicidal acts. She recalls her sister's death as one of the triggers for her deterioration.

At the age of 18, she was admitted to Burghölzli for negativism, mutism, aggressiveness, irritability, and provocative behavior. Mood swings and feelings of depersonalization. Her condition worsened when she received news from her family or when Jung, her psychiatrist, was absent and Bleuler had to take over her care. The diagnosis reflected in her medical history: Hysteria.

She wrote: "I am alone, alone in the world. No father, no mother, no home. I have no one to trust. I am alone with my sorrows."

When Sabina began treatment, Jung and Riklin were interested in conducting verbal association experiments; she was the first patient Jung approached using this model over a few months. The relationship with Jung began to take on importance. Establishing a good therapeutic alliance with her was a slow and complicated process.

She wrote in her diary, "I wish for a good friend to whom I could expose every trait of my soul. I wish for the love of an older person who loves and understands me, as parents love their child."

Bleuler and Jung lent her books on philosophy and psychoanalysis. They encouraged her to study medicine at the University of Zurich. She felt intellectually supported. She was finally discharged on June 1, 1905. She continued to see Jung for consultations until 1909 when they began a romantic relationship that ended when the relationship became public that year.

Dear Mamochka:

I am a little tired now, but completely at peace. I am deliriously happy like never before in my life. At the same time, it hurts and I would like to cry with happiness. You have probably guessed that the cause of all this is Jung. Today I visited him.

A stormy encounter took place between Jung and Sabina. Jung wrote to Freud stating that his first psychoanalytic patient had betrayed him, causing a scandal, for "not giving him a child."

Freud's response: he made no explicit references to the issue, commenting in passing that "being defamed was a price to pay in the psychoanalytic profession."

Indignant about the course of events, Sabina turned to Freud requesting a brief interview, to which Freud responded that such experiences had also happened to him and that they helped toughen the skin to control countertransference. The ultimate responsibility for the facts lies with hysterical patients; "these women can bring out, as charms, all imaginable psychic perfections, until they have achieved their goal." There is a clear attempt to justify and protect Jung, advising Sabina to repress all those experiences, without believing her account.

Sabina replied that repression was not the right path, as she would lose the possibility of loving another man. She chose to confront Jung and set certain conditions to end the matter: restore her reputation to her parents and to Freud.

Jung finally admitted his share of responsibility in the affair, although without mentioning that they had had sexual relations.

> I am largely to blame for my former patient's exalted hopes. My behavior was despicable. (Jung to Freud, June 21, 1909)

> Accept my heartfelt sympathy for the elegant way you resolved the conflict. (Freud to Sabina, June 24, 1909)

However, in Sabina's personal diary, the word poetry constantly appears as a synonym for sexual encounters she had with him. She began studying Medicine in 1905 at the University of Zurich. "It's a pity I'm not a man. Everything is easier for them." In 1911, she graduated with the reading of her thesis "The Psychological Content of a Case of Schizophrenia," supervised by Bleuler. Her thesis dealt with experiments on verbal associations to "decipher" the disorganized and delusional language of a schizophrenic patient, comparing the patient's thought mechanisms with mythology. This is the first academic text in which the term "schizophrenia" is used for the first time.

She joined the Vienna Psychoanalytic Association and read her second-most important work. She began practicing psychoanalysis in various European capitals, and publishing articles on Child Psychology: she published works with Piaget (being her psychoanalyst), Vygotsky, and Luria. She was offered a chair at the University of Moscow and the direction of a child psychoanalytic clinic.

She wrote about early childhood development, especially language, recording observations of her first daughter, comparing them with those of other writers.

In her conclusions, she valued language as an innate ability, albeit in need of stimuli to develop. She authored 29 publications on child psychology, linguistics, and language development and had a fluid correspondence with Jung and Freud.

Some of Jung's main ideas: anima (the unconscious part of man that personifies the feminine nature and vice versa) and shadow are believed to have been original ideas of Sabina Spielrein.

The concept of death drive originates from her. In 1912, Spielrein anticipated Freud by nine years in developing the concept of death drive or destruction in her article "Destruction as the Cause of Becoming."

Sabina Spielrein played a particularly important role in the development of Freud's theory of the death drive by presenting her work (after obtaining her medical degree the previous year with a case of schizophrenia) in 1912 under the title "Destruktion alsursadre des werdens" (Destruction as Cause of Becoming).

The novelty of Sabina Spielrein's theory lies in relating the death drive to the life drive. She argues that these two forces not only maintain balance but are a condition for each other that both are primary. So, the existence of one is unthinkable without the other. And what stands out is that Sabina Spielrein shows above all how myths, legends, and sacred texts from different cultures relate death and birth. There is a certain logical connection, she says, between returning to the original matter and being reborn. She also shows how the same myths and legends reveal a knowledge of the aggressive and destructive element in the erotic, and how self-destruction is within us as an instinct, both because it paves the way for the new and because it is related to the feeling of pleasure.

Sabina Spielrein argues in her work: "You feel the enemy within you (...). It is the fervent love, which with an urgent need forces you to do what you do not desire; you feel the end, the ephemeral, but you do not wish to escape or flee far away."

In the twentieth century, other psychoanalysts like Karen Horney denied the existence of a Thanatos or death drive, arguing that adverse situations in society would create in each person a drive against the self.

It is from the analysis of schizophrenia and neurosis, from the artistic realization of loving surrender, she states, that the conflict between the sexual drives of life and the drives of destruction and death merge in the creation of becoming, of creative movement. Destruction as the cause of birth, for some authors, constitutes what will be Freud's death drive. Freud himself acknowledges, in a footnote in his book *Beyond the Pleasure Principle*, the anticipation that Sabina had in her ideas.

> The list of the top ten psychoanalysts of the 20th century is a matter of fashion and taste, but in any list, five names would inevitably appear: Freud, Jung, Piaget, Luria, and Vygotsky. Sabina met each and every one of them. Both Jung, Freud, Piaget, and Vygotsky benefited from Sabina Spielrein's ideas. [5]

In 1924, she moved to Berlin with her 11-year-old daughter Renata and her husband, Dr. Paul Scheftel, and took a train to Moscow. She took with her the most recent book by Freud *The Ego and the Id. Language and Thought in the Child*, the first book in which her former patient, a 27-year-old young man, Jean Piaget, outlines the genesis of child thought from sensorimotor skills to abstract reasoning based on the ideas she provided and on Renata's spontaneous observations, her daughter.

The ten luminous poems on time and death from the "Duino Elegies" dedicated to her by Rainer Maria Rilke. Martin Buber's "I and Thou." Thomas Mann's "The Magic Mountain." "The Surrealist Manifesto" with which André Breton believes he affiliates art with psychoanalysis. She became the director of the White Nursery in Moscow. Psychoanalysis was banned in the Soviet Union in 1936. Sabina was executed in a synagogue in Rostov in 1942 along with her two daughters.

Sabina represents what in the Nordic countries we call the volva, a chosen, exceptional person who, through the fate of her people and her own suffering, was able to penetrate the depths of the soul, the depth of the human being.

> In any case, what I want to highlight from my work is the image of Sabina Spielrein that has remained fixed in my mind after writing the book, from which I have not yet been able to free myself. It is the image of the Sibyl, of a person who is never accepted in her time, no one believes her, she is systematically rejected by all. Rejected and exploited. (Alnaes 1996)

It was two Russian women, Sabina Spielrein (1885–1941) and Tatiana Rosenthal (1885–1921) who participated in the psychoanalytic circle, with the former contributing an excellent work entitled Destruction as the Cause of Birth, where she presented an elegant theory of repression and not, as traditionally held, the first ideas regarding the death drive in the case of Sabina Spielrein.

7.2 Marguerite Anzieu

The Aimée case, known for "curing" delirium, may perhaps be the least followed one. Aimée, who gained fame for her "self-punitive paranoia" as Lacan termed it, was meant to be known in asylums as "the delirium pensioner." With the real name of Marguerite, she ended up working as a cook and governess, without displaying any further signs of madness. She even worked in the house of Lacan's father. Marguerite's son, who subsequently became a psychoanalyst, learned on the couch of his teacher, Lacan, that his mother was the subject of the famous case of Aimée ("the loved one") [6].

7.3 Karen Horney (1885–1952)

Karen Danielsen was born in Germany in 1885. She studied Medicine at the universities of Freiburg, Göttingen, and Berlin, which had only recently started accepting women, and graduated in 1913. During her studies, she met Oskar Horney, whose last name she adopted after marrying him in 1909 and with whom she had three daughters before they divorced. A few years after Horney graduated, her parents died, and she fell into a prolonged state of depression. It was then that she began training as a psychoanalyst while undergoing therapy with Karl Abraham, a pioneer of psychoanalysis who Freud said was his best student. In 1915, she was appointed secretary of the German Psychoanalytic Association, founded by Abraham.

Abraham attributed Horney's symptoms to the repression of incestuous desires toward her father; Horney rejected his hypothesis and abandoned therapy. She would later become one of the main critics of the dominant psychoanalytic current and its emphasis on male sexuality.

Horney rejected the early psychoanalytic emphasis on sexuality and aggression as determining factors in personality development and neurosis. This author found particularly absurd Freud's and other male psychiatrists' obsession with the penis.

Horney believed that "penis envy" was explained by the social inequality between genders; what women envied in men was not their sexual organ, but their social role, and the same could happen in the opposite direction. She also believed that these roles were largely determined by culture, not just biological differences.

She was one of the main representatives of neo-Freudianism, a movement that was able to challenge psychoanalysis at the time, allowing for openness. She was the first female psychiatrist to publish essays on women's mental health and question the biologicalist approaches to gender differences of her predecessors. Between 1922 and 1937, Horney made various theoretical contributions on female psychology, becoming the first feminist psychiatrist, and is considered the founder of feminist psychology.

Among the topics she wrote about were the overvaluation of the male figure, the difficulties of motherhood, and the inherent contradictions of monogamy.

According to Horney, neurosis is a disturbance in a person's relationship with themselves and others. The key factor in the appearance of symptoms is how parents handle a child's anxiety during their development.

Neurotic personality or character neurosis arises when parents do not provide their children with a loving and secure environment, generating feelings of isolation, helplessness, and hostility. This blocks normal development and prevents the person from becoming their "real self."

In Horney's work, the real self is equivalent to identity. If an individual's personal growth is healthy, their behaviors and relationships develop properly, leading to self-realization. For Horney, this is a natural human tendency; later humanists like Rogers and Maslow would hold the same belief. She dedicated herself to therapy, training, and the development of her theory until 1952, the year of her death [7].

Gladys Swain (1945–1992) was a French psychiatrist. She was known especially for two books: *Le Sujet de la folie*, which revisits and reworks the pages of her doctoral thesis from 1974, and *La Pratique de l'esprit humain*, written with Gauchet, essayist and editor-in-chief of Le Debat. Her reflection, according to some, is the result of the 1968 generation that had to assess the questioning of the psychiatric discipline. Her *Dialogue with the Insane*, very significant, was written between 1977 and 1987. It is divided into four parts, which dialogue or complement her previously mentioned texts. She advocated for a commitment to care that led her to question the psychiatric discipline (from within her own practice), valuing the contributions of the anti-psychiatric movement, from which she always kept a prudent distance, and those of the "new" psychoanalysis embodied in Jacques Lacan. This is her starting point to understand this kind of reclamation of moral treatment, at least in its origins, from the psychotherapy that required for her practice a psychopathological doctrine in which the subjectivity of the madman appeared as crucial. An attempt to "think the present" from the conviction that "every history is contemporary." For Foucault, as we have seen, madness is "imprisoned in a moral world," but also, the asylum is a "religious domain without religion, a domain of pure morality, of ethical uniformity." On the contrary, G. Swain criticizes, as simplistic, this idea, which she considers very widespread among her colleagues. Moral treatment thus emerges as a specific therapeutic method aimed at subjects with mental alienation, in any of its forms. A treatment that required an adequate infrastructure and that had to be applied in institutions specially designed for this purpose. Our author gives a capital importance to the Pinelian revolution in the birth of psychiatry, not because it freed the mad from their chains, but because with Pinel, the birth of the clinic (psychiatric) takes place. This occurs in the context of the so-called "Moral Treatment" imported by Pinel and instituted in asylums such as the Salpêtriére. The aim of this therapy was to moderate passions and destroy delusions through gentle treatment, persuasion, and respect. It is here where moral treatment takes on an unprecedented importance, because it constitutes, at least in the thought and practices of the early alienists, a possibility of cure for mental patients. The asylum is understood by Swain as a therapeutic institution, not necessarily repressive. Naturally, it is not exempt from contradictions or bad practices, but "conceptually," and at least on paper, it would not be originally designed as an institution of social control and defense. The interpretive model proposed by Gladys Swain aims to explain the birth of psychiatry understanding the asylum and moral treatment as a "therapeutics of the person" not necessarily based, despite its contradictions or failures, on disciplinary power, or the imposition of knowledge or a "regime of truth," or obtaining amendment through repentance, but on the reconstruction of the individuality of the subject. However, it is Gladys Swain, once again, who with great solidity has insisted on this crucial aspect. For her, "moral treatment, at least as understood by Pinel and Esquirol, is a treatment that gives more importance to appealing to intellectual faculties and to feelings or passions. This subjectivity of madness is shared by most authors who have dealt, with greater or lesser insistence, with the birth of alienism. Disagreements or differences in approaches are sometimes noticeable, but the backdrop of subjectivity is present in most approaches. Both in the therapeutic and integrative hypothesis, as well as in the regulatory and/or exclusionary, subjectivity, reflexivity, and internalization of patients are taken into account. It is somewhat surprising the little attention that psychiatric historiography has paid to the process of constitution of mental medicine from the development and diffusion of modern culture around the self or subjectivity [8]".

7.4 Rita Levi Montalcini

The researcher Riva Levi Montalcini, in her autobiographical book *In Praise of Imperfection*, wrote: "I moved forward while the world was collapsing, thanks to the desperate and, in part, unconscious will to ignore what was happening, because full awareness would have prevented us from continuing to live. Each bombing protected her life as if it were her microscope. Those studies, conducted against the grain, would lead to the discovery of the nerve growth factor (NGF), which earned her the Nobel Prize in Medicine in 1968. NGF is the protein that stimulates the growth and renewal of nerve cells and, therefore, their survival; it plays an essential role in the formation of the nervous system. Hence, the discovery from many years of research with chicken embryos and mouse tumors continues to inspire new lines of research on other growth factors, due to their regenerative power for damaged neurons, whether from Alzheimer's or other degenerative diseases. As the researcher herself described: "Embryonic cells offer huge possibilities to researchers seeking cures for the worst diseases. Seventy years ago, I was already working with embryonic brains and perceiving all that we could learn from them."

In her work, she takes stock of her professional and personal trajectory. After receiving the Nobel Prize in Medicine, she always tried to reconcile two irreconcilable aspirations: perfection in life or perfection in work. She achieved this by opting for a certain imperfection in both life and work. And by discovering the pleasure both activities gave her, she realized that imperfection was the aspect that most aligned with human nature. And more so in the case of women. She fought for equality throughout her life. In Rome, where young women continue to research NGF, she said: "They are all women, yes, and that proves that talent has no gender. Women and men have the same mental capacity."

In fact, she said: "The future of the planet depends on the possibility of giving all women access to education and leadership" [9]".

References

1. Jausoro C, Marino M. Women Mental Health all over the world: Socio-political aspects of gender discrimination and violence. Immigration and transnational motherhood. In: Saenz-Herrero M, editor. Psychopathology in women. A gender perspective. Cham: Springer; 2015. ISBN 978-3-319-05869-6.
2. Chesler P. Women and madness. Palgrave Macmillan; 2005. ISBN 10: 1403968977.
3. Pappenheim B. http://www.heroinas.net/2019/05/bertha-pappenheim-defensora-y-pionera.html.
4. Didi-Huberman G. La invención de la Histeria. Ensayo Arte Cátedra. 2007.
5. Alnaes K. La verdadera historia de Sabina Spielrein. Madrid: Siruela Eds; 2010.
6. Lacan L. De la Psicosis paranoicas en sus relaciones con la personalidad; 1976 Mexico Siglo XXI ed.
7. Horney K. https://psicologiaymente.com/biografias/karen-horney.
8. Huertas R. Historia cultural de la Psiquiatría. Madrid: Editorial Catarata; 2012.
9. Levi-Montalcini R. Elogio de la imperfección. Barcelona: Círculo de Lectores; 1990. ISBN: 84-226-3079-6.

Part III

Gender and Psychopathology

Introduction

8

Margarita Sáenz-Herrero

The main aim of this book is to introduce the gender paradigm perspective in a narrative format to offer a different understanding of symptoms from the way they are usually presented in psychopathology [1].

The term feminism, as defined in the Oxford Dictionary, refers to the advocacy of women's rights on the grounds of gender equality. Etymologically, the word feminism comes from the French féminisme (1893). Alexandre Dumas (son of the famous writer Alexandre Dumas) used the term to describe men who defended women's rights. At the end of the nineteenth century and the early twentieth century, suffragettes fought for the right to vote and for equal participation in public life.

In France, the Panthéon in Paris—where many notable French figures such as Voltaire and Victor Hugo are buried—contains the tombs of only five women: Sophie Berthelot ("Cette distinction lui a été attribuée en hommage à sa vertu conjugale, étant morte à quelques heures de son mari"), Marie Curie, Simone Veil, Geneviève de Gaulle-Anthonioz, and Josephine Baker. Even in 2025, this number remains strikingly low. Moreover, in the French language, the term Droits de l'homme ("Rights of Man") is still commonly used to refer to human rights, illustrating the persistence of androcentric language.

In the United Kingdom, significant political change did not occur until the emergence of the suffragette movement in the late nineteenth century. A 'second wave' of feminism arose in the 1960s, emphasizing unity and sisterhood.

It is important to clarify that gender is not a feminist concept. The term was first used by Dr. John Money, a sexuality researcher and pediatrician at Johns Hopkins University, to distinguish intersex conditions as another natural variation of human sexuality. Gender anthropology, as part of critical reflection, raises questions about both universal and culturally specific aspects of human societies, challenging

M. Sáenz-Herrero (✉)
Acute Unit, Cruces University Hospital, Barakaldo, Spain

M. López-Atanes, M. Sáenz-Herrero (eds.), *Applying the Gender Perspective in Psychiatry and Psychotherapy*, https://doi.org/10.1007/978-3-032-17883-1_8

androcentric biases and ethnocentric structures. This led to a revision of theoretical models and their consequences.

The distinction between sex and gender as biological identity versus the social and cultural construction of identity, brought about a significant epistemological shift in the understanding of female identity. The philosophical contributions of Simone de Beauvoir and the anthropological studies of Margaret Mead played a crucial role in shaping this discourse.

Feminism is for everybody: To be a feminist is to seek liberation for all people—both men and women—from sexist patterns of domination and oppression. Yet, even after 40 years, the world continues to grapple with gender inequality and sexism. Health systems and scientific research are no exceptions, and neither is psychopathology [2].

Most doctors, psychiatrists, and psychologists still study descriptive psychopathology based on Karl Jaspers' model, without incorporating the gender dimension in the understanding of symptoms. Jaspers, in his Phenomenological Approach in Psychopathology, emphasized the meaningful connections between life history and psychosis. His most influential work, General Psychopathology (Allgemeine Psychopathologie), was published in 1913 at a time when psychiatry was dominated by neurobiological approaches. Jaspers' primary goal was to reestablish psychiatry within the domain of the human sciences. Today, descriptive psychopathology and clinical psychiatry still largely rely on his framework [3].

Professor Berrios has consistently argued that every generation of psychiatrists should contribute to the ongoing construction of psychopathology, as historical, cultural, and social factors influence mental health worldwide. While the biopsychosocial model is widely recognized, the social component is often overlooked. Likewise, the gender paradigm has been omitted from the history of psychiatry.

This book is an attempt to integrate gender into the way psychopathology is understood and expressed in human experience [1].

Gender is without any doubt, a nuclear fact that distinguishes human beings even before birth. The first thing asked when a baby is born, and even before, is whether it's a boy or a girl. Despite biological diversity and the existence of Turner Syndrome (X0); Klinefelter Syndrome (XXY); intersexual human beings, a binary model is usually presented and where gender is one of the most difficult taboos to break in western culture.

Gender commences at birth; it is learnt; it is interpreted, with values in our families, social contexts and cultures. It is necessary to broaden the area in which Psychopathology is built. As in science, it is necessary to include gender in research and in Psychopathology too; not to do so is to do bad science.

In its 2001 report *Exploring the Biological Contributions to Human Health: Does sex matter?* the Institute of Medicine called on biomedical researchers to step up their investigations of sex and gender as critical variables affecting health. Wizeman in 2001 proposed that increased understanding of the roles of gender and sex at every level of existence, from the sociological level down to the molecular level in health and disease, could advance preventive, diagnostic, and therapeutic healthcare practices [4] Gender (subsuming masculinity and femininity) appears to possess its own significance in the study of health and disease. In fact, several studies suggest that individual differences in degree of masculine and feminine gender characteristics assessed in early adulthood were significantly related to morbidity, mortality and health behaviors. For instance, a large longitudinal study demonstrated that greater levels of masculine gender characteristics assessed in early adulthood were significantly related to increased mortality over the next several decades, even after adjusting for unhealthy lifestyle habits (e.g., smoking, obesity, risk-taking). Importantly, this finding held true for both sexes, i.e., female and male participants who manifested higher levels of masculine gender characteristics than did their same-sex peers were also more likely to die at any given age. In the Terman study (2000) *is masculinity hazardous to your health?* mortality rates were highest for the most masculine males and lowest for the most feminine females.

An updated History of Gender needs to be included in Psychiatry and Mental Health. When dynamics change, symptoms change through History. A discourse should be created, not only for historians, anthropologists and sociologists but for Public Mental Health overall including Gender in Psychopathology.

During the 1950s and 1960s, physicians were still taught that women suffer from "penis envy," were "morally inferior to men," and were innately "masochistic," "dependent," "passive," "heterosexual," and "monogamous." According to the prevailing belief at the time, neuroses and psychoses were caused by mothers—never fathers, genetic predisposition, accidents, or poverty. This view was widely disseminated, including in the 2005 edition of Phyllis Chesler's book.

Chesler writes [5] "None of my teachers ever said that women or men suffer oppression, or that oppression causes trauma, especially when the sufferers are blamed for their own misfortune and it is diagnosed as a pathology."

Chesler combined patient interviews with an analysis of women's roles in history, society, and myth, documenting the double standard by which women were judged psychologically and psychiatrically. This work highlights the ways in which gender biases have shaped psychiatric diagnoses and the treatment of women.

The first question we must ask ourselves when constructing our understanding of reality is: How do we know what we think we know? To challenge traditional discourse, we must open fissures to include what has been excluded. Public spaces should be dynamic, reflecting a changing world and evolving symptoms.

A return to the definition of gender as a term that encompasses both masculinity and femininity (male versus female) would help clear up confusion and could have important implications for the study of health and disease. In this sense, gender relates to biological sex, rather than to masculinity or femininity as they pertain to behavior and psychology—traits that have traditionally been associated with males and females, respectively. However, it is crucial to note that both males and females differ widely in the extent to which they express gender characteristics typically considered masculine (e.g., aggression, stoicism) or feminine (e.g., nurturing, expressiveness) [6].

Sex and gender are related, but they are not the same. Each variable warrants its own independent study. Gender is a continuous variable, not a categorical one, when examining various health outcomes. Research into the relationships between gender characteristics and health outcomes could yield insights into the mechanisms that underlie broader differences between the sexes in terms of morbidity, mortality, and health behaviors.

This is not an attempt to criticize current psychopathology, but rather a call to approach it from a critical perspective that incorporates a gender lens. Semiological and clinical aspects involve symptoms rooted in an individual's biography, and these cannot be decontextualized from the social, historical, and cultural contexts in which they arise. However, we face the challenge of objectifying human subjectivity while addressing these complexities.

Gender has been identified as a critical determinant of Mental Health and well-being. In this sense, gender inequality acts as a powerful engine of stratification, determining the distribution of health, power, and risk factors for both physical and mental well-being by WHO in 2022 [7] From a biopsychosocial perspective, both strictly biological aspects and socioeconomic factors, including gender, are relevant sources of variation in the appearance of certain risk factors, disease prevalence, age of onset, prognosis, and treatment effectiveness [8–10] Addressing social reality from this paradigm includes women and men, seeks to make visible, identify, and take into account the differences, needs, and specific problems that constitute a unit of analysis. This allows for the incorporation of social aspects to design health actions, strategies, interventions, and policies.

Gender bias in research could be defined as a systematically erroneous gender-dependent approach related to social construct, which incorrectly regards women and men as similar/different. Most gender bias can be found in the context of discovery (development of hypotheses), but it has also been found in the context of justification (methodological process), which must be improved. In fact, one of the main effects of gender bias in research is partial or incorrect knowledge contained in the results, which are systematically different from the real values. This is a serious mistake in scientific research. The problem is not only with gender and different role gender but masculine gender is still considered superior than female gender.

Gender is one of the most powerful social determinants in the construction of our identity as human beings. It is crucial to incorporate this perspective in the construction of symptoms and signs that constitute Psychopathology and Mental Health. It is not about criticizing current Psychopathology but it does imply the need to approach psychopathology from a critical perspective that incorporates a Gender Perspective. The semiology and clinical aspects involve a list of symptoms that are present in each individual's biography and cannot be decontextualized from the social, historical, and cultural context in which they occur. However, we face the difficulty of objectifying human subjectivity.

Addressing social reality from this paradigm includes women and men, seeks to make visible, identify, and take into account the differences, needs, and specific problems that constitute a unit of analysis. This allows for the incorporation of social aspects to design health actions, strategies, interventions, and policies.

A paradigm, constitutes a theory or set of theories that are accepted and serve as a model for solving problems. The biomedical paradigm is crossed by social and gender factors in a nuclear way. Mental health problems after the pandemic have been made visible and placed on the political agenda. The consequences of the pandemic are present in our society. Social isolation, social networks as a means of communication, have led to an increase in mental health problems and disorders. This translates into an increase in the demand for mental health consultations, especially among adolescents and women.

Sex and gender are terms that are often used interchangeably, but in practice, although related, they are different. In this sense, sex refers to the biological differences between men and women. It encompasses the characteristics of an individual that are biologically defined (sex chromosomes, phenotypic factors, and physical and physiological characteristics of individuals).

Gender refers to the social construction of biological sex that occurs in each era, culture, and moment, and determines to a greater or lesser extent the construction of our identity and subjectivity. The differential socialization between men and women implies that health problems are expressed and manifested differently, and structural inequality between them results in more mental health problems in women.

The dominant paradigm until the seventies was that of the major psychopathological structures, arising from Gestalt theory, linguistics, and neurology, and following the phenomenological currents of the work of Minkowsky and Binswanger, psychoanalysis on the other hand, and the French school of Henry Ey. For some authors, we are in a paradigm crisis in terms of Thomas Kuhn as referred to by the historian of Psychiatry.

The crisis of the scientific paradigm for Lanteri Laura [11] is that psychiatry consists of an articulated set of semiological and clinical data, without hierarchical independence, related to other disciplines such as anatomy, neurophysiology, psychoanalysis, psychology, sociology.

For German Berrios, psychopathology is a set of languages developed by societies to describe, explain, and manage deviations or behavioral disorders that fundamentally depend on a neurophysiological or psychological deviation.

In a critical article, Professor Jean Garrabé [12] wondered if psychiatry was going to disappear by merging with neuroscience or if it was going to integrate the contributions of these sciences that are foreign to it but that can enrich its practice as therapists such as psychology, sociology, anthropology, pharmacology, knowledge of brain function, human behavior, evolutionary psychology, behaviorism, etc. Psychiatry place a nuclear space at the crossroads of many other disciplines.

Women are twice as likely to be diagnosed with depression. This has been related from the biomedical paradigm to genetic and hormonal factors, on the one hand, and environmental factors, on the other hand. Women's vulnerability to mental health problems may be a stereotype, but it also constitutes a reality in the current world. Sexual abuse in girls and women is more common, as well as gender-based violence, sexual assaults, and traumatic events [13].

It must be recognized that psychiatry and psychology have an enormous debt to the victims of sexual abuse. If we review the history of the treatment given to sexual abuse and trauma, we will find references that have justified, from biology, science and psychoanalysis, the naturalization of sexual violence through "natural" male aggressiveness and female "passivity." There are also numerous references in the psychotherapeutic tradition that relate "fantasy" and "daydreaming" to women's stories (unconscious fantasies).

Women who resist sexual intercourse have been stigmatized as "inhibited," "repressed" and "asexual." Women's "reticence," "aversion," and "frigidity" have been labeled as "puritanism" and "prudishness" in the face of sexual relations. It could be "a rebellion of women against male domination and power as Emilce dio Bleichmar explain in *The spontaneous feminism of hysteria* [14].

Structural inequality implies that women are much more likely to live in poverty, have greater inequality in access to resources and power status, and generate greater concern about the future, low self-esteem, lack of control over life itself, which constitutes the "depressive cognitive triad" described by Beck, which could be interpreted as depressive realism in the case of many women, if we include the gender paradigm in its interpretation.

There is an incomprehension of women mental health issues including questioning.

the veracity of the story or dismissing its semiological expression and comparing it with male standard. There is a thinking that their pathology is banal. They are not taking into account social conditioning factors, not offering all diagnostic and therapeutic possibilities. There is a failure to consider the relationship between mental health and a history of multiple violence.

Depressive disorders represent the most common cause of disability according to WHO information. And it affects women twice as much as men. Finding an explanation for these results is complex, as it may result from a double paradoxical process in which women may be experiencing overdiagnosis and overmedicalization of their mental health, while men may be experiencing underdiagnosis and undermedicalization [15] (Bacigalupe, Cabezas, Martin, 2021). Some authors have called this process of possible over-treatment, on the one hand, and insufficient recognition, on the other, the paradox of mental health [16, 17] This fact could be the result of the differential socialization of emotionality in men and women, which implies that traditionally feminine attributes such as sensitivity, expression through crying, or emotional lability favor their identification as depression. Consequently, healthcare professionals may find it easier to associate symptoms constituting the classic diagnosis in women (Ussher, 2010). Likewise, there may also be underdiagnosis in men, since the social requirements of traditional male identity reward a lack of emotional expressiveness, making the diagnosis of depression in men difficult. Men commit suicide much more often, although suicide attempts are more frequent in women. This equating of the feminine with the pathological is closely linked to how knowledge has been constructed. There is no room for the social aspect and no response is provided to women's distress, expressed more diffusely from their own experience [17].

Throughout the history of Psychiatry, women have been identified as more vulnerable to mental illnesses, attributing characteristics such as weakness, sensitivity, and influenceability to their character. The term "hysteria" even carries the word "uterus" in its etymology, directly relating it to women. Hysteria has been interpreted as a way for women to escape the reality they have to live in.

Emilce Bleichmar, in her book *The Spontaneous Feminism of Hysteria*, explained that hysteria is a form of masquerade—a way for women to break free from the reality imposed upon them. María Zambrano also stated that metamorphosis is a way for all living beings to avoid suffering and that humans constantly strive to become something more or different than what they are.

In psychiatry, it is crucial to consider the differences between men and women, not only in terms of biology and their response to treatments but also in relation to the social inequalities they face. Gender differences in mental health and health care must be recognized and addressed to ensure equitable and effective care for everyone. It is not enough for a resident to simply master the language of psychopathology and correctly identify a patient's symptoms. The true challenge lies in understanding how this knowledge is applied in daily psychiatric practice and how it can benefit the patient in a meaningful way.

Although the biopsychosocial model of disease still prevails, the gender paradigm has yet to be integrated into the model of human illness. Men's and women's health is different and unequal, shaped by both biological factors—such as genetic and physiological differences that expose individuals to specific risks—and by the roles society assigns based on gender. These roles affect opportunities, life experiences, and overall health outcomes.

Gender has become a significant ideological battleground. Media attention on issues like social and economic justice, sexual harassment, gender violence, and the influence of social media has pushed these topics to the forefront globally. The economic crisis has deepened inequalities between men and women in the European Union, particularly increasing female unemployment and rolling back gender equality policies. Growing populism and political polarization have made gender a dividing issue in society.

In medicine, it is essential to consider both sex and gender in research, as they impact the causes of illness, how different pathologies manifest, and how diagnoses and treatments are approached. This is vital for scientific rigor and is not an ideological stance. Ignoring these factors leads to flawed science.

A critical perspective, with a clear look at the past, is necessary for progress. Gender-related mental health issues, such as anxiety and mood disorders, are often tied to social factors, the burden of care placed on women, and the construction of our subjectivity. It is particularly difficult to objectify subjectivity, especially for women, whose sense of agency is often centered around seeking love rather than pursuing personal goals. Reflecting on these internal representations and making changes is essential for personal growth and empowerment.

Psychiatry is concerned with meaning as much as with physiological facts. Understanding individuals is central to psychiatry, but it is a different kind of understanding compared to identifying causal or etiological reasons for diseases. This understanding must also consider psychosocial, cultural, and historical aspects.

However, gender and sex have often been used as synonymous concepts in medical literature. In fact, there are few studies where gender is the primary lens through which we explore how psychopathology is differently expressed in relation to it. Gender studies have emerged as a growing field, incorporating gender as a central object of study especially in social studies and the humanities in doctoral theses, articles, books, and university curricula. However, this remains a controversial area in medicine. Medical studies need to integrate a gender perspective.

The diagnosis of mental health conditions or psychiatric disorders is based on criteria that are inherently linked to the sociocultural context of the individual and should account for gender as well as the social context of the person being diagnosed. These criteria include factors that define what is considered rational or irrational, compulsive or voluntary, expected or unexpected, and they are closely tied to specific circumstances. However, identifying internal dysfunction is rarely done independently of the personal condition of the individual. The presence of a mental health disorder implies an alteration in the internal mechanisms responsible for normal functioning.

It is time to advocate for equality that respects biological differences, particularly those of women. This book aims to serve as a comprehensive review that we hope will have a significant impact on psychiatrists and psychologists. We believe that it is possible to shift perspectives and that is our goal.

Recent societal changes and evolving lifestyles demand a shift in priorities when evaluating clinical symptoms and psychopathology. It is essential that we address new priorities for mental health disorders, but this can only happen if we change our approach to include the gender perspective as a core paradigm and work to convince others to do the same.

References

1. Sáenz-Herrero M. Foreward. Psychopathology in women: incorporating gender perspective into descriptive psychopathology. Springer; 2015. ISBN 978-3-319-05869-6.
2. The Lancet. Feminism is for everybody. Lancet. 2019;393(10171):493. https://doi.org/10.1016/S0140-6736(19)30239-9.
3. Jaspers K. Psicopatología general. Buenos Aires: Editorial Beta; 1977.
4. Wizeman TM, et al. Exploring the biological contributions to human health: does sex matter? Washington, DC: National Academies Press (US); 2001.
5. Chesler P. Women and madness. Palgrave Macmillan; 2005. ISBN 10: 1403968977.
6. Risvedt SL. The evolution of gender. JAMA. 2014;71(1):13–4. https://doi.org/10.1001/jamapsychiatry.2013.3199.
7. World Health Organization. Gender and health [Internet]. who.int. [cited July 17]. Available from: https://www.who.int/health-topics/gender.
8. Valls-Llobet C, Banqué M, Fuentes M, Ojuel J. Morbilidad diferencial entre mujeres y hombres. Anuario de psicología/UB J Psychol. 2008;39(1):9–22.
9. Riecher-Rössler A. Sex and gender diferences in mental disorders. Lancet Psychiatry. 2017;4(1):8–9. https://doi.org/10.1016/S2215-0366(16)30348-0.
10. Seeman MV. Men and women respond differently to antipsychotic drugs. Neuropharmacology. 2020;163:107631. https://doi.org/10.1016/j.neuropharm.2019.05.008.
11. Lanteri-Laura G. Ensayo sobre los paradigmas de la psiquiatría moderna. Editorial Triacastela; 2000. Archivos de Neurobiología 9788493091460.
12. Garrabé J. La Psiquiatría del siglo XXI. Atopos N2 Diciembre, 2003. 2002.
13. Sáenz-Herrero M. Gender violence and mental health: a gap between clinical assistance and research. Actas Esp Psiquiatr. 2018;46(1):29.

14. Dio Bleichmar E. El feminism espontáneo de la histeria (The spontaneous feminism of hysteria). Madrid: SIGLO XXI; 1991. ISBN 9788432307324.
15. Bacigalupe A, Martín U. Gender inequalities in depression/anxiety and the consumption of psychotropic drugs: are we medicalising women's mental health? Scand J Public Health. 2021;49(3):317–24. https://doi.org/10.1177/1403494820944736.
16. PLOS Medicine Editors. The paradox of mental health: overtreatment and under-recognition. PLoS Med. 2013;10(5):e1001456. https://doi.org/10.1371/journal.pmed.1001456.
17. Martin LA, Neighbors HW, Griffith DM. The experience of symptoms of depression in men vs wom analysis of the National Comorbidity Survey Replication. JAMA. Psychiat, 2013;70: 1100–1106.

Gender Bias in Mental Health Disorders and Epidemiology of Psychiatric Disorders

9

María Recio-Barbero, Rodrigo Romero-Jiménez, and Margarita Sáenz-Herrero

9.1 Introduction

The contemporary understanding of mental disorders has undergone a paradigmatic shift in recent decades, recognizing gender as a determinant of mental health that goes beyond the mere reductionism of biological differences. This chapter provides a comprehensive analysis of how social constructs of gender interact with neurobiological, psychological, and sociocultural factors to shape differentiated epidemiological patterns, persistent diagnostic biases, and therapeutic inequalities in psychiatry.

Current scientific evidence shows that gender operates as a critical modulator of mental health through multiple mechanisms. Functional neuroimaging studies reveal sex differences in amygdala activation in response to emotional stimuli [1],

M. Recio-Barbero
Early Phases of Psychosis Group, Biobizkaia Health Research Institute, Cruces University Hospital, Barakaldo, Spain

Department of Psychiatry, Cruces University Hospital, Barakaldo, Spain

R. Romero-Jiménez
Early Phases of Psychosis Group, Biobizkaia Health Research Institute, Cruces University Hospital, Barakaldo, Spain

Department of Psychiatry, Cruces University Hospital, Barakaldo, Spain

Faculty of Medicine and Nursing, University of the Basque Country (EHU), Leioa, Spain

M. Sáenz-Herrero (✉)
Department of Psychiatry, Cruces University Hospital, Barakaldo, Spain

University of the Basque Country (UPV/EHU), Leioa, Spain

Early Phases of Psychosis Group, Department of Psychiatry, Biobizkaia Health Research Institute, Cruces University Hospital, Barakaldo, Spain
e-mail: margarita.saenzherrero@osakidetza.eus

M. López-Atanes, M. Sáenz-Herrero (eds.), *Applying the Gender Perspective in Psychiatry and Psychotherapy*, https://doi.org/10.1007/978-3-032-17883-1_9

while epigenetic research shows how gender roles can influence gene expression related to the stress response [2]. Simultaneously, the theoretical framework of intersectionality has enabled an understanding of how gender interacts with other social categories such as class, ethnicity, or sexual orientation to produce unique experiences of psychological distress [3, 4].

9.2 Epidemiology and Clinical Presentation of Mental Disorders

International epidemiological studies have consistently documented significant gender-based differences in the prevalence, clinical presentation, and course of mental disorders. The Global Burden of Disease Study 2019 [5] provides revealing data on these disparities, identifying a female-to-male ratio of 1.7:1 for depressive disorders in Western countries, increasing to 2.3:1 in low-income contexts. This geographical variation suggests that social determinants interact with biological factors to modulate gender-differentiated risk. Conversely, substance use disorders display the opposite pattern, with a global male-to-female ratio of 2.8:1, though with major regional variations; for instance, in some Eastern European countries, this difference reaches 4:1 [6]. Schizophrenia, although with similar prevalence across sexes, presents key differences in clinical expression: men tend to have earlier onset (ages 18–25 vs. 25–35 in women) and more severe cognitive impairment, while women show more affective symptoms and better initial response to antipsychotics [7].

9.2.1 Influence of Gender-Differentiated Factors in the Development and Maintenance of Psychiatric Disorders

- *Biological Factors*
- Neurobiological sex differences are fundamental to understanding epidemiological disparities. Research on the hypothalamic-pituitary-adrenal (HPA) axis reveals that women exhibit a more prolonged and less adaptable stress response than men, potentially predisposing them to internalizing disorders such as depression [8]. This is linked to estrogen's regulation of glucocorticoid receptors, modulating stress resilience. In pharmacology, pharmacokinetic studies show that women metabolize many psychotropic drugs more slowly due to differences in CYP450 enzyme activity, increasing the risk of adverse effects [9]. For instance, benzodiazepines have a longer half-life in women, partly explaining higher prescription and dependency rates. Hormonal influences also vary neurotransmission in serotonin and dopamine systems throughout the menstrual cycle, affecting both symptomatology and treatment response [10].
- *Psychosocial Factors*
- Traditional gender roles create differential burdens that impact mental health. The caregiving overload, predominantly carried out by women (73% of informal

caregivers per WHO), is associated with higher risks of emotional exhaustion and anxiety disorders [11]. This is exacerbated in poverty contexts, where women face a "double shift" of paid and domestic work without adequate support. Gender-based violence is another critical factor: 1 in 3 women globally has suffered physical or sexual violence, tripling the risk of PTSD and major depression [12]. On the other hand, hegemonic masculinity stereotypes ("men don't cry") discourage men from seeking psychological help, delaying diagnosis of internalizing disorders and increasing suicide risk [13]. Men are 40% less likely than women to access mental health services, even when experiencing severe symptoms [14].

9.2.2 Intersectionality and Structural Determinants

Gender analysis in mental health must consider its intersection with other social categories. Migrant women, for instance, show higher depression rates than native women, not only due to acculturative stress but also due to increased exposure to labor exploitation and violence [15]. Similarly, young men from ethnic minorities in marginalized urban contexts are at higher risk of substance use disorders, linked to economic exclusion and normalization of substance use in their environments [16]. These findings highlight that mental health inequalities are not merely biological, but influenced by socio-environmental factors that shape both the emergence and persistence of mental illness.

9.3 Gender Biases in the Diagnostic Process and Therapeutic Approach in Psychiatry: A Critical Analysis

Although psychiatric diagnostic systems are designed with standardized criteria, they may still reflect social constructs that warrant critical examination. Various studies suggest that implicit biases—both individual and institutional—can influence how symptoms are interpreted based on the patient's gender. An analysis of 2347 clinical records showed differentiated diagnostic tendencies: while 73% of women received a diagnosis of depression for a specific symptom profile, 62% of men with similar manifestations were diagnosed with work-related stress [17]. These differences prompt reflection on how psychosocial factors and gender expectations may interact with diagnostic processes.

9.3.1 Differential Medicalization of Distress

Chronic pain is a paradigmatic example of these differences. Longitudinal studies show that 70% of women presenting with chronic pain are prescribed anxiolytics as a first-line treatment, whereas men with identical symptoms are more frequently directed toward organic diagnostic protocols [18]. This disparity reflects what some authors refer to as "the somatic versus psychological bias" in clinical practice [19]. The phenomenon is exacerbated when intersectional variables are considered. Women from ethnic minorities and low-income backgrounds are 40% more likely to receive a personality disorder diagnosis rather than a mood disorder when presenting with mixed symptomatology [20]. This pattern suggests the existence of a "double diagnostic standard" based on gender, class, and ethnicity.

9.3.2 Gender Bias in Assessment Instruments

Standardized questionnaires commonly used in clinical practice have important limitations. The Hamilton Depression Rating Scale, for instance, places greater emphasis on symptoms more typically associated with men (such as irritability) than on those more frequently reported by women (such as feelings of worthlessness) [21]. This imbalance leads to an underestimation of depression severity in women and an overestimation of milder cases in men.

9.4 Pathologization of Femininity: From Hysteria to BPD

9.4.1 Historical Evolution of Diagnostic Constructs

The trajectory of premenstrual syndrome in diagnostic manuals clearly illustrates this phenomenon. From its conception as "uterine hysteria" in the nineteenth century to its current classification as premenstrual dysphoric disorder in the DSM-5, this construct has served to medicalize normal physiological experiences [22]. Epidemiological data show that while 80% of women experience some premenstrual symptoms, only 3–8% would meet criteria for the disorder, raising debates on the boundaries between pathology and physiology [23].

9.4.2 The Case of Borderline Personality Disorder (BPD) and Antisocial Personality Disorder

Diagnostic patterns for borderline personality disorder (BPD) and antisocial personality disorder show significant gender-based variations that merit reflection. Epidemiological studies indicate similar prevalence of BPD in men and women (1.6% vs. 1.7%), yet women are three times more likely to receive this diagnosis in clinical practice [24]. This may be linked to how current diagnostic criteria emphasize certain clinical manifestations: emotional lability (more often recognized in women) versus externalized impulsivity (more frequently identified in men).In a parallel but opposite trend, antisocial personality disorder is disproportionately diagnosed in men. This divergence in diagnostic patterns raises important questions about:

- The potential influence of gender stereotypes in symptom identification.
- The limitations of current diagnostic systems in capturing the diverse expression and broad symptomatic spectrum of mental disorders.
- The need to consider how gender can modulate the manifestation of psychopathology.

9.5 Implicit Biases in the Diagnostic Approach to Psychiatric Emergencies: Evidence from Clinical Practice

Gender biases in psychiatric care are a well-documented phenomenon, but their clinical manifestations in urgent mental healthcare settings remain insufficiently explored. A study by our group [25], which analyzed 9789 emergency mental health episodes (53.9% involving women), reveals patterns that prompt critical reflection on diagnostic and therapeutic processes. Key findings include:

- Prevalence rates of mental health conditions were primarily represented in populations with higher socioeconomic deprivation. The study found that socioeconomic quintile distribution varied significantly by gender, with lower income women overrepresented in consultations for internalizing problems.
- Data showed clear gender segregation in consultation reasons: women were overrepresented in anxiety and mood disorders (up to 65% of cases), as well as in personality disorders (82.5% of episodes), whereas men accounted for 70% of substance use disorder cases. This distribution not only confirms previous epidemiological findings but also raises questions about the underlying social mechanisms driving these differences.

The analysis revealed significant disparities in pharmacological management, with women receiving more anxiolytic treatment than men across three diagnostic categories:

- Common mental disorders, including anxiety and adjustment disorders (PR = 1.122; $p = 0.025$).
- Severe mental disorders, including schizophrenia spectrum disorders, bipolar disorder, and major depressive episodes (PR = 1.217; $p = 0.007$).
- Personality disorders (PR = 1.398; $p = 0.028$).
- A differential pattern was observed in the request for diagnostic tests for the same symptomatic grouping in emergency care:
  - In the common mental disorder group, women were less likely than men to undergo imaging (PR = 0.76 [0.65–0.89]; $p = 0.001$) or laboratory tests (PR = 0.81 [0.70–0.94]; $p = 0.005$).

These results suggest that the greater medicalization of emotional distress in women and the externalization of symptoms in men may reflect deeply rooted gender stereotypes. The findings point to a possible "gender-conditioned prescribing reflex," where similar symptoms lead to different pharmacological approaches. The persistence of these differences even in diagnostic categories lacking biological justification for distinct treatments indicates the influence of implicit biases in clinical practice.

9.6 Therapeutic Approach and Pharmacology

9.6.1 Disparities in Pharmacological Prescription

The analysis of 1.2 million prescriptions within the Spanish National Health System [26] revealed differentiated patterns in psychopharmacological prescribing that raise questions about potential biases in clinical practice. Women received 1.8 times more benzodiazepine prescriptions for similar symptoms—a finding that persisted even after adjusting for symptom severity and comorbidities. This phenomenon may be linked to what some authors call the "differential medicalization of emotional distress" [27], where symptoms such as anxiety or insomnia are more frequently managed pharmacologically in women.

Conversely, men were more likely to receive higher initial doses of antipsychotics during first psychotic episodes (OR = 1.34, $p < 0.01$), particularly in those under age 35 [28]. This difference may reflect both greater initial severity of psychotic symptoms in males and potential biases in the clinical perception of psychomotor agitation.A particularly concerning finding was the higher rate of psychiatric polypharmacy among women over age 65 (2.3 times more likely), a phenomenon associated with an increased risk of drug interactions and adverse effects [29]. These patterns persist even after controlling for relevant clinical variables, highlighting the need for critical review of therapeutic decision-making processes.

9.6.2 Differential Response to Psychotropic Treatments and Non-pharmacological Interventions

The meta-analysis by Zucker and Prendergast [30], covering 143 clinical trials, offers robust evidence of significant gender differences in therapeutic response:

- Differential efficacy of pharmacological and non-pharmacological interventions: The meta-analysis showed that women respond better to certain drugs, such as selective serotonin reuptake inhibitors (SSRIs) (d Cohen = 0.32), especially during reproductive years (ages 25–45). This phenomenon seems related to the modulatory action of estrogens on the serotonergic system, as these sex hormones have been shown to increase serotonin transporter availability and enhance serotonergic neurotransmission [31]. By contrast, men showed better outcomes

with cognitive-behavioral therapy for substance use disorders (OR = 1.42), a difference that could be attributed not only to motivational and adherence factors [32] but also to neurobiological variations in reward and inhibitory control circuits.
- Differences in drug safety profiles: Gender differences in safety profiles are particularly notable. Women experience 1.5 times more adverse effects with equivalent doses of antipsychotics, especially metabolic effects (such as weight gain and dyslipidemia) and extrapyramidal symptoms [7]. This increased vulnerability can be explained by several key physiological differences: first, women have a higher proportion of body fat (25–31% of body weight vs. 18–24% in men), significantly affecting the distribution and accumulation of lipophilic drugs [9]. Second, women present a lower volume of distribution and higher plasma peaks for many psychotropic drugs, increasing the risk of toxicity. In addition, differences in hepatic CYP450 enzyme activity (particularly CYP3A4 and CYP2D6) significantly alter the metabolism of many psychotropic agents.
- Hormonal variability and the role of estrogens: Hormonal variability represents another critical factor. Numerous studies have documented significant fluctuations in the efficacy and tolerability of psychotropic drugs throughout the menstrual cycle, particularly during the luteal phase, when higher progesterone levels may alter the activity of various neurotransmitter systems [33]. During perimenopause, abrupt hormonal changes can affect both therapeutic response and the occurrence of side effects—an aspect traditionally underestimated in clinical trials. This variability is exacerbated by the fact that many studies systematically exclude women of reproductive age or fail to properly control for menstrual cycle phase in their assessments.

These intrinsic physiological differences, together with psychosocial factors and prescribing biases, underscore the urgent need to develop personalized therapeutic protocols that take these variables into account to optimize both the efficacy and safety of psychopharmacological treatments. Implementing therapeutic monitoring strategies that consider these differences could significantly reduce treatment-related morbidity in vulnerable populations.

9.7 New Proposals Toward Gender-Sensitive Clinical Practice: From the Micro (Education) to the Macro (Health System)

9.7.1 Incorporating Gender-Sensitive Initiatives into Educational Reform

Mental health training requires a structural transformation to address the gender disparities identified in clinical practice. Evidence-based proposals highlight the need for a transversal curricular integration that includes specific modules on sex–gender differences in pharmacology [34]. These contents should encompass three core pillars: the study of pharmacokinetic and pharmacodynamic variations according to biological sex, the systematic identification of implicit biases in prescribing patterns, and the clinical management of hormonal fluctuations across the life cycle. Integrating these topics into medical training curricula can improve healthcare professionals' competence and reduce gender disparities in clinical care. The implementation of specific modules in these areas, as suggested by evidence-based proposals, represents a necessary step toward more inclusive and equitable medical education [35].

9.7.2 Inclusion of Gender Perspective in Psychopathology, Clinical Approach, and Psychopharmacological and Psychotherapeutical Treatment in Common Mental Health

It is estimated that one in four people in Europe will experience some form of mental health issue during their lifetime, with similar figures in Spain [36]. However, the distribution of this morbidity by gender is not balanced. Gender differences in mental health are well known. Women suffer more from mood disorders, depression, anxiety, somatization disorders, and eating disorders, while men are more affected by substance abuse disorders [37–39]. There is no evidence that genetic or biological factors alone explain these differences, and these disparities, which are minimal during childhood, become more evident during adolescence. Therefore, it is essential to analyze which factors related to socialization and the specific needs of men and women contribute to the mental health process. To do so, it is crucial to have sex-disaggregated data to compare and then ask questions, applying a gender perspective.

To explain these differences, we can consider the role society has assigned to men and women, gender roles; the ideal constructed for each, gender stereotypes, and the gender mandates—social norms that both women and men must adhere to in society [40, 41]. Violating these norms has had and continues to have very high costs, especially for women.

Gender stereotypes intersect with other social determinants, such as social class, ethnicity, race, and immigration status, which are socially shared. Understanding this concept is important because stereotypes are also defined as beliefs about specific social groups that shape our attitudes.

Social gender stereotypes are closely linked to the prevalence of so-called common mental disorders (CMDs): depression, anxiety, and somatizations, which affect approximately one in three people, particularly women. These conditions represent a serious public health problem, and it is important to remember that there is evidence supporting the role of gender determinants in mental health [25, 40].

According to the World Health Organization (WHO), mental health problems are the leading cause of disability worldwide, and major depression, the second leading cause of disability, is twice as common among women as among men [42].

Primary care serves as the entry point for many people experiencing mental health disorders who require effective treatment to improve their health and quality of life. There are factors that reduce proper detection and diagnosis: the limited time during consultations or the presence of comorbid disorders, among other emotional or physical conditions [43, 44], which can lead to an inaccurate diagnosis [45, 46], and difficulties in detecting and referring individuals to appropriate treatment in primary care or other social-health settings, including social prescribing.

Common Mental Disorders (CMDs) represent the most frequently addressed mental health issue in primary care centers, general emergency departments, and mental health centers, being much more common in women. Gender is a risk factor for the presentation of depressive symptoms across all age groups.

Regarding diagnostic approaches, most mental illnesses and mental health disorders only require a clinical history and a proper psychopathological examination, where knowledge, attitude, and personal and professional experience can sometimes lead to misinterpretation of symptoms and signs. As German Berrios, Professor of Psychopathology affirmed, each generation of psychiatrists must participate in constructing psychopathology that evaluates behaviors perceived as dysfunctional at each historical moment. Often, the recording of symptoms in the medical history does not align with what women report (influenced by what has been studied in medicine and by the scientific literature according to sex) [47].

At times, for women, sharing a complaint or emotional discomfort has translated into more frequent visits to consultations, where, instead of listening and understanding, medicalization takes place, and medications are prescribed [48]. This may be one reason why the use of medication, particularly psychotropic drugs, is much higher in women. In somatization disorders, it is quite common for women to be labeled and prescribed medication, while men are investigated for potential causes and undergo tests [47].

Another gender bias is the undervaluation of women's symptoms and unnecessary medicalization. This leads to situations where the veracity of their reports is questioned or their semiological expressions are dismissed, as they are compared to the male standard (the androcentric model of medicine) [49].

This type of common mental disorder is labeled as having a trivial pathology. Healthcare personnel often do not take into account the underlying social determinants. Frequently, not all diagnostic and therapeutic options are offered, as shown in a study conducted by our group in psychiatric emergency and mental health departments [25] where more tests were requested for men, and women were prescribed more anxiolytics.

Lastly, and equally important is the failure to consider the relationship between mental health and a history of multiple forms of violence that women suffer, especially those who frequently visit healthcare facilities with various somatic or mental symptomatology.

For women who accept situations of gender violence, it is necessary to work with them with their internal resources. These women need to be able to construct an internal representation and a sense of agency, and their self-worth should not be based on attachment but on having resources and capabilities. "Feeling that the world is valid despite failures, despite disappointments, even though things may not be as we would like them to be, or we may not be who we would like to be," as Jessica Benjamin pointed out [50]. This means accepting that human beings are dependent, that our psyche is fragile, that we rely on each other, and that everyone can depend on someone else who, in turn, may not be well. In the case of women suffering from gender violence, it is relevant what we have internalized, what has happened with our significant family relationships, and the representations we have of them. Being able to include the idea that disappointments and failures are part of life and adopting a different attitude toward failures and disappointments in meaningful relationships without affecting one's sense of agency. It is not the same to be raised by a mother who defines her identity through motherhood as it is to be raised by a mother who sees motherhood as just one role among many others. Similarly, it is different to be raised by a father who has internalized masculine values compared to being raised by a father who can express emotional vulnerability and tenderness. To transform subjugated identities, they must be modified in order to transform ourselves. As Celia Amorós says, "It has to do with a new individuality" [51].

The difficulty in expressing and communicating emotions is another barrier for men, who also face challenges in asking for help. These reasons are connected to gender stereotypes: admitting weakness is seen as unacceptable, and the stigma surrounding mental health issues may cause them to reject help. Men have fewer opportunities for diagnosis because they attend primary care and mental health consultations less frequently. Therefore, it is possible that depression in men is underdiagnosed, likely in relation to gender biases.

9.7.3 Inclusion of Gender Perspective in Biomedical Research

Research designs in mental health must evolve to adequately capture the complexity of sex and gender-related differences. The implementation of SGBA (Sex and Gender-Based Analysis) protocols represents a critical step in this direction [52]. These protocols require three essential components: standardization in reporting results disaggregated by sex and gender, a priori calculation of the statistical power needed for meaningful subgroup analyses, and the systematic incorporation of relevant sociocultural variables into study designs.

At the same time, clinical guidelines and care protocols require significant updates to reflect the latest scientific findings. The CANMAT guidelines model for depression [53] offers a valuable example by including sex-specific recommendations that differentiate preferred pharmacological options, optimal titration strategies, and adverse effect monitoring protocols. Complementarily, the implementation of smart monitoring systems in electronic health records [54] could transform clinical practice through automated alerts that detect potentially biased prescribing patterns, suggest gender-informed therapeutic alternatives, and prevent dangerous drug interactions in particularly vulnerable populations.

These proposals represent a concrete path toward a more equitable clinical practice, where diagnostic and therapeutic decisions are based on rigorous scientific evidence and sensitivity to gender differences—rather than stereotypes or unconscious biases. Their implementation will require sustained institutional commitment and the allocation of specific resources, but the potential benefits for care quality and health outcomes amply justify the effort.

References

1. Stevens JS, Hamann S. Sex differences in brain activation to emotional stimuli. NeuroImage. 2012;59(3):2425–32. https://doi.org/10.1016/j.neuroimage.2011.08.099.
2. Bale TL, Epperson CN. Sex differences and stress across the lifespan. Nat Neurosci. 2015;18(10):1413–20. https://doi.org/10.1038/nn.4112.
3. Bowleg L. The problem with the phrase women and minorities: intersectionality-an important theoretical framework for public health. Am J Public Health. 2012;102(7):1267–73. https://doi.org/10.2105/AJPH.2012.300750.
4. Vu M, Li J, Haardörfer R, et al. Mental health and substance use among women and men at the intersections of identities and experiences of discrimination: insights from the intersectionality framework. BMC Public Health. 2019;19(1):108. https://doi.org/10.1186/s12889-019-6430-0.
5. GBD 2019 Mental Disorders Collaborators. Global, regional, and national burden of 12 mental disorders in 204 countries and territories, 1990-2019: a systematic analysis for the Global Burden of Disease Study 2019. Lancet Psychiatry. 2021;9(2):137–50.
6. White A, Castle IJ, Chen CM, et al. Gender differences in substance use disorders. Curr Opin Psychiatry. 2015;28(4):264–70. https://doi.org/10.1097/YCO.0000000000000169.
7. Seeman MV. Gender differences in antipsychotic treatment. Schizophr Res. 2021;228:456–63. https://doi.org/10.1016/j.schres.2020.12.025.
8. Bangasser DA, Valentino RJ. Sex differences in stress-related psychiatric disorders: neurobiological perspectives. Front Neuroendocrinol. 2014;35(3):303–19. https://doi.org/10.1016/j.yfrne.2014.03.008.
9. Soldin OP, Mattison DR. Sex differences in pharmacokinetics and pharmacodynamics. Clin Pharmacokinet. 2009;48(3):143–57. https://doi.org/10.2165/00003088-200948030-00001.
10. Gillies GE, McArthur S. Estrogen actions in the brain and the basis for differential action in men and women. Neurosci Biobehav Rev. 2010;34(7):979–1000. https://doi.org/10.1016/j.neubiorev.2009.11.015.
11. Hahmann TE, Hamilton-Wright S, Ziegler C, et al. Gender differences in caregiver burden. J Womens Health (Larchmt). 2022;31(4):543–51. https://doi.org/10.1089/jwh.2021.0234.
12. World Health Organization. Violence against women prevalence estimates, 2018. 2021. https://doi.org/10.1016/S0140-6736(21)02664-7.
13. Addis ME, Mahalik JR. Men, masculinity, and the contexts of help seeking. Am Psychol. 2003;58(1):5–14. https://doi.org/10.1037/0003-066X.58.1.5.
14. Oliffe JL, Ogrodniczuk JS, Gordon SJ, et al. Men's health help-seeking behaviors. Am J Mens Health. 2016;10(6):NP155–64. https://doi.org/10.1177/1557988315586979.
15. Bhugra D, Gupta S, Bhui K, et al. Mental health of migrants and refugees. Lancet Psychiatry. 2021;8(1):76–87. https://doi.org/10.1016/S2215-0366(20)30434-5.
16. Villatoro JA, Duarte-Vélez Y, Delva J, et al. Substance use among urban minority youth. Drug Alcohol Depend. 2018;182:86–92. https://doi.org/10.1016/j.drugalcdep.2017.10.011.
17. Loring M, Powell B. Gender, race, and DSM-III. J Health Soc Behav. 1988;29(1):1–22. https://doi.org/10.2307/2137179.
18. Hoffmann DE, Tarzian AJ. The girl who cried pain. J Law Med Ethics. 2001;29(1):13–27. https://doi.org/10.1111/j.1748-720X.2001.tb00037.x.
19. Gijsbers van Wijk CM, Kolk AM, van den Bosch WJ, et al. Gender perspectives and quality of care. Soc Sci Med. 1999;48(6):707–17. https://doi.org/10.1016/S0277-9536(98)00396-8.

20. Lewis B, Williams DR, Tamene M, et al. Intersectional disparities in mental health diagnosis. Am J Psychiatry. 2021;178(6):511–9. https://doi.org/10.1176/appi.ajp.2020.20071034.
21. Martin LA, Neighbors HW, Griffith DM. Gender differences in depression symptoms. J Affect Disord. 2013;151(3):1133–41. https://doi.org/10.1016/j.jad.2013.06.058.
22. Figert AE. The women's health movement and the rise of the premenstrual syndrome. Soc Sci Med. 2013;41(6):781–9. https://doi.org/10.1016/0277-9536(95)00347-F.
23. Epperson CN, Steiner M, Hartlage SA, et al. Premenstrual dysphoric disorder: evidence for a new category for DSM-5. Am J Psychiatry. 2012;169(5):465–75. https://doi.org/10.1176/appi.ajp.2012.11081302.
24. Paris J, Chenard-Poirier MP, Biskin R. Gender differences in borderline personality disorder. J Personal Disord. 2013;27(6):734–46. https://doi.org/10.1521/pedi_2013_27_109.
25. Sáenz-Herrero M, López-Atanes M, Recio-Barbero M, et al. Gender differences in psychiatric emergencies. Arch Womens Ment Health. 2024;27(1):45–56. https://doi.org/10.1007/s00737-023-01360-x.
26. Ruiz-Cantero MT, Vives-Cases C, Artazcoz L, et al. Gender bias in clinical medicine. Gac Sanit. 2020;34(3):286–92. https://doi.org/10.1016/j.gaceta.2019.09.007.
27. Haussman M, Riecher-Rössler A, Seeman MV. Gendered medicalization of distress. Soc Sci Med. 2022;292:114541. https://doi.org/10.1016/j.socscimed.2021.114541.
28. González-Rodríguez A, Labad J, Seeman MV. Gender differences in first-episode psychosis treatment. Schizophr Res. 2021;228:474–81. https://doi.org/10.1016/j.schres.2021.01.008.
29. Maust DT, Strominger J, Kim HM, et al. Psychotropic polypharmacy in older adults. JAMA Intern Med. 2020;180(2):283–5. https://doi.org/10.1001/jamainternmed.2019.5264.
30. Zucker I, Prendergast BJ. Sex differences in pharmacokinetics predict adverse drug reactions in women. Biol Sex Differ. 2020;11(1):32. https://doi.org/10.1186/s13293-020-003.
31. Albert PR, Lemonde S, Gharbi N, et al. Estrogen modulation of serotonin pathways in depression. Biol Psychiatry. 2021;89(1):15–24. https://doi.org/10.1016/j.biopsych.2020.08.018.
32. Worley MJ, Tate SR, McQuaid JR, et al. Gender differences in CBT for substance use disorders. J Subst Abus Treat. 2022;132:108491. https://doi.org/10.1016/j.jsat.2021.108491.
33. Petersen N, London ED, Liang L, et al. Menstrual cycle effects on psychotropic medications. Psychoneuroendocrinology. 2022;136:105608. https://doi.org/10.1016/j.psyneuen.2021.105608.
34. Farkas RH, Bonifacino E, Yu A, et al. Gender medicine in medical education. Acad Med. 2023;98(3):345–52. https://doi.org/10.1097/ACM.0000000000005021.
35. Becher E, Oertelt-Prigione S. The impact of sex and gender in medicine and pharmacology. Handb Exp Pharmacol. 2023;282:3–23. https://doi.org/10.1007/164_2023_688.
36. World Health Organization Regional Office for Europe. Mental health: prevalence and gender disparities. 2018. Available from: https://www.euro.who.int/en/health-topics/noncommunicable-diseases/mental-health.
37. Boyd A, Van de Velde S, Vilagut G, de Graaf R, O'Neill S, Florescu S, et al. Gender differences in mental disorders and suicidality in Europe: results from a large cross-sectional population-based study. J Affect Disord. 2015;173:245–54. https://doi.org/10.1016/j.jad.2014.11.002.
38. Seedat S, Scott KM, Angermeyer MC, et al. Cross-national associations between gender and mental disorders in the World Health Organization world mental health surveys. Arch Gen Psychiatry. 2009;66(7):785–95. https://doi.org/10.1001/archgenpsychiatry.2009.36.
39. Riecher-Rössler A. Sex and gender differences in mental disorders. Lancet Psychiatry. 2017;4(1):8–9. https://doi.org/10.1016/S2215-0366(16)30348-0.
40. Christiansen DM, McCarthy MM, Seeman MV. Where sex meets gender: how sex and gender come together to cause sex differences in mental illness. Front Psych. 2022;13:856436. https://doi.org/10.3389/fpsyt.2022.856436.
41. Hankivsky O. Women's health, men's health, and gender and health: implications of intersectionality. Soc Sci Med. 2012;74(11):1712–20. https://doi.org/10.1016/j.socscimed.2011.11.029.
42. World Health Organization. World mental health report: transforming mental health for all. 2022. Available from: https://www.who.int/publications/i/item/9789240049338.

43. Castro-Rodríguez JI, Olariu E, Garnier-Lacueva C, et al. Diagnostic accuracy and adequacy of treatment of depressive and anxiety disorders: a comparison of primary care and specialized care patients. J Affect Disord. 2015;172:462–71. https://doi.org/10.1016/j.jad.2014.10.020.
44. Fernández A, Haro JM, Codony M, et al. Treatment adequacy of anxiety and depressive disorders: primary versus specialised care in Spain. J Affect Disord. 2006;96(1–2):9–20. https://doi.org/10.1016/j.jad.2006.05.005.
45. Aragonès E, Piñol JL, Labad A. The overdiagnosis of depression in non-depressed patients in primary care. Fam Pract. 2006;23(3):363–8. https://doi.org/10.1093/fampra/cmi120.
46. Olariu E, Rodrigo M, Alvarez Lopez P, et al. Diagnosing anxiety disorders in primary care: a systematic review and meta-analysis. Value Health. 2014;17(7):A325. https://doi.org/10.1016/j.jval.2014.08.578.
47. Malterud K. Symptoms as a source of medical knowledge: understanding medically unexplained disorders in women. Fam Med. 2000;32(9):603–11.
48. Organisation for Economic Co-operation and Development. Health at a glance 2023: OECD indicators [Internet]. Paris: OECD Publishing; 2023 [cited 2024 Jan 15]. Available from: https://www.oecd.org/en/publications/health-at-a-glance-2023_7a7afb35-en.html.
49. Risberg G, Johansson EE, Hamberg K. Gender disparities in medical assessments. Scand J Public Health. 2003;31(2):113–9.
50. Távora A, Esteban ML. El amor romántico y la subordinación social de las mujeres: revisiones y propuestas. Anu Psicol. 2008;39(1):59–74.
51. Amorós C, Tiempo de feminismo. Sobre feminismo, proyecto ilustrado y posmodernidad. Madrid: Cátedra; 1997.
52. Heidari S, Babor TF, De Castro P, et al. Sex and gender equity in research (SAGER guidelines). Lancet. 2016;387(10026):1717–8. https://doi.org/10.1016/S0140-6736(16)30380-7.
53. Kennedy SH, Lam RW, McIntyre RS, et al. Canadian Network for Mood and Anxiety Treatments (CANMAT) guidelines. J Affect Disord. 2021;279:474–88. https://doi.org/10.1016/j.jad.2020.10.022.
54. Bushnell GA, Stürmer T, Gaynes BN, et al. Sex differences in psychotropic medication use. JAMA Psychiatry. 2021;78(4):369–77. https://doi.org/10.1001/jamapsychiatry.2020.4064.

The Medicalization of Women's Mental Health: Examining Depression and Anxiety

10

Amaia Bacigalupe, Andrea Cabezas-Rodríguez, and Maite Campo Iparragirre

10.1 Introduction

Internationally, numerous studies have consistently demonstrated that women exhibit higher rates of poor mental health, anxiety, and depression diagnoses, as well as greater consumption of psychotropic drugs than men—in some cases, with nearly twice the prevalence [1–3]. In recent years, there has been a sustained increase in anxiety and depression diagnoses, alongside a rise in the use of anxiolytics and antidepressants, which remain consistently more prevalent among women across all age groups. The data presented in Fig. 10.1 clearly illustrate this trend in Spain.

Gender inequalities in mental health have been so extensively reported across the psychiatric epidemiological literature that we have become accustomed to considering them essential or natural, typically through biological explanations linked to hormonal variability across women's life cycles [4]. However, understanding gender differences requires a more nuanced approach to the deeper and interrelated reasons underlying the differences that quantitative indicators reveal about men's and women's mental health. These differences result from the convergence of a diverse range of phenomena, such

A. Bacigalupe · M. Campo Iparragirre
Department of Sociology and Social Work, University of the Basque Country (UPV/EHU), Leioa, Biscay, Spain

Research Group in Social Determinants of Health and Demographic Change-OPIK, University of the Basque Country (UPV/EHU), Leioa, Biscay, Spain

A. Cabezas-Rodríguez (✉)
Research Group in Social Determinants of Health and Demographic Change-OPIK, University of the Basque Country (UPV/EHU), Leioa, Biscay, Spain

Department of Nursing 2, University of the Basque Country (UPV/EHU), Leioa, Biscay, Spain
e-mail: andrea.cabezas@ehu.eus

M. López-Atanes, M. Sáenz-Herrero (eds.), *Applying the Gender Perspective in Psychiatry and Psychotherapy*, https://doi.org/10.1007/978-3-032-17883-1_10

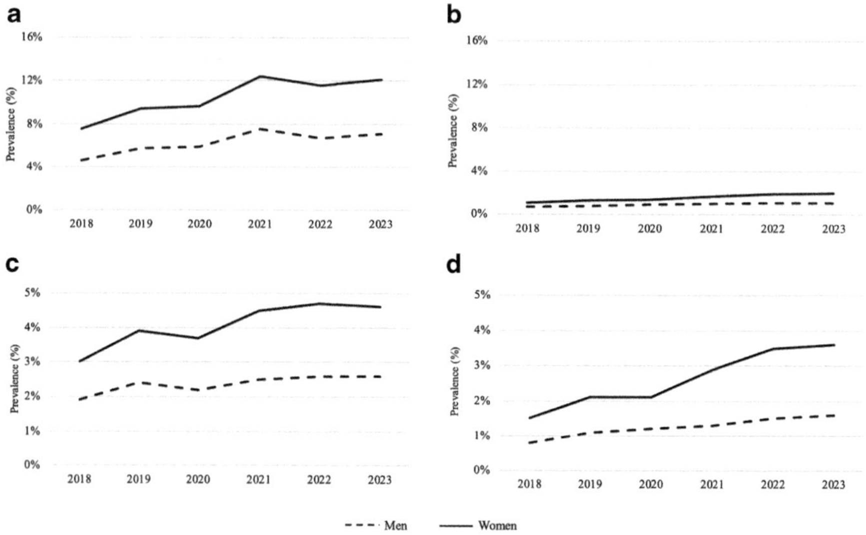

Fig. 10.1 Temporal trend of the prevalence (%) of diagnosis of anxiety (**a**) and depression (**b**), and anxiolytic (**c**) and antidepressant (**d**) consumption by gender in Spain. BDCAP, 2018–2023. (Created using data extracted from BDCAP (Spain), 2018–2023)

as the material and symbolic subordination of women in a patriarchal society, the androcentric roots of biomedical science, and the broader trends in *medicalization of society* and contemporary *diagnostic cultures* [5, 6] (Fig. 10.1).

Structural gender inequalities impose more adverse living conditions on women—including lower social class, greater responsibility for caregiving and domestic tasks, and multiple forms of discrimination and violence—which contribute to their higher rates of mental distress. Additionally, hegemonic gender mandates influence the construction of social group identities. In the case of women, this translates into the attribution of traits such as self-sacrifice, emotional dependence, and even an expectation of finding satisfaction in such roles. This undermines autonomy, generates feelings of guilt, and ultimately deteriorates emotional health.Without overlooking the relevance of all these factors, this chapter focuses on the role that healthcare professionals play in the higher frequency of depression and anxiety diagnoses and the prescription of psychotropic drugs to women throughout their life cycles. The hypothesis we propose is that part of this gender gap which is due to a biased clinical practice that disproportionately medicalizes women's mental health.

10.2 The Medicalization of Life, Diagnostic Cultures, and Mental Health

The concept of medicalization of life has been a subject of academic discussion since at least the early 1970s, when scholars began examining how "medicine and diagnostic labels were becoming increasingly relevant to human existence" [7]. In

Peter Conrad's classic definition, medicalization is the process through which human conditions or problems—related to behaviors, emotions, and other non-medical aspects—are redefined and treated as medical issues, typically in terms of diseases or disorders [6].

Broader interpretations of the concept even suggest that an aspect of life becomes medicalized as soon as it is framed within a biomedical perspective and characterized through a medical lexicon. We live in diagnostic cultures that use diagnostic categories to interpret, regulate, and mediate various understandings of distress, not only among healthcare professionals but also among patients and society at large [5].

Although early discussions of medicalization referred to "intensive medicalization" or "medical imperialism"—exerted unidirectionally by professionals onto patients—medicalization has been redefined as a more extensive or bottom-up process. This means that the focus should not be placed solely on the control exerted by the healthcare institution, but also on patients and the public, who actively seek medicalization and even engage in self-medicalization [5, 6].

Although medicalization occurs across different social groups, it is plausible to argue that they have been particularly intense concerning women's bodies throughout history [8]. The longstanding association of women with their reproductive function has led to medical interventions in physiological processes such as menstruation, pregnancy, childbirth, and menopause—which have often been interpreted in terms of pathology, disorder, or deficiency [9]. Beyond reproduction, other aspects of women's lives, including their mental health, have also been subjected to medicalization. The "psi sciences," in general, and psychiatry, in particular, have historically pathologized traits considered traditionally feminine, thereby reinforcing the association of women with the socio-symbolic realm of madness [10].

Psychiatry has historically classified symptoms of psychological distress differently in men and women, aligning them with dominant gender norms. Traits associated with the female role—such as dependency, vulnerability, and emotionality—have been more frequently pathologized, whereas those traditionally linked to masculinity—independence, rationality, leadership, or even selfishness—are often regarded as non-pathological. This phenomenon is what Phyllis Chesler termed the "double standard" in mental health [1].

As a consequence of the androcentric foundations of biomedicine and the psi sciences, evidence suggests that clinical practice is often biased. Mental health practitioners are more likely to diagnose depression and other mental health disorders and prescribe psychotropic drugs at higher rates in women, even when their symptoms and mental health needs are identical to those of men [11–13]. Conversely, depression in men may be underdiagnosed, as physicians tend to be more attuned to or responsive to mental health concerns when they arise in women [13, 14].

Moreover, diagnostic and mental health screening tools may also be gender-biased, as they tend to prioritize symptoms more commonly associated with women over those typically expressed by men. These tools often emphasize internalizing symptoms—such as sadness and loss of interest or pleasure in previously enjoyed activities—while overlooking symptoms that align more closely with traditional masculine role norms, such as anger, substance misuse, emotional suppression, and risk-taking [15]. A meta-analysis found that women with depression reported symptoms listed as diagnostic criteria in the DSM-V or ICD-10 more frequently and with greater intensity than men [16]. However, research on the extent and impact of this potential measurement bias remains inconclusive [17].

From the patients' perspective, qualitative evidence on depression suggests that men have greater difficulty discussing their emotions compared to women. This reluctance stems from the belief that expressing sadness, crying, or displaying other depressive symptoms is less socially acceptable for men than for women [18]. Indeed, gender differences in symptom reporting have been extensively documented and are largely shaped by societal constructions of masculinity and femininity [19].

These gender biases in mental health care, which contribute to the dynamics of medicalization, may vary in intensity depending on intersecting axes of inequality, such as social class, race, or age. As predicted by intersectionality theory, various studies have shown that as educational level or socioeconomic status declines, gender disparities in depression diagnoses and antidepressant use become more pronounced. This pattern persists even after controlling for women's overall poorer mental health status, older age, higher frequency of primary care visits, and greater number of diagnoses [12, 20].

In the following sections of this chapter, we analyze the medicalization of mental health through a gender lens, drawing on multiple databases covering Spain. Our analysis takes a life-course perspective, which entails examining this phenomenon separately across different age groups: adolescents and young people, adults, and older individuals. We follow the analyses by discussing the results obtained and making key recommendations for action. Despite its purely quantitative approach, the analyses in this chapter are grounded in a critical-realist epistemology [21], which acknowledges both the material and objective determinants of mental distress, as well as the culturally and socially constructed nature of depression and anxiety as diagnostic categories. These conditions are understood as products of cultural practices that define suffering as pathological within specific contextual and temporal frameworks. As Janne Marecek [22] stated, "depression is not something people have, but a set of practices authorized by the culture through which people express to others that they are suffering."

10.3 Medicalization of Women's Mental Health in Spain

In the following sections, we present an analysis of the medicalization of mental health from a gender perspective, taking Spain as the context of analysis. Our study adopts a life-course approach and draws on various data sources.

1. For the adult population aged 25–64, we used data from Spanish sample of the 2020 European Health Interview Survey (EHIS). This survey collects information on a range of health indicators, socioeconomic characteristics, and the use of health services, based on a randomly selected sample of Spanish households [23].
2. For the population aged 65 and over, our analysis is also based on data from the EHIS, supplemented by the 2018 Survey of Health, Ageing, and Retirement in Europe (SHARE). SHARE provides detailed information on health status, socio-

economic conditions, and social and family networks among individuals aged 50 and over across several European countries: Austria, Germany, Sweden, Netherlands, Spain, Italy, France, Denmark, Greece, Switzerland, Belgium, Czech Republic, Poland, Luxembourg, Hungary, Slovenia, Estonia, Croatia, Lithuania, Bulgaria, Finland, Romania [24].

3. Finally, our analysis of adolescents and young people aged 10–25 draws on data from the 2023 Primary Care Clinical Database (BDCAP). This database includes clinical records from the Spanish National Health System (NHS), covering visits to primary care services, diagnoses, and the dispensing of prescribed medications [25].

To evaluate the extent of mental health medicalization from a gender perspective, we analyzed the likelihood of women receiving a diagnosis of anxiety or depression compared to men, by calculating prevalence ratios (PRs). These ratios were adjusted for differences in mental health status between sexes, as such differences could contribute to a higher number of diagnoses among women. To examine potential over-prescription of psychotropic medications in women, we calculated the likelihood of receiving a prescription, taking into account not only differences in mental health status but also differences in diagnostic rates between men and women, meaning that for the same diagnosis, we will assess if men and women get prescribed differently. All analyses control for age because our outcomes have strong age patterns and because women in these data sets are, on average, older (due mostly to the female survival advantage), which may increase their probability of receiving a diagnosis or a prescription. We also control for frequency of primary care visits, given that women tend to attend more regularly for a host of reasons, thereby increasing their likelihood of receiving any diagnosis, including psychiatric ones. It is worth noting that mental health status data were not available in the BDCAP database, which means that only the potential over-prescription of psychotropic medications given diagnosis could be assessed, but not the over-diagnosis of depression.

10.3.1 Adult Population Aged 25–64

In 2020, adult women in Spain showed poorer mental health than men, both in terms of depressive and anxiety symptoms, as well as in the higher prevalence of diagnoses and psychotropic drug prescriptions—showing levels twice as high as those observed in men for several indicators. Indeed, the likelihood of receiving a diagnosis of depression was 34% higher in women, a difference that could not be explained by variations in age, mental health status, or the number of medical consultations between the sexes. In the case of prescribed antidepressants and stimulants, women were 29% more likely to receive psychotropic medication, even after adjusting for the aforementioned factors and for differences in diagnostic rates between men and women (Table 10.1). These findings suggest a potential gender bias in the labelling and therapeutical management of mental health, whereby adult women may be receiving more diagnoses and prescriptions than men, despite comparable mental health status and apparent clinical need.

Table 10.1 Prevalence ratio (PR) (IC 95%) of diagnosis of depression and antidepressant/stimulant consumption according to different adjustments[a] (reference category: men)

	Model 1	Model 2	Model 3	Model 4
Diagnosis of depression	1.93 (1.65–2.27)	1.39 (1.19–1.62)		1.34 (1.15–1.56)
Antidepressants/stimulants consumption	2.04 (1.73–2.42)	1.59 (1.34–1.87)	1.32 (1.14–1.53)	1.29 (1.12–1.50)

European Health Interview Survey (Spain), 2020
[a]Model 1: Adjusted by age; Model 2: Adjusted by age and depressive symptoms; Model 3: Adjusted by age, depressive symptoms and diagnosis of depression; Model 4: Adjusted by age, depressive symptoms and number of visits to Primary Care in the case of the variable "Diagnosis of depression"; and adjusted by age, depressive symptoms, diagnosis of depression and number of visits to Primary Care in the case of the variable "Antidepressants/stimulants consumption". Created using data extracted from EHIS (Spain), 2020

As mentioned, from an intersectional perspective, gender inequalities are expected to vary depending on other axes of social stratification, and may be more pronounced, for example, among socioeconomically disadvantaged groups, individuals of racial and ethnic minorities, or older populations. Findings from Spain support this pattern since the data show that gender inequalities in the medicalization of mental health are lower among the higher educated, even disappearing among those with university-level education. This pattern holds true for both depression diagnoses and the prescription of antidepressants and stimulants (Fig. 10.2). We see a similar pattern across social class, with no gender inequalities found in depression diagnoses or psychotropic prescriptions among individuals in the highest social classes (I–II) (Data not shown).

When considering place of birth, the data reveal that women—both Spanish-born and foreign-born—have higher rates of depression diagnosis and psychotropic drug use than men, even after adjusting for multiple factors (age, depressive symptoms, prior diagnosis, and use of primary care services). Notably, foreign-born women exhibit the highest risk of receiving a diagnosis of depression, suggesting a potential interaction between gender and migrant status in the medicalization of mental health. Regarding psychotropic consumption, the gender pattern was similar in both the Spanish-born and foreign-born populations, although the model only detected statistically significant differences for the Spanish-born group. (Table 10.2).

Finally, age also appears to be a relevant factor in the analysis of gender inequalities in the medicalization of mental health. Among the adult population aged 25–64 (results for the population over 64 are discussed in the following section), the magnitude of gender disparities in depression diagnosis was similar across the two age groups analyzed (Table 10.3). However, inequalities in the prescription of psychotropic medications were only significant in the older one (50–64 years). In this group, women were 45% more likely than men to have received an antidepressant or stimulant prescription, after accounting for equivalent mental health needs between sexes.

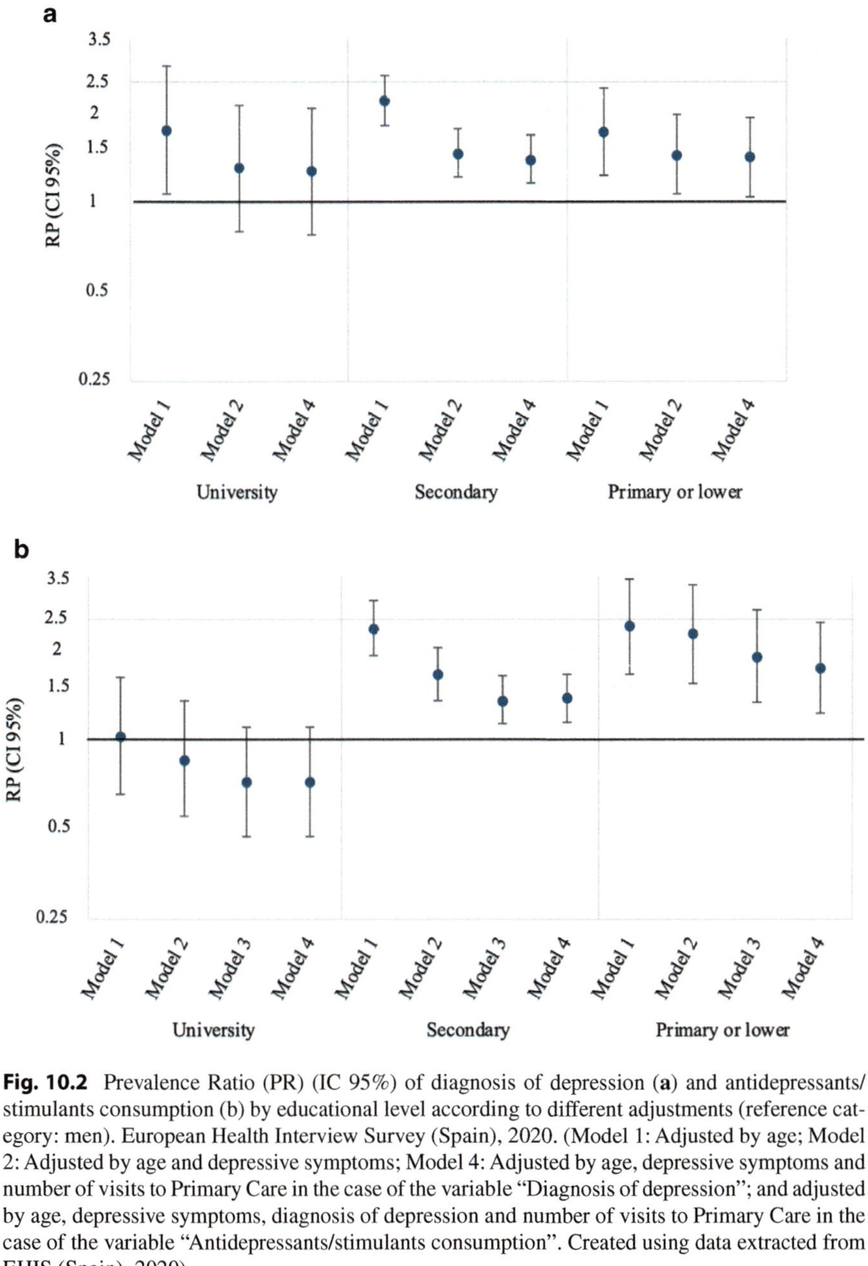

Fig. 10.2 Prevalence Ratio (PR) (IC 95%) of diagnosis of depression (**a**) and antidepressants/stimulants consumption (b) by educational level according to different adjustments (reference category: men). European Health Interview Survey (Spain), 2020. (Model 1: Adjusted by age; Model 2: Adjusted by age and depressive symptoms; Model 4: Adjusted by age, depressive symptoms and number of visits to Primary Care in the case of the variable "Diagnosis of depression"; and adjusted by age, depressive symptoms, diagnosis of depression and number of visits to Primary Care in the case of the variable "Antidepressants/stimulants consumption". Created using data extracted from EHIS (Spain), 2020)

Table 10.2 Prevalence ratio (PR) (IC 95%) of diagnosis of depression and antidepressants/stimulants consumption by birth country according to different adjustments[a] (reference category: men)

	Model 1	Model 2	Model 3	Model 4
Diagnosis of depression				
Spain	*1.79 (1.50–2.12)*	*1.35 (1.15–1.59)*		*1.32 (1.12–1.55)*
Foreign	*3.15 (1.97–5.03)*	*1.85 (1.17–2.90)*		*1.73 (1.10–2.74)*
Antidepressants/stimulants consumption				
Spain	*1.91 (1.59–2.28)*	*1.56 (1.31–1.85)*	*1.33 (1.14–1.55)*	*1.31 (1.12–1.53)*
Foreign	*3.61 (2.10–6.19)*	*2.21 (1.28–3.79)*	1.45 (0.89–2.35)	1.33 (0.79–2.22)

European Health Interview Survey (Spain), 2020
[a]Model 1: Adjusted by age; Model 2: Adjusted by age and depressive symptoms; Model 3: Adjusted by age, depressive symptoms and diagnosis of depression; Model 4: Adjusted by age, depressive symptoms and number of visits to Primary Care in the case of the variable "Diagnosis of depression"; and adjusted by age, depressive symptoms, diagnosis of depression and number of visits to Primary Care in the case of the variable "Antidepressants/stimulants consumption". Created using data extracted from EHIS (Spain), 2020

Table 10.3 Prevalence ratio (PR) (IC 95%) of diagnosis of depression and antidepressant/stimulant consumption by age according to different adjustments[a] (reference category: men)

	Model 1	Model 2	Model 3	Model 4
Diagnosis of depression				
25–49	*1.89 (1.49–2.38)*	*1.42 (1.13–1.78)*		*1.34 (1.06–1.68)*
50–64	*1.98 (1.58–2.46)*	*1.36 (1.11–1.68)*		*1.33 (1.08–1.64)*
65–79	*2.83 (2.18–3.69)*	*1.82 (1.41–2.34)*		*1.81 (1.41–2.33)*
80 and over	*2.17 (1.48–3.18)*	*1.83 (1.21–2.76)*		*1.82 (1.21–2.75)*
Antidepressants/stimulants consumption				
25–49	*1.82 (1.43–2.33)*	*1.47 (1.16–1.88)*	1.19 (0.95–1.47)	1.16 (0.94–1.45)
50–64	*2.28 (1.80–2.88)*	*1.70 (1.35–2.14)*	*1.48 (1.21–1.80)*	*1.45 (1.19–1.78)*
65–79	*3.34 (2.45–4.56)*	*2.28 (1.67–3.10)*	*1.71 (1.30–2.26)*	*1.70 (1.29–2.25)*
80 and over	*1.91 (1.30–2.82)*	*1.59 (1.04–2.45)*	1.28 (0.89–1.83)	1.28 (0.89–1.84)

European Health Interview Survey (Spain), 2020
[a]Model 1: Crude; Model 2: Adjusted by depressive symptoms; Model 3: Adjusted by depressive symptoms and diagnosis of depression; Model 4: Adjusted by depressive symptoms and number of visits to Primary Care in the case of the variable "Diagnosis of depression"; and adjusted by depressive symptoms, diagnosis of depression and number of visits to Primary Care in the case of the variable "Antidepressants/stimulants consumption". Created using data extracted from EHIS (Spain), 2020

10.3.2 Population Aged 65+

Some studies suggest that gender inequalities in mental health and its clinical management may be more pronounced in older populations; however, few have explored these disparities in depth or examined their underlying causes [26]. This appears to be the case in Spain, where data from the 2020 EHIS show that women over the age of 64 were approximately 80% more likely than men of the same age to receive a diagnosis of depression, even after adjusting for age, mental health status, and the number of primary care visits. Regarding the use of antidepressants and stimulants, gender inequalities were also evident: women aged 65–79 had a 70% higher likelihood of using psychotropic medication for the same level of clinical need (Table 10.3).

Taking a broader, comparative perspective, the same analyses have been replicated with data from the 2018 SHARE survey for 22 European countries. In 32% of the countries analyzed, significant gender gaps in depression diagnoses were observed. France and Italy stood out with the most pronounced differences, where women were more than twice as likely as men to receive a diagnosis—differences that could not be explained by greater clinical need (Data not shown). Likewise, significant gender inequalities in the use of psychotropic medication were found in 73% of the countries studied, even after accounting for differences in age, mental health status, diagnosis rates, and primary care utilization. France again emerged as the country with the largest gender gap in this regard (Data not shown).

10.3.3 Youth and Adolescents Aged 10–25

As seen in the adult and older population, several studies also show that there is a clear gender pattern in mental health and psychotropic drug use in the adolescent and young adult population [27]. According to clinical records from a 2023 extract of the BDCAP database, girls aged 10–25 in Spain had a higher likelihood of being prescribed anxiolytics, hypnotics, and sedatives (AHS), as well as antidepressants. These differences were not fully explained by the higher prevalence of depression and anxiety diagnoses among girls nor by their greater use of health services. Specifically, girls were 31% more likely to be prescribed an AHS and 60% more likely to receive an antidepressant than boys of the same age. These findings suggest, again, a potential gender bias in the clinical management of mental health among adolescents and young adults, leading to greater medicalization of emotional distress in girls (Table 10.4).

Gender differences in the frequency of anxiety and depression diagnoses, as well as in the use of AHS and antidepressants, first seems to become noticeable around age 13, and increased progressively with age (Fig. 10.3). From this age onwards, even when controlling for the number of diagnoses and primary care visits in both sexes, girls were more likely than boys to receive prescriptions for AHS or antidepressants. This gender bias in clinical practice peaked between the ages of 16 and

Table 10.4 Prevalence ratio (PR) (CI 95%) of AHS and Antidepressant consumption, according to different adjustments[a] (reference category: men)

	Model 1	Model 2	Model 3
Anxiolytics, hypnotics, and sedatives	1.75 (1.74–1.77)	1.50 (1.48–1.51)	1.31 (1.30–1.32)
Antidepressant	2.30 (2.24–2.31)	1.83 (1.81–1.85)	1.60 (1.59–1.62)

BDCAP (2023)

[a]Model 1: adjusted by age; Model 2: adjusted by age, and diagnosis of depression and anxiety; Model 3: adjusted by age, diagnosis of depression and anxiety, and visits to Primary Care

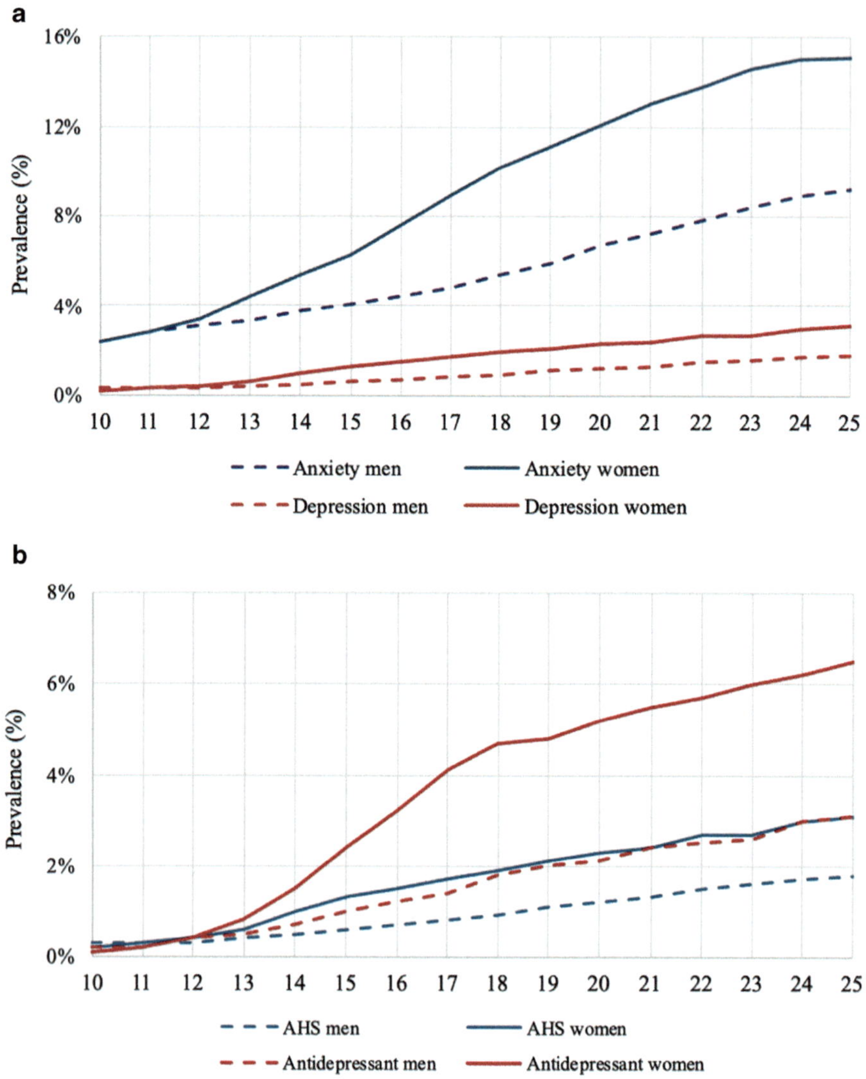

Fig. 10.3 Prevalence (%) of Diagnosis of Anxiety and Depression (**a**) and AHS and Antidepressant consumption (**b**) by age. BDCAP (Spain), 2023. (Created using data extracted from BDCAP (Spain), 2023)

17, a period characterized by particularly intense medicalization of emotional distress during mid-to-late adolescence (Fig. 10.4).

As already shown with EHIS data for old age groups, gender intersects with other social factors—such as migration status and socioeconomic level—in shaping the extent of inequalities in mental health medicalization. For young people in Spain, according to BDCAP data, gender disparities in the medicalization of mental health were more pronounced among those from middle- and high-income

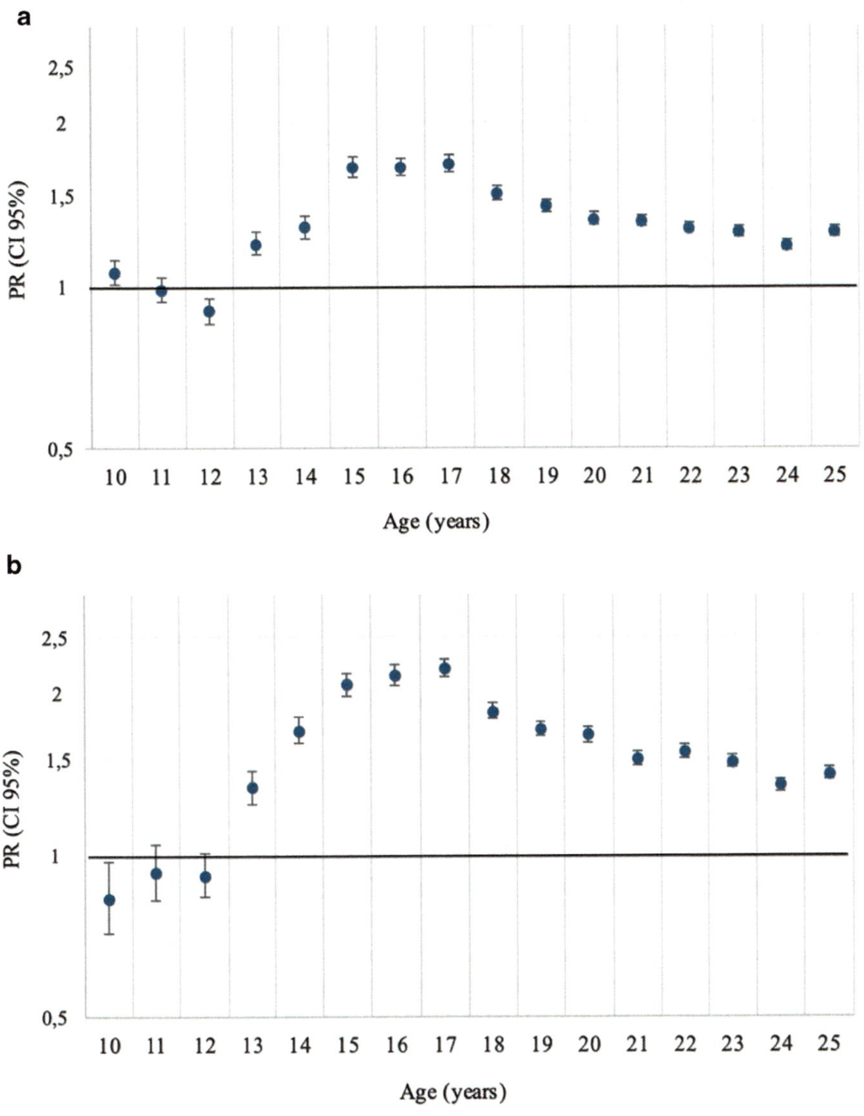

Fig. 10.4 Prevalence ratio (PR) (IC 95%) of AHS (**a**) and antidepressant (**b**) consumption by age (reference category:men). BDCAP (Spain), 2023. (Adjusted by diagnosis of anxiety and depression and number of visits to Primary Care. Created using data extracted from BDCAP (Spain), 2023)

backgrounds—an inverse pattern compared to the general population (Table 10.5). In this case, this is not due to a greater medicalization of emotional distress in girls from higher socio-economic backgrounds, but rather to less intervention in the emotional problems of boys from higher socio-economic backgrounds, thereby exacerbating gender inequality at higher socio-economic levels, as has also been documented in other populations and contexts [13]. Regarding place of birth, girls

Table 10.5 Prevalence ratio (PR) (CI 95%) of AHS and antidepressant consumption by socioeconomic status, according to different adjustments[a] (reference category: men)

	Model 1	Model 2	Model 3
Anxiolytics, hypnotics, and sedatives			
≥100.000 €	2.00 (1.80–2.22)	1.79 (1.62–1.99)	1.66 (1.50–1.84)
18.000–99.999 €	1.80 (1.76–1.83)	1.57 (1.54–1.60)	1.42 (1.40–1.45)
<18.000 €	1.87 (1.85–1.89)	1.56 (1.55–1.58)	1.34 (1.33–1.35)
Very low	1.49 (1.46–1.51)	1.32 (1.30–1.34)	1.16 (1.14–1.18)
Antidepressant			
≥100.000 €	2.26 (2.05–2.49)	1.98 (1.80–2.17)	1.83 (1.67–2.01)
18.000–99.999 €	2.49 (2.44–2.55)	2.06 (1.02–2.10)	1.85 (1.81–1.88)
<18.000 €	2.47 (2.44–2.50)	1.91 (1.89–1.93)	1.66 (1.64–1.68)
Very low	1.74 (1.71–1.78)	1.47 (1.44–1.50)	1.26 (1.24–1.29)

BDCAP (2023)

The income level variable is derived from each individual's pharmaceutical co-payment, considering factors such as age, income, and illness severity. The "Very Low" category applies to individuals exempt from co-payment, while the remaining categories are based on income. Consequently, the "<18,000" category does not have a defined lower limit

[a]Model 1: adjusted by age; Model 2: adjusted by age, and diagnosis of depression and anxiety; Model 3: adjusted by age, diagnosis of depression and anxiety, and visits to Primary Care

born in EU countries were more likely than boys to be prescribed AHS or antidepressants. However, after adjusting for diagnostic and consultation differences, gender inequalities were greater among young people born in Spain (Data not shown). Thus, gender bias in clinical practice appeared to be more pronounced in the Spanish-born population, although differences with the foreign-born population remained relatively small.

10.4 Interpretation of Results and Conclusions

Gender inequalities in mental health likely stem from a complex interplay of multiple, interconnected factors. In this chapter, we explore patterns of overdiagnosis and overprescription, which have been relatively understudied to date. The overdiagnosis of depression and anxiety, along with the overprescription of psychotropic medication to women driven by gender-biased healthcare practices, may help explain the persistent gender gap in mental health observed across clinical data and population-based health surveys.

To frame the hypothesis of the medicalization of women's health alongside other relevant contributing factors, we draw on Brickmann's cultural approach to the pathologization of everyday life [5], adding gender nuance to the framework to better understand this phenomenon. According to Brickmann, the increasing psychiatric framing of everyday life in modern society can be attributed to a set of social changes; the progressive adoption of diagnostic cultures as a new lens through which human suffering is interpreted and communicated; shifts in medical practices; and the growing influence of the pharmaceutical industry. We briefly describe all three dimensions, but our analysis will place particular emphasis on the second—diagnostic cultures—scrutinizing it through a gender lens to better understand the medicalization of women's mental health.

First, the *sociological perspective* points to the role played by the current phase of capitalist development in the rise of psychological distress. In its neoliberal form of governmentality, this system produces and relies upon individuals subjected to chronic pressure to increase their productivity, while simultaneously holding them personally accountable for their actions. At the same time, the neoliberal era has led to a deterioration in living conditions for large sectors of the population, whose life trajectories have become increasingly precarious, while the resources and services provided by many welfare states have been progressively weakened. Within this broader context, women are in a particularly vulnerable position, as the heteropatriarchal nature of the system intensifies pressures on them. Women are routinely relegated to subordinate positions in society—not only in terms of socioeconomic status; but also through a lack of visibility and social recognition. These dynamics give rise to harmful living conditions—such as discrimination, gender-based violence, horizontal and vertical segregation in the labor market, and a disproportionate burden of domestic and caregiving responsibilities—all of which have adverse effects on women's mental health [28].

Second, the *perspective of diagnostic cultures* highlights the many ways that individuals use psychiatric categories to make sense of their distress, to express it to others, and to manage it. Increasingly, the psychiatric language to name human suffering has displaced other ways of conceptualizing pain and anguish, becoming the dominant lens through which such experiences are interpreted. People are actively seeking this language in search of conceptual tools that allow them to explain their personal problems and make sense of their suffering. From a gender perspective, it seems plausible that if, traditionally, women have had more contact with health services, and health services have more often applied biomedical language to explain their emotions, women have internalized this framework of interpretation more intensely than men. Women may tend to express their suffering through psychiatric labels, not because their distress is biological, but because psychiatric and patriarchal culture has shaped this way of understanding their mental suffering [29]. In this way, women become consumers of diagnostic labels more often than men, as these can be key in the constitution of their identity. Several qualitative studies highlight the importance of women's agency in managing their own mental health [30]. Women's active involvement in the diagnostic process and in the use of psychotropic medication not only serves to legitimize the suffering that stems from the material and symbolic inequalities they face but also provides a justification for not meeting socially imposed expectations or for finding ways to cope with expectations while continuing to fulfill their responsibilities. Women's active involvement in the diagnostic process may also open a path toward recognizing and interrogating the structural dimensions underlying their mental suffering [10]. This may contribute to a higher demand for diagnoses among women, as, compared to men, diagnostic labels play a more significant role in activating their agency. Additionally, once in a healthcare setting, women may be more likely to passively accept diagnostic and therapeutic proposals from professionals, ultimately resulting in a greater likelihood of undergoing processes of medicalization of their mental health [31].

Lastly, and particularly relevant for the results of this chapter, is the interpretation pointing to the role of medical practices in the clinical management of mental health. While Brickmann focuses on the historical process that has resulted in an expanded range of diagnostic labels in manuals such as the DSM or the ICD, thus expanding the possibilities of pathologizing aspects of everyday life perceived as maladaptive, our approach centers on the gender biases inherent in medical practice and the processes of medicalization it entails, particularly in relation to women's mental health. As mentioned in the introduction, a 'double standard' has historically been applied to define good mental health for men and women, in accordance with social expectations that reinforce normative gender roles. For women, good mental health has been associated with conformity to traits such as submissiveness, dependence, vulnerability, and emotionality. In contrast, men's mental well-being has been linked to opposite traits such as independence, strength, rationality, and leadership. This asymmetry may contribute to biased clinical practices [32]. Gender norms and the clinical descriptions of psychiatric diagnoses are closely bound. Indeed, the construction of these diagnoses based on male and female subjectivities may have influenced the gender-biased nature of clinical assessment tools and psychometric instruments used in mental health. Characteristics traditionally associated with women, such as apathy or crying, are often included in these instruments, whereas typically masculine ones, such as aggressiveness or risk-taking behaviors, rarely appear—potentially leading to gender biases in the identification of mental disorders [33].

This may have significant diagnostic implications by giving rise to a paradoxical dynamic: while women's mental health tends to be medicalized, men may be underdiagnosed or undertreated [34]. Hegemonic masculinity norms promote the suppression of emotional expression, particularly of emotions deemed feminine, due to fear of stigma, which can obscure the recognition and diagnosis of depression in men [33]. One study found that substituting traditional depression symptoms (typically associated with female presentations) with alternative symptoms more common among men led to an increase in depression diagnoses in male participants [15]. Moreover, when both traditional and alternative symptoms were included, gender differences in the prevalence of individuals meeting diagnostic criteria for depression disappeared [15]. These findings suggest that health professionals, trained within a biomedical and androcentric framework, may more readily pathologize women's mental health [35].

Adopting a life-course perspective reveals that certain population groups—such as older adults and adolescents—can also experience gender disparities in the medicalization of mental health, shaped by age-specific dynamics. Among individuals over the age of 64, research remains scarce; however, existing evidence points to a gender bias in the diagnosis and treatment of depression: women are 44% more likely to receive a diagnosis and 31% more likely to use antidepressants than men, even after adjusting for age, severity of depressive symptoms, and healthcare utilization [13]. These findings align with previous studies conducted in the Spanish context [12, 20, 36]. The limited research available on gender inequalities in the medicalization of mental health among older adults hinders a deeper understanding of the mechanisms involved. Nevertheless, it is likely that some of the explanatory factors identified in the adult population also apply to this age group.

Regarding adolescence and youth, literature consistently highlights gender inequalities in mental health [27], with higher rates of diagnosis and psychotropic drug use among girls compared to boys of the same age, a pattern replicated for Spain in our findings. In these ages, common experiences such as family conflicts or interpersonal conflicts often give rise to intense but transitory emotional distress, which may be pathologized as depressive disorders, particularly among girls [37]. Adolescence is a critical stage for the internalization of gender roles, and the pronounced expression of femininity during this period may contribute to the increased medical labeling of emotional suffering through diagnoses of depression and anxiety. Moreover, as observed in adult women, the prescription of psychotropic medication to young people can serve to legitimize their distress and facilitate a sense of normalcy in their lives [38], which may help explain the increased demand for such medications in clinical settings. It is important to note, however, that other agents such as schools, families, and social media also play a significant role in the medicalization of everyday life among adolescents and young people. These milieus likewise reproduce gender biases in how distress is labeled. For instance, in school settings, teachers are more likely to identify symptoms related to depression and withdrawal in girls and behavioral problems in boys [39].

While building on Brikmann's hypotheses, a fuller understanding of the findings presented in this chapter benefits from showing of how multiple axes of inequality, such as gender, age, social class, ethnicity, and sexuality, intersect to shape differentiated experiences of psychological distress, as well as the processes of diagnosis and medicalization in mental health [40]. However, most published research on mental health medicalization does not address the intersecting nature of multiple axes of inequality remains limited. The limited studies that do take this analytic perspective support the patterns identified in our findings [12, 20, 36]. Our analysis suggests that, among the adult population, having a disadvantaged socioeconomic status, a low level of education, being foreign-born, or being older are factors that exacerbate gender disparities in depression diagnoses and the use of prescribed psychotropic medications. These results reinforce the idea that intersecting forms of discrimination place disadvantaged women in a particularly vulnerable position, increasing their exposure to biased clinical practices. Evidence shows that patients with lower income and educational levels tend to receive less information about their diagnosis and are more likely to experience less participatory clinical encounters, which in turn limits their ability to engage in decision-making about their treatment [41]. Beyond inequalities in the doctor–patient relationship, wider gender disparities in diagnosis and prescribing among more disadvantaged groups may also be linked to the persistence of traditional masculine norms among men with lower socioeconomic status [42] and from older cohorts [18]. These norms may contribute to the minimization or avoidance of symptoms, leading to lower rates of help-seeking and, consequently, under-treatment among men. Conversely, women with fewer socioeconomic resources may be more likely to seek immediate pharmacological solutions that enable them to recover quickly and resume their caregiving responsibilities, given the limited availability of external support [10].

Among children and adolescents, the intersectional impact of various axes of inequality on the medicalization of mental health may follow a different pattern. While the use of psychotropic medication is generally higher among those from lower income backgrounds [43], when levels of need are held constant, gender disparities appear to be more pronounced within more privileged social groups. This pattern may be attributed to a lower degree of medicalization among boys from socioeconomically advantaged backgrounds. as they face a reduced risk of having everyday behaviors pathologized as mental health issues [44]. Research on older populations in the Swedish context has revealed a similar class-based dynamic, with greater gender disparities in the overdiagnosis of depression and the overprescription of antidepressants observed among individuals from more affluent socioeconomic backgrounds [13]. Given the diversity of intersectional effects across different age groups, there is a clear need for further research to better identify whether women from certain social groups are more intensely exposed to processes of medicalization.

Based on the preceding points, it can be concluded that reducing the medicalization of women's mental health will require action at multiple levels. Although clinical interventions are useful on an individual basis, they do not address the root causes of suffering and its medicalization, which often stem from structural determinants. Political intervention is essential for addressing the issue collectively, and adopting a feminist perspective could help prevent the pathologization of suffering and promote fairer and more equitable social policies.

References

1. Bandelow B, Michaelis S. Epidemiology of anxiety disorders in the 21st century. Dialogues Clin Neurosci. 2015;17(3):327–35. https://doi.org/10.31887/DCNS.2015.17.3/bbandelow.
2. Alonso J, Angermeyer MC, Bernert S, Bruffaerts R, Brugha TS, Bryson H, et al. Psychotropic drug utilization in Europe: results from the European Study of the Epidemiology of Mental Disorders (ESEMeD) project. Acta Psychiatr Scand Suppl. 2004;109(420):55–64. https://doi.org/10.1111/j.1600-0047.2004.00331.x.
3. Van de Velde S, Bracke P, Levecque K. Gender differences in depression in 23 European countries. Cross-national variation in the gender gap in depression. Soc Sci Med. 2010;71(2):305–13. https://doi.org/10.1016/j.socscimed.2010.03.035.
4. Labaka A, Goñi-Balentziaga O, Lebeña A, Pérez-Tejada J. Biological sex differences in depression: a systematic review. Biol Res Nurs. 2018;20(4):383–92. https://doi.org/10.1177/1099800418776082.
5. Brinkmann S. Culturas del diagnóstico. Barcelona: Herder; 2021.
6. Conrad P. The medicalization of society: on the transformation of human conditions into treatable disorders. Baltimore: Johns Hopkins University Press; 2007.
7. Zola IK. Medicine as an institution of social control. Sociol Rev. 1972;20(4):487–504.
8. Bell SE, Figert AE. Gender and the medicalization of healthcare. In: Kuhlmann E, Annandale E, editors. The Palgrave handbook of gender and healthcare. London: Palgrave Macmillan; 2012. https://doi.org/10.1057/9781137295408_8.

9. Amoretti MC. Gender as a category of analysis in medical knowledge. In: Schramme T, Walker M, editors. Handbook of the philosophy of medicine. Dordrecht: Springer; 2024. https://doi.org/10.1007/978-94-017-8706-2_95-1.
10. Bacigalupe A, González-Rábago Y, Jiménez-Carrillo M. Desigualdad de género y medicalización de la salud mental: factores socioculturales determinantes desde el análisis de percepciones expertas. Aten Primaria. 2022;54(7):102378. https://doi.org/10.1016/j.aprim.2022.102378.
11. Potts MK, Burnam MA, Wells KB. Gender differences in depression detection: a comparison of clinical diagnosis and standardized assessment. Psychol Assess. 1991;3(4):609–15.
12. Cabezas-Rodríguez A, Bacigalupe A, Martín U. Diagnosis and treatment of depression in Spain: are there gender inequalities? Int J Environ Res Public Health. 2020;17(24):9232. https://doi.org/10.3390/ijerph17249232.
13. Bacigalupe A, Martín U, Triolo F, Sjöberg L, Sterner TR, Dekhtyar S, Fratiglioni L, Calderón-Larrañaga A. Is the diagnosis and treatment of depression gender-biased? Evidence from a population-based aging cohort in Sweden. Int J Equity Health. 2024;23(1):252. https://doi.org/10.1186/s12939-024-02320-2.
14. Borowsky SJ, Rubenstein LV, Meredith LS, Camp P, Jackson-Triche M, Wells KB. Who is at risk of nondetection of mental health problems in primary care? J Gen Intern Med. 2000;15(6):381–8.
15. Martin LA, Neighbors HW, Griffith DM. The experience of symptoms of depression in men vs women: analysis of the National Comorbidity Survey Replication. JAMA Psychiatry. 2013;70(10):1100–6. https://doi.org/10.1001/jamapsychiatry.2013.1985.
16. Cavanagh A, Wilson CJ, Kavanagh DJ, Caputi P. Differences in the expression of symptoms in men versus women with depression: a systematic review and meta-analysis. Harv Rev Psychiatry. 2017;25(1):29–38. https://doi.org/10.1097/HRP.0000000000000128.
17. Jane JS, Oltmanns TF, South SC, Turkheimer E. Gender bias in diagnostic criteria for personality disorders: an item response theory analysis. J Abnorm Psychol. 2007;116(1):166–75. https://doi.org/10.1037/0021-843X.116.1.166.
18. Rydberg Sterner T, Dahlin-Ivanoff S, Gudmundsson P, Wiktorsson S, Hed S, Falk H, et al. 'I wanted to talk about it, but I couldn't': an H70 focus group study about experiencing depression in early late life. BMC Geriatr. 2020;20(1):528. https://doi.org/10.1186/s12877-020-01908-x.
19. Luppa M, Sikorski C, Luck T, Ehreke L, Konnopka A, Wiese B, et al. Age- and gender-specific prevalence of depression in latest life: a systematic review and meta-analysis. J Affect Disord. 2012;136(3):212–21. https://doi.org/10.1016/j.jad.2010.11.033.
20. Bacigalupe A, Martín U. Gender inequalities in depression/anxiety and the consumption of psychotropic drugs: are we medicalising women's mental health? Scand J Public Health. 2021;49(3):317–24. https://doi.org/10.1177/1403494820944736.
21. Ussher JM, Perz J. Disruption of the silenced-self: the case of pre-menstrual syndrome. In: Jack DC, Ali A, editors. The depression epidemic: international perspectives on women's self-silencing and psychological distress. Oxford: Oxford University Press; 2010. p. 435–58.
22. Marecek J. Social suffering, gender, and women's depression. In: Keyes CL, Goodman SH, editors. Women and depression: a handbook for the social, Behavioral and biomedical sciences. Cambridge: Cambridge University Press; 2006. p. 283–308.
23. Spanish National Statistics Institute (INE). Encuesta Europea de Salud en España 2020. Metodología. Madrid: Instituto Nacional de Estadística; 2020. Available online: https://www.sanidad.gob.es/estadEstudios/estadisticas/EncuestaEuropea/EncuestaEuropea2020/Metodologia_EESE_2020.pdf.
24. Bergmann M, Börsch-Supan A. SHARE Wave 8 Methodology: Collecting cross-national survey data in times of COVID-19. Munich: MEA, Max Planck Institute for Social Law and Social Policy; 2021.
25. Ministerio de Sanidad. Statistics of the Spanish National Health System Primary Care dataset 2023. [Portal Estadístico del SNS – Base de Datos Clínicos de Atención Primaria]—BDCAP. Available online: https://www.sanidad.gob.es/estadEstudios/estadisticas/estadisticas/estMinisterio/SIAP/home.htm.

26. Kiely KM, Brady B, Byles J. Gender, mental health and ageing. Maturitas. 2019;129:76–84. https://doi.org/10.1016/j.maturitas.2019.09.004.
27. Campbell OLK, Bann D, Patalay P. The gender gap in adolescent mental health: a cross-national investigation of 566,829 adolescents across 73 countries. SSM Popul Health. 2021;13:100742. https://doi.org/10.1016/j.ssmph.2021.100742.
28. Fraser N. From redistribution to recognition? Dilemmas of justice in a 'post-socialist' age. New Left Rev. 1995;212:68–93.
29. Halliday P. What sort of mental health problems are experienced by women in contemporary British society? What do different feminist perspectives offer as alleviation? J Int Womens Stud. 2005;6(2):8–23. Available online: https://vc.bridgew.edu/cgi/viewcontent.cgi?article=1516&context=jiws.
30. Martinez-Mendia X, González-Rábago Y, Jiménez-Carrillo M, Bacigalupe A. From vulnerability to agency: the management and medicalization of mental health in women and men. Womens Stud Int Forum. 2024;105:102953. https://doi.org/10.1016/j.wsif.2024.102953.
31. Doblytė S. 'Women are tired and men are in pain': gendered habitus and mental healthcare utilization in Spain. J Gend Stud. 2020;29(6):694–705. https://doi.org/10.1080/09589236.2020.1780420.
32. Chesler P. Mujeres y locura. Madrid: Continta Me Tienes; 2019.
33. Smith DT, Mouzon DM, Elliott M. Reviewing the assumptions about men's mental health: an exploration of the gender binary. Am J Mens Health. 2018;12(1):78–89. https://doi.org/10.1177/1557988316630953.
34. PLOS Medicine Editors. The paradox of mental health: over-treatment and under-recognition. PLoS Med. 2013;10(5):e1001456. https://doi.org/10.1371/journal.pmed.1001456.
35. Pujal M, Calatayud M, Amigot P. Subjetividad, desigualdad social y malestares de género: una relectura del DSM-V. Rev Int Sociol. 2020;72:e155. https://doi.org/10.3989/ris.2020.78.2.18.113.
36. Bacigalupe A, Cabezas A, Bueno MB, Martín U. El género como determinante de la salud mental y su medicalización. Informe SESPAS 2020. Gac Sanit. 2020;34 Suppl 1:61–7. https://doi.org/10.1016/j.gaceta.2020.06.013.
37. Horwitz AV, Wakefield JC. Should screening for depression among children and adolescents be demedicalized? J Am Acad Child Adolesc Psychiatry. 2009;48(7):683–7. https://doi.org/10.1097/CHI.0b013e3181a5e3ad.
38. Wills C, Gibson K, Cartwright C, Read J. Young women's selfhood on antidepressants: "not fully myself". Qual Health Res. 2020;30(2):268–78. https://doi.org/10.1177/1049732319877175.
39. Green JG, Guzmán J, Didaskalou E, Harbaugh AG, Segal N, LaBillois J. Teacher identification of student emotional and Behavioral problems and provision of early supports: a vignette-based study. J Emot Behav Disord. 2017;26(4):225–42. https://doi.org/10.1177/1063426617740879.
40. Crenshaw K. Demarginalizing the intersection of race and sex: a black feminist critique of anti-discrimination doctrine, feminist theory and antiracist politics. Univ Chic Leg Forum; 1989.
41. Verlinde E, De Laender N, De Maesschalck S, Deveugele M, Willems S. The social gradient in doctor-patient communication. Int J Equity Health. 2012;11:12. https://doi.org/10.1186/1475-9276-11-12.
42. Courtenay WH. Constructions of masculinity and their influence on men's well-being: a theory of gender and health. Soc Sci Med. 2000;50(10):1385–401. https://doi.org/10.1016/s0277-9536(99)00390-1.
43. Mar J, Larrañaga I, Ibarrondo O, González-Pinto A, Las Hayas C, Fullaondo A, Izco-Basurko I, Alonso J, Zorrilla I, Vilagut G, Mateo-Abad M, de Manuel E, UPRIGHT Consortium. Incidence of mental disorders in the general population aged 1-30 years disaggregated by gender and socioeconomic status. Soc Psychiatry Psychiatr Epidemiol. 2023;58(6):961–71. https://doi.org/10.1007/s00127-023-02425-z.
44. Fagrell Trygg N, Gustafsson PE, Månsdotter A. Languishing in the crossroad? A scoping review of intersectional inequalities in mental health. Int J Equity Health. 2019;18(1):115. https://doi.org/10.1186/s12939-019-1012-4.

Gender Differences in Clinical Research and Diagnostic Criteria

11

María Recio-Barbero and Rodrigo Romero-Jiménez

11.1 Introduction

Historically, medicine has advanced under a research model that has largely taken males as the universal reference. This androcentric view has resulted in significant knowledge gaps about how diseases affect women and men differently, both in clinical presentation and in diagnosis and treatment. Incorporating a gender perspective in medical research is not only a matter of equity but also a necessary condition for more precise, effective, and safer medicine for the entire population.

This chapter aims to analyze how gender influences the design and execution of clinical research, the interpretation of its results, and the development of diagnostic criteria. It examines concrete examples across various medical specialties, explores the effects of gender biases in health care, and proposes strategies to promote more inclusive and rigorous science.

M. Recio-Barbero (✉)
Early Phases of Psychosis Group, Biobizkaia Health Research Institute, Cruces University Hospital, Barakaldo, Spain

Department of Psychiatry, Cruces University Hospital, Barakaldo, Spain
e-mail: Maria.reciobarbero@bio-bizkaia.eus

R. Romero-Jiménez
Early Phases of Psychosis Group, Biobizkaia Health Research Institute, Cruces University Hospital, Barakaldo, Spain

Department of Psychiatry, Cruces University Hospital, Barakaldo, Spain

Faculty of Medicine and Nursing, University of the Basque Country (EHU), Leioa, Spain

M. López-Atanes, M. Sáenz-Herrero (eds.), *Applying the Gender Perspective in Psychiatry and Psychotherapy*, https://doi.org/10.1007/978-3-032-17883-1_11

11.2 Gender Biases in Clinical Research

Contemporary medicine is undergoing a paradigm shift that challenges the epistemological foundations that have guided clinical research for over a century. The traditional androcentric model, which conceived the male organism as the universal prototype of human physiology [1], is being progressively replaced by a biopsychosocial approach that recognizes the complex interaction between biological (sex), psychological, and sociocultural (gender) factors in determining health–disease processes [2, 3].

This change has not been merely theoretical but has been driven by three fundamental factors:

(a) Accumulated scientific evidence about significant sexual differences in aspects such as pharmacokinetics [4], symptomatic presentation of pathologies [5], and differential progression of disease processes [6].
(b) Pressure from social movements, particularly scientific feminisms that since the 1970s have denounced the systematic exclusion of women from medical studies [7, 8], revealing how researchers' implicit biases profoundly influence research protocol design [9]. These biases, defined as attitudes or stereotypes that unconsciously affect our understanding, actions, and decisions, have been shown to significantly impact clinical practice. Recent studies indicate that 72% of healthcare professionals lack specific training in gender perspective [10], contributing to the perpetuation of diagnostic and therapeutic errors.
(c) The development of regulatory frameworks that have institutionalized gender perspective in research, notably the EU Gender Equality Strategy (2020–2025) and U.S. NIH policies [11].

11.3 Historical Evolution of Gender Bias in Clinical Research

11.3.1 The Androcentric Phase: The Twentieth Century as an Exclusionary Paradigm

Androcentrism in medicine has its roots in Western scientific tradition, which has historically considered males as the biological norm. From Vesalius's early anatomical studies in the sixteenth century to twentieth-century animal models, research has predominantly focused on male organisms, arguing that females introduced "experimental noise" due to their hormonal cycles [12].

This view translated into concrete research practices: throughout much of the twentieth century, 80% of preclinical animal studies exclusively used male specimens [13], ignoring documented sexual differences in metabolism, immune response, and pharmacodynamics [14].

In the clinical realm, this bias became institutionalized through policies like the exclusion of women of childbearing age from trials [15], based on the myth that male data were sufficient for generalization [8]. Throughout much of the twentieth century, women were systematically excluded from clinical trials due to concerns about hormonal fluctuations and potential pregnancy risks [16]. This exclusion led to classifying women as "vulnerable populations," resulting in treatments and dosages based almost exclusively on data from men [17]. This approach erroneously assumed results would be applicable to women without adjustments, ignoring key differences in pharmacokinetics and therapeutic response [4].

Only in the 1990s, with evidence of sexual differences in cardiovascular diseases [18] and drug responses [4], did this paradigm begin to be questioned, leading to regulatory reforms requiring systematic inclusion of both sexes in basic and clinical research [11]. However, as recent studies warn, the bias persists: even today, 75% of neuroscience research uses only male animals [19], and only 35% of European Medicines Agency (EMA) protocols include systematic gender analyses [20], perpetuating critical gaps in medical knowledge.

- The "Yentl Effect" in Medical Diagnosis: The term "Yentl syndrome," coined by cardiologist Bernadine Healy in 1991, describes how women must present identical symptoms to men to be correctly diagnosed [21]. This phenomenon is particularly evident in cardiovascular diseases, where female symptoms (fatigue, nausea, back pain) are often attributed to psychological causes or diagnosed late [5].

11.3.2 Current Problems in Clinical Research

Despite regulatory advances in recent decades, women's representation in clinical trials remains insufficient. A meta-analysis of studies published between 2016 and 2020 revealed that only 41% of participants were women, with notable disparities across medical specialties [22]. In areas like cardiology, women represent less than 35% of subjects in heart failure and acute myocardial infarction trials [23], despite these conditions significantly affecting both sexes. Similarly, in oncology, lung cancer trials—traditionally considered a "male disease"—include only 30–40% women, even as incidence rates among women have risen dramatically in recent years [24]. This underrepresentation directly impacts the external validity of results, as biological differences in metabolism, immune response, and pharmacodynamics can alter treatment efficacy and safety [25]. Moreover, in diseases with marked gender differences, such as autoimmune disorders (lupus, multiple sclerosis) or chronic pain conditions, the lack of specific data limit treatment personalization [6].

11.3.3 Lack of Sex-Disaggregated Analyses

Perhaps more concerning than numerical underrepresentation is the persistent lack of sex-differentiated analyses in studies that do include women. Research published in *The Lancet* [26] analyzing over 11.5 million scientific articles found that less than 30% of high-impact journal studies reported sex-stratified analyses. This methodological omission has direct clinical consequences: women experience 50–75% more adverse drug reactions than men at equivalent doses [25], including severe reactions to anticoagulants, psychotropic drugs, and antiarrhythmics.

In neurology, for example, women metabolize triptans (used for migraines) more slowly, potentially requiring dosage adjustments [27]. However, most clinical guidelines do not incorporate these differences, perpetuating a one-size-fits-all therapeutic approach based predominantly on male data [28]. The lack of transparency in sex-disaggregated reporting also hinders the identification of specific biomarkers, such as in colon cancer, where tumors in women present distinct genetic mutations that may influence immunotherapy response [29].

11.3.4 Implicit Biases in Clinical Practice

Healthcare professionals' unconscious biases present an additional barrier to equitable care. Controlled studies show physicians attribute cardiac symptoms in women to psychological causes 30% more frequently than identical symptoms in men [5]. Similarly, in chronic pain management, 40% of women experience significant diagnostic delays compared to men [30]. These biases are closely related to lack of specific training: a European survey revealed less than 15% of medical schools systematically include sex and gender differences in their curricula [10].

11.3.5 Initiatives to Correct Gender Biases in Clinical Research

In response to accumulated evidence about gender biases in research, various institutions have developed policies to integrate gender considerations at all methodological levels:

- In the United States, the National Institutes of Health (NIH) established in 2016 a cross-cutting requirement: all funded studies must include sex as a fundamental biological variable [11]. This policy mandates not only equitable inclusion of women but also differentiated reporting of results, marking a milestone in biomedical research.
- The European Union integrated gender perspective as a cross-cutting axis in its Horizon 2020 program, requiring all funded projects to systematically consider sex and gender variables in methodological design [31].
- A complementary advance is the SAGER Guidelines (Sex and Gender Equity in Research), published in 2016, which establish international standards for reporting disaggregated data in scientific publications, now adopted by over 100 indexed journals [32].

11.4 Implications of Gender Biases: From Biomedical Research to Clinical Reality

The impact of gender biases in medicine transcends research to manifest in tangible clinical consequences that differentially affect women's health. This section briefly analyses and highlights four paradigmatic areas where these disparities are particularly relevant, revealing how sociocultural factors and methodological limitations translate into healthcare inequities.

- *Cardiovascular Diseases:*

  Gender bias in cardiovascular disease (CVD) significantly impacts the diagnosis, treatment, and outcomes for women. Despite CVD being the leading cause of mortality for both men and women, it is often underdiagnosed and undertreated in women. This bias stems from multiple factors, including provider, patient, and societal levels.

  Provider bias is evident in the under-recognition of female-predominant cardiovascular conditions such as nonobstructive coronary artery disease and heart failure with preserved ejection fraction. These conditions are less researched, leading to fewer treatment options for women [33]. Additionally, women are less likely to undergo diagnostic procedures like exercise ECGs and coronary angiography, and they receive less aggressive treatment for conditions like acute coronary syndrome (ACS) [34, 35].

  Patient-level factors also contribute to gender bias. Women are less likely to seek urgent medical attention for cardiovascular symptoms, partly due to societal expectations to prioritize others' needs over their own. This delay in seeking care can result in worse outcomes [33]. Furthermore, women often do not perceive themselves to be at risk for heart disease, leading to fewer discussions about risk factors with healthcare providers [33].

  Societal biases further exacerbate these disparities. Women are underrepresented in clinical trials, which limits the applicability of research findings to female patients. This underrepresentation is partly due to systemic sexism in research leadership, where women are less likely to lead cardiovascular trials [36]. The American Heart Association has called for increased efforts to address these gaps in knowledge and care delivery to achieve equity in cardiovascular health [37].

  To mitigate these biases, it is essential to increase the visibility and involvement of women in cardiovascular research and clinical leadership. Additionally, healthcare providers should be educated on gender biases and encouraged to offer patient-centered care tailored to women's needs. Addressing these issues requires a multifaceted approach, including more inclusive research and targeted health promotion efforts [38, 39].

- *Autoimmune diseases:*

  Gender bias in autoimmune diseases is a well-documented phenomenon, with a significant preponderance of these conditions occurring in females. Approximately 80% of autoimmune disease patients are women, a disparity that is influenced by a complex interplay of genetic, hormonal, and environmental factors [40–42].

Sex hormones, particularly estrogen and progesterone, play a crucial role in modulating immune responses. Estrogen generally enhances immune activity, leading to a more robust inflammatory response, which can predispose women to autoimmune diseases. Conversely, testosterone tends to have immunosuppressive effects, which may offer some protection against these conditions in men [40, 41]. The cyclical nature of female sex hormones, particularly during reproductive years, further influences immune function and disease susceptibility [43].

Genetic factors also contribute to the gender bias in autoimmunity. The presence of two X chromosomes in females is significant, as the X chromosome contains numerous immune-related genes. Although one X chromosome is typically inactivated in females, about 25% of X-linked genes escape this inactivation, leading to higher expression levels of these genes in women [44, 45]. This phenomenon can contribute to the heightened immune responses observed in females. Additionally, the role of regulatory T cells (Tregs), which are crucial for maintaining immune tolerance, is influenced by gender. The X-linked gene FOXP3, essential for Treg function, may be differentially regulated in males and females, contributing to the observed sex differences in autoimmune disease prevalence [46].

Environmental and lifestyle factors, including diet, microbiota, and sociocultural influences, also play a role in the gender disparity seen in autoimmune diseases. These factors can interact with genetic and hormonal influences to modulate immune responses differently in men and women [40, 47].

Stressful life events have a significant impact on the disease activity of systemic lupus erythematosus (SLE), particularly in women [48, 49]. Psychosocial factors influence autoimmune diseases differently depending on gender. In women, chronic stress, adverse life events, and caregiving responsibilities increase the risk of developing SLE and rheumatoid arthritis (RA) [50]. In contrast, men with RA are more likely to receive greater social support, such as being accompanied to medical appointments, which may positively influence disease management [51]. These gender differences in the effects of stress and social support can shape the progression and overall experience of autoimmune illness.

In conclusion, the gender bias in autoimmune diseases is multifactorial, involving hormonal, genetic, and environmental components. Understanding these differences is crucial for developing gender-specific therapeutic strategies and improving disease management for both men and women.

- *Oncologic diseases:*

Gender bias in oncologic diseases is a multifaceted issue that impacts various aspects of cancer research, clinical trials, and patient outcomes. Historically, female patients have been underrepresented in clinical trials, which has led to a significant data gap in understanding the efficacy and safety of oncologic treatments for women. This underrepresentation persists despite the increased burden of certain cancers in women, such as gynecologic malignancies [52].

Clinical trials leading to FDA oncology drug approvals have shown a consistent underrepresentation of women. Between 2014 and 2019, women comprised only 39.7% of trial participants, despite the national cancer incidence being 44.6% for women [53]. This disparity is particularly pronounced in specific tumor types, such as thyroid cancer, where women are significantly underrepresented [53]. The lack of gender-specific data can lead to suboptimal treatment regimens for women, as dosing and side effect profiles may differ between sexes.

Gender bias also extends to the professional environment in oncology. Female oncologists report higher rates of gender bias in clinical practice, research activities, and balancing work and non-work responsibilities compared to their male counterparts [54]. This bias contributes to burnout and hinders career advancement, further perpetuating gender disparities in leadership roles within oncology [55].

Biological differences between sexes also play a role in cancer incidence and treatment outcomes. Men generally have higher cancer incidence and poorer outcomes for non-reproductive organ cancers. However, women often experience more severe adverse events to immunotherapies [56]. These differences are influenced by sex hormones, chromosome-encoded gene products and epigenetic mechanisms [57].

In conclusion, addressing gender bias in oncology requires a multifaceted approach that includes equitable representation in clinical trials, targeted funding, and promotion of gender equity in professional environments. These efforts are essential to improve the diagnosis, treatment, and outcomes for all patients, regardless of gender.

- *Psychiatric Disease:*

  Gender bias in psychiatric disease is a multifaceted issue that impacts diagnosis, treatment, and outcomes. Research indicates significant sex and gender differences in the prevalence, symptomatology, and treatment responses of various psychiatric disorders. For instance, internalizing disorders such as depression and anxiety are more commonly diagnosed in women, whereas externalizing disorders like conduct disorder and antisocial personality disorder are more frequently diagnosed in men [58, 59].

  Biological factors, including genetic predispositions and hormonal influences, play a crucial role in these differences. Gonadal hormones, such as estrogen and testosterone, have been shown to affect brain function and behavior, contributing to sex-specific vulnerabilities in psychiatric conditions [60]. Additionally, psychosocial factors, including gender roles, societal expectations, and cultural traditions, further influence the expression and management of mental illnesses. Women often face unique stressors related to reproductive health, caregiving responsibilities, and gender-based violence, which can exacerbate psychiatric symptoms [61, 62].

  Diagnostic biases also contribute to gender disparities in mental health care. Studies have shown that clinicians may be more likely to diagnose certain disorders based on gender stereotypes, potentially leading to misdiagnosis or underdiagnosis. For example, autism spectrum disorder and attention deficit hyperactivity disorder are often underdiagnosed in females due to their atypical presentation compared to males [59, 63]. Conversely, disorders like histrionic personality disorder may be overdiagnosed in women due to gender-biased diagnostic criteria [59, 64].

  To address these biases, it is essential to incorporate gender-specific approaches in psychiatric research and clinical practice. This includes using gender-sensitive diagnostic tools, providing training in cultural competence, and ensuring equitable representation of both sexes in clinical trials [59, 65]. Furthermore, understanding the interplay between biological sex and sociocultural gender variables can enhance the accuracy of diagnoses and the effectiveness of treatments [64, 66].

In conclusion, gender bias in psychiatric disease is a complex issue influenced by biological, psychological, and social factors. Recognizing and addressing these biases through research, education, and clinical practice is crucial for improving mental health outcomes for all individuals.

References

1. Laqueur T. Making sex: body and gender from the Greeks to Freud. Harvard University Press; 1990.
2. Engel GL. The need for a new medical model: a challenge for biomedicine. Science. 1977;196(4286):129–36. https://doi.org/10.1126/science.847460.
3. Regitz-Zagrosek V. Sex and gender differences in health. EMBO Rep. 2012;13(7):596–603. https://doi.org/10.1038/embor.2012.87.
4. Soldin OP, Mattison DR. Sex differences in pharmacokinetics and pharmacodynamics. Clin Pharmacokinet. 2009;48(3):143–57. https://doi.org/10.2165/00003088-200948030-00001.
5. Bairey Merz CN, Andersen H, Sprague E, Burns A, Keida M, Walsh MN, Greenberger P, Campbell S. The Yentl syndrome in the 21st century. J Am Coll Cardiol. 2016;67(2):139–47. https://doi.org/10.1016/j.jacc.2015.10.078.
6. Mazure CM, Jones DP. Twenty years and still counting: including women as participants and studying sex and gender in biomedical research. BMC Womens Health. 2015;15:94. https://doi.org/10.1186/s12905-015-0251-9.
7. Hammarström A, Johansson K, Annandale E, Ahlgren C, Aléx L, Christianson M, Elwér S, Eriksson C, Fjellman F, Gilenstam K, Gustafsson PE, Harryson L, Lehti A, Stenberg G, Verdonk P. Central gender theoretical concepts in health research: the state of the art. J Epidemiol Community Health. 2014;68(2):185–90. https://doi.org/10.1136/jech-2013-202572.
8. Merton V. The exclusion of pregnant, pregnable, and once-pregnable people (a.k.a. women) from biomedical research. Am J Law Med. 1993;19(4):369–451. https://doi.org/10.1017/S009885880000394X.
9. FitzGerald C, Hurst S. Implicit bias in healthcare professionals: a systematic review. BMC Med Ethics. 2017;18(1):19. https://doi.org/10.1186/s12910-017-0179-8.
10. European Institute for Gender Equality. Gender equality index 2022: health. Publications Office of the European Union; 2022. https://eige.europa.eu/publications/gender-equality-index-2022-health.
11. Clayton JA, Collins FS. Policy: NIH to balance sex in cell and animal studies. Nature. 2014;509(7500):282–3. https://doi.org/10.1038/509282a.
12. Beery AK, Zucker I. Sex bias in neuroscience and biomedical research. Neurosci Biobehav Rev. 2011;35(3):565–72. https://doi.org/10.1016/j.neubiorev.2010.07.002.
13. Prendergast BJ, Onishi KG, Zucker I. Female mice liberated for inclusion in neuroscience and biomedical research. Neurosci Biobehav Rev. 2014;40:1–5. https://doi.org/10.1016/j.neubiorev.2014.01.001.
14. Zucker I, Beery AK. Males still dominate animal studies. Nature. 2010;465(7299):690. https://doi.org/10.1038/465690a.
15. National Institutes of Health. Guidelines on the inclusion of women in clinical research. NIH; 1977.
16. Merkatz RB. Inclusion of women in clinical trials: a historical overview of scientific, ethical, and legal issues. J Obstet Gynecol Neonatal Nurs. 1993;22(2):161–70. https://doi.org/10.1111/j.1552-6909.1993.tb01797.x.

17. Kim AM, Tingen CM, Woodruff TK. Sex bias in trials and treatment must end. Nature. 2010;465(7299):688–9. https://doi.org/10.1038/465688a.
18. Bairey Merz CN, Shaw LJ, Reis SE, Bittner V, Kelsey SF, Olson M, Johnson BD, Pepine CJ, Mankad S, Sharaf BL, Rogers WJ, Pohost GM, Sopko G. Insights from the NHLBI-sponsored women's ischemia syndrome evaluation (WISE) study. J Am Coll Cardiol. 2006;47(3 Suppl):S21–9. https://doi.org/10.1016/j.jacc.2005.01.072.
19. Woitowich NC, Beery A, Woodruff T. Opinion: gender equality from a European perspective. eLife. 2020;9:e54503. https://doi.org/10.7554/eLife.54503.
20. European Medicines Agency. Gender considerations in clinical trials. EMA; 2023. https://www.ema.europa.eu/en/documents/scientific-guideline/guideline-gender-considerations-clinical-trials_en.pdf.
21. Healy B. The Yentl syndrome. N Engl J Med. 1991;325(4):274–6. https://doi.org/10.1056/NEJM199107253250408.
22. Liu KA, DiPietro Mager NA. Women's involvement in clinical trials: historical perspective and future implications. Pharm Pract. 2016;14(1):708. https://doi.org/10.18549/PharmPract.2016.01.708.
23. Scott PE, Unger EF, Jenkins MR, Southworth MR, McDowell TY, Geller RJ, Elahi M, Temple RJ, Woodcock J. Participation of women in clinical trials supporting FDA approval of cardiovascular drugs. J Am Coll Cardiol. 2020;71(18):1960–9. https://doi.org/10.1016/j.jacc.2018.02.070.
24. Unger JM, Vaidya R, Hershman DL. Sex differences in cancer immunotherapy. Nat Rev Clin Oncol. 2021;18(2):75–9. https://doi.org/10.1038/s41571-020-00434-4.
25. Zucker I, Prendergast BJ. Sex differences in pharmacokinetics predict adverse drug reactions in women. Biol Sex Differ. 2020;11(1):32. https://doi.org/10.1186/s13293-020-00308-5.
26. Westergaard D, Moseley P, Sørup FKH, Baldi P, Brunak S. Population-wide analysis of differences in disease progression patterns in men and women. Nat Commun. 2019;10(1):666. https://doi.org/10.1038/s41467-019-08475-9.
27. Mauvais-Jarvis F, Bairey Merz N, Barnes PJ, Brinton RD, Carrero JJ, DeMeo DL, De Vries GJ, Epperson CN, Govindan R, Klein SL, Lonardo A, Maki PM, McCullough LD, Regitz-Zagrosek V, Regensteiner JG, Rubin JB, Sandberg K, Suzuki A. Sex and gender: modifiers of health, disease, and medicine. Lancet. 2020;396(10250):565–82. https://doi.org/10.1016/S0140-6736(20)31561-0.
28. Liu KA, Gutierrez E, Jones MR. Reporting of sex and gender in clinical trials. JAMA Netw Open. 2022;5(2):e220152. https://doi.org/10.1001/jamanetworkopen.2022.0152.
29. O'Connor MJ, Paley K, Bale TL. Sex differences in the tumor microenvironment. Nat Rev Cancer. 2021;21(3):151–61. https://doi.org/10.1038/s41568-020-00322-2.
30. Hoffmann DE, Tarzian AJ. The girl who cried pain: a bias against women in the treatment of pain. J Law Med Ethics. 2001;29(1):13–27. https://doi.org/10.1111/j.1748-720X.2001.tb00037.x.
31. European Commission. A Union of Equality: gender equality strategy 2020–2025. Publications Office of the European Union; 2020. https://eur-lex.europa.eu/legal-content/EN/TXT/?uri=CELEX:52020DC0152.
32. Heidari S, Babor TF, De Castro P, Tort S, Curno M. Sex and gender equity in research (SAGER guidelines). Lancet. 2016;387(10026):1717–8. https://doi.org/10.1016/S0140-6736(16)30380-1.
33. Kim I, Field TS, Wan D, Humphries K, Sedlak T. Sex and gender bias as a mechanistic determinant of cardiovascular disease outcomes. Can J Cardiol. 2022;38(12):1865–80. https://doi.org/10.1016/j.cjca.2022.09.009.
34. Daly C, Clemens F, Lopez Sendon JL, Tavazzi L, Boersma E, Danchin N, Delahaye F, Gitt A, Julian D, Mulcahy D, Ruzyllo W, Thygesen K, Verheugt F, Fox KM. Gender differences in the management and clinical outcome of stable angina. Circulation. 2006;113(4):490–8. https://doi.org/10.1161/CIRCULATIONAHA.105.561647.

35. Haider A, Bengs S, Luu J, Osto E, Siller-Matula JM, Muka T, Gebhard C. Sex and gender in cardiovascular medicine: presentation and outcomes of acute coronary syndrome. Eur Heart J. 2020;41(13):1328–36. https://doi.org/10.1093/eurheartj/ehz898.
36. Van Spall HGC, Lala A, Deering TF, Casadei B, Zannad F, Kaul P, Mehran R, Pearson GD, Shah MR, Gulati M, Grines C, Volgman AS, Revkin JH, Piña IL, Lam CSP, Hochman JS, Simon T, Walsh MN, Bozkurt B. Ending gender inequality in cardiovascular clinical trial leadership: JACC review topic of the week. J Am Coll Cardiol. 2021;77(23):2960–72. https://doi.org/10.1016/j.jacc.2021.04.038.
37. Wenger NK, Lloyd-Jones DM, Elkind MSV, Fonarow GC, Warner JJ, Alger HM, Cheng S, Kinzy C, Hall JL, Roger VL. Call to action for cardiovascular disease in women: epidemiology, awareness, access, and delivery of equitable health care: a presidential advisory from the American Heart Association. Circulation. 2022;145(23):e1059–71. https://doi.org/10.1161/CIR.0000000000001071.
38. Gauci S, Cartledge S, Redfern J, Gallagher R, Huxley R, Lee CMY, Vassallo A, O'Neil A. Biology, bias, or both? The contribution of sex and gender to the disparity in cardiovascular outcomes between women and men. Curr Atheroscler Rep. 2022;24(9):701–8. https://doi.org/10.1007/s11883-022-01046-2.
39. Tayal U, Pompei G, Wilkinson I, Adamson D, Sinha A, Hildick-Smith D, Cubbon R, Garbi M, Ingram TE, Colebourn CL, Camm CF, Guzik TJ, Anderson L, Page SP, Wicks E, Jenkins P, Rosen SD, Eftychiou S, Roberts E, et al. Advancing the access to cardiovascular diagnosis and treatment among women with cardiovascular disease: a joint British Cardiovascular Societies' consensus document. Heart. 2024;110(22):e4. https://doi.org/10.1136/heartjnl-2024-324625.
40. Dodd KC, Menon M. Sex bias in lymphocytes: implications for autoimmune diseases. Front Immunol. 2022;13:945762. https://doi.org/10.3389/fimmu.2022.945762.
41. Rubtsova K, Marrack P, Rubtsov AV. Sexual dimorphism in autoimmunity. J Clin Invest. 2015;125(6):2187–93. https://doi.org/10.1172/JCI78082.
42. Xing E, Billi AC, Gudjonsson JE. Sex bias and autoimmune diseases. J Invest Dermatol. 2022;142(3 Pt B):857–66. https://doi.org/10.1016/j.jid.2021.06.008.
43. Keestra SM, Male V, Salali GD. Out of balance: the role of evolutionary mismatches in the sex disparity in autoimmune disease. Med Hypotheses. 2021;151:110558. https://doi.org/10.1016/j.mehy.2021.110558.
44. Lovell CD, Anguera MC. More X's, more problems: how contributions from the X chromosomes enhance female predisposition for autoimmunity. Curr Opin Immunol. 2025;93:102543. https://doi.org/10.1016/j.coi.2025.102543.
45. Sakkas LI, Chikanza IC. Sex bias in immune response: it is time to include the sex variable in studies of autoimmune rheumatic diseases. Rheumatol Int. 2024;44(2):203–9. https://doi.org/10.1007/s00296-023-05446-8.
46. Nie J, Li YY, Zheng SG, Tsun A, Li B. FOXP3+ Treg cells and gender bias in autoimmune diseases. Front Immunol. 2015;6:493. https://doi.org/10.3389/fimmu.2015.00493.
47. Goulmamine S, Chew S, Aninye IO. Autoimmune health crisis: an inclusive approach to addressing disparities in women in the United States. Int J Environ Res Public Health. 2024;21(10):1339. https://doi.org/10.3390/ijerph21101339.
48. Katz P, Patterson SL, DeQuattro K, Lanata CM, Barbour KE, Greenlund KJ, Gordon C, Criswell LA, Dall'Era M, Yazdany J. The association of trauma with self-reported flares and disease activity in systemic lupus erythematosus (SLE). Rheumatology. 2023;62(8):2780–8. https://doi.org/10.1093/rheumatology/keac690.
49. Patterson S, Trupin L, Hartogensis W, DeQuattro K, Lanata C, Gordon C, Barbour KE, Greenlund KJ, Dall'Era M, Yazdany J, Katz P. Perceived stress and prediction of worse disease activity and symptoms in a multiracial, multiethnic systemic lupus erythematosus cohort. Arthritis Care Res. 2023;75(8):1681–9. https://doi.org/10.1002/acr.25076.
50. Parks CG, Pettinger M, de Roos AJ, Tindle HA, Walitt BT, Howard BV. Life events, caregiving, and risk of autoimmune rheumatic diseases in the Women's Health Initiative Observational Study. Arthritis Care Res. 2023;75(12):2519–28. https://doi.org/10.1002/acr.25164.

51. Flurey CA, White A, Rodham K, Kirwan J, Noddings R, Hewlett S. 'Everyone assumes a man to be quite strong': men, masculinity and rheumatoid arthritis: a case-study approach. Sociol Health Illn. 2018;40(1):115–29. https://doi.org/10.1111/1467-9566.12628.
52. Karpel HC, Zambrano Guevara LM, Rimel BJ, Hacker KE, Bae-Jump V, Castellano T, Curtin J, Pothuri B. The missing data: a review of gender and sex disparities in research. Cancer. 2025;131(6):e35769. https://doi.org/10.1002/cncr.35769.
53. Dymanus KA, Butaney M, Magee DE, Hird AE, Luckenbaugh AN, Ma MW, Hall ME, Huelster HL, Laviana AA, Davis NB, Terris MK, Klaassen Z, Wallis CJD. Assessment of gender representation in clinical trials leading to FDA approval for oncology therapeutics between 2014 and 2019: a systematic review-based cohort study. Cancer. 2021;127(17):3156–62. https://doi.org/10.1002/cncr.33533.
54. Balanchivadze N, Mckay C, Nasser Z, Passalacqua KD, Li P, Chino F, Duma N. Exploring perceptions of gender bias in oncology: a survey study. J Clin Oncol. 2022;40(16 Suppl):11056. https://doi.org/10.1200/JCO.2022.40.16_suppl.11056.
55. Krischak MK, Nam CS, Luckenbaugh AN, Herrel LA. Gender equity in oncology: Progress, challenges, and the path forward in urologic oncology and oncologic specialties. Cancer. 2025;131(1):e35690. https://doi.org/10.1002/cncr.35690.
56. Wagner AD, Oertelt-Prigione S, Adjei A, Buclin T, Cristina V, Csajka C, Coukos G, Dafni U, Dotto GP, Ducreux M, Fellay J, Haanen J, Hocquelet A, Klinge I, Lemmens V, Letsch A, Mauer M, Moehler M, Peters S, Özdemir BC. Gender medicine and oncology: report and consensus of an ESMO workshop. Ann Oncol. 2019;30(12):1914–24. https://doi.org/10.1093/annonc/mdz414.
57. Xiao T, Lee J, Gauntner TD, Velegraki M, Lathia JD, Li Z. Hallmarks of sex bias in immuno-oncology: mechanisms and therapeutic implications. Nat Rev Cancer. 2024;24(5):338–55. https://doi.org/10.1038/s41568-024-00680-z.
58. Christiansen DM, McCarthy MM, Seeman MV. Where sex meets gender: how sex and gender come together to cause sex differences in mental illness. Front Psych. 2022;13:856436. https://doi.org/10.3389/fpsyt.2022.856436.
59. Garb HN. Race bias and gender bias in the diagnosis of psychological disorders. Clin Psychol Rev. 2021;90:102087. https://doi.org/10.1016/j.cpr.2021.102087.
60. Franceschini A, Fattore L. Gender-specific approach in psychiatric diseases: because sex matters. Eur J Pharmacol. 2021;896:173895. https://doi.org/10.1016/j.ejphar.2021.173895.
61. Almeida M, Fletcher SJ. Serious mental illness in women. Curr Opin Psychiatry. 2022;35(3):157–64. https://doi.org/10.1097/YCO.0000000000000786.
62. Balta G, Dalla C, Kokras N. Women's psychiatry. Adv Exp Med Biol. 2019;1192:225–49. https://doi.org/10.1007/978-981-32-9721-0_11.
63. Santos S, Ferreira H, Martins J, Gonçalves J, Castelo-Branco M. Male sex bias in early and late onset neurodevelopmental disorders: shared aspects and differences in autism spectrum disorder, attention deficit/hyperactivity disorder, and schizophrenia. Neurosci Biobehav Rev. 2022;135:104577. https://doi.org/10.1016/j.neubiorev.2022.104577.
64. Sáenz-Herrero M, Recio-Barbero M, López-Atanes M, Santorcuato A, Bacigalupe A, Segarra R. Gender differences in the management of acute psychiatric episodes in the emergency department: a cross-sectional analysis of the 2017-2019 triennium. Arch Womens Ment Health. 2023;26(6):777–83. https://doi.org/10.1007/s00737-023-01360-x.
65. DuMont M, Agostinis A, Singh K, Swan E, Buttle Y, Tropea D. Sex representation in neurodegenerative and psychiatric disorders' preclinical and clinical studies. Neurobiol Dis. 2023;184:106214. https://doi.org/10.1016/j.nbd.2023.106214.
66. Cipriani E, Samson-Daoust E, Giguère CE, Kerr P, Consortium, Lepage C, Juster R. A step-by-step and data-driven guide to index gender in psychiatry. PLoS One. 2024;19(1):e0296880. https://doi.org/10.1371/journal.pone.0296880.

Part IV

Gendered Interventions in Psychotherapy

Introduction to Gender Perspective in Psychotherapy

12

Margarita Sáenz-Herrero, Cristina Díez-Alegría Gálvez, Leire Fernández-Arregui, Clara Martinez-Mateo, and Violeta Pintor-Martinez

12.1 Introduction

The concept of *gender* is addressed by various fields of knowledge, and although there is still no unanimity regarding its conceptual delimitation, it is undeniable that, as a historical-cultural social construct, both its subjectivation and its expression have been and continue to be mutable across different contexts and periods [1]. It constitutes a variable that inevitably permeates the individuality of each human being, and at the social level, it has historically been used as a pseudo-natural segregating factor to legitimize power hierarchies that have normalized the male standard and devalued anything that does not conform to it.

Gender inequality is represented in the field of health. Biases and false assumptions in this area, which have promoted an androcentrism implicitly understood as neutral, have been widely exposed [2–7], revealing that women experience epistemic injustices and barriers to accessing health care. This highlights medicine as another field where patriarchal discrimination is evident.

Mental health, as an integral part of general health, is not exempt from such biases; in fact, it is subject to even greater stigma, especially for women, who face prejudices and discriminatory practices in Mental Health Care, which reproduces the same gender stereotypes that persist in society. The diagnosis of Post-Traumatic Stress Disorder [PTSD] in particular serves as a paradigmatic example. Its initial conceptualization was based on clinical observations of male war veterans, disregarding other groups such as women and child survivors of abuse [8], under the

M. Sáenz-Herrero (✉) · L. Fernández-Arregui · C. Martinez-Mateo · V. Pintor-Martinez
Cruces University Hospital, Basque Country University, Bilbao, Spain

C. D.-A. Gálvez
San Carlos Clinic Hospital, Complutense University, Madrid, Spain

M. López-Atanes, M. Sáenz-Herrero (eds.), *Applying the Gender Perspective in Psychiatry and Psychotherapy*, https://doi.org/10.1007/978-3-032-17883-1_12

presumption that the world is inherently safe unless one is exposed to a traumatic event. This assumption could only hold true for white, heterosexual, middle-class men [9], overlooking the political nature of traumatic experiences.

12.2 Trauma as a Particular Form of Distress in Women

By addressing women's suffering cannot ignore their experience of traumatic events, which remains alarmingly prevalent [10]. Psychiatry and psychology owe a significant debt, particularly to victims of sexual abuse, as prevailing trauma models have failed to account for or integrate the complexity of women's traumatic experiences within a gender-divided society.

A significant aspect of sexual violence is its close link to psychopathology. When studying the prevalence of certain disorders, it is very common to find a history of traumatic events in women's lives: there is an association between a history of sexual abuse and diagnoses of various psychiatric and somatic disorders [including anxiety, depression, eating disorders, PTSD, sleep disturbances, suicide attempts, widespread chronic pain, and chronic fatigue, among others] [11, 12]. Beyond diagnoses, and following Germán Berrios' perspective [13], psychopathology is understood as a set of languages developed to describe, explain, and manage behavioral deviations that evolve across different contexts and historical periods. This reveals it as a type of knowledge subsumed within the omnipresent patriarchal social structure, further exposing the negative impact of discrimination on women's lives [including gender inequality, power dynamics, and exposure to traumatic experiences].

Feminist theorists De la Hermosa and Polo [14] focus on power dynamics in sexual relationships, where men are granted a dominant position and women the submissive counterpart. From this perspective, sexuality is constructed based on the male gaze, and any desire or eroticism that deviates from it is punished, whether through direct aggression or symbolic violence that permeates all narratives about female sexuality. In this sense, women's reluctance, aversion, and frigidity in the sexual sphere could even be understood as a rebellion against male dominance and power.

Writer Virginie Despentes [15], in her book *King Kong Theory*, recounts her own experience of sexual assault and highlights a central aspect of rape culture. She presents rape as a form of control over women's bodies that keeps them subordinate and confined to private spaces (where most abuses occur) by historically representing them as helpless victims of men who want to rape them. This creates the illusion that women cannot defend themselves against sexual violence and are powerless against men's uncontrolled sexual appetites and greater physical strength.

Victims of sexual violence bear witness to these heteropatriarchal narratives. Yapp [16], from a feminist perspective, provides a concise and incisive review of the evolution of the dominant discourse on sexual trauma, even within the "psy" disciplines. She examines the illustrative example of "hysteria" as a paradigm of both sexual violence and its denial and silencing, as well as the popular conceptualization of trauma as a "scar" or "wound" with its double-edged implications for victims. Herman's [8] contributions have been highly influential in this regard: her critique of Personality Disorder and PTSD diagnoses, understood as modern hysteria, articulates an alternative explanation of the psychological experience of trauma and sexual violence, linking it to the social sphere.

Additionally, from an intersectional feminist approach, abuse and violence are shaped not only by gender but also by variables such as social class, ethnicity, sexuality, disability, and psychiatric diagnosis, making them deeply connected to social context, status, and identity. Marginalized groups are more exposed to these forms of violence and yet are absent from educational materials on sexual violence. As De la Hermosa and Polo [14] point out, this compels us to reflect on whether we react the same way to accounts of sexual abuse from a migrant or racialized woman, someone diagnosed with a severe mental disorder, a trans woman, or a woman with a disability [p. 354].

12.3 Conceptualization of Subjectivity and Women's Suffering

Sexual violence is just one of the many adversities women endure. When women speak of their suffering, they do so not only through words. The structural violence imposed both directly and indirectly on female identity has shaped a subjectivity rooted in this identity, manifesting as a bodily mask—like an eggshell—filled with barriers, interruptions, falsehoods, and pain. For example, anthropologist Kimberly Theidon's [17] work with women during the armed conflict in Ayacucho, Peru, highlights the ways in which social and political contexts, along with their fractures, inhabit women's bodies. It also challenges the rigidity and limited applicability of the category of "post-traumatic stress" in Indigenous cultural contexts.

The consequence of reducing women's ways of life to their corporeality—meaning, to functions biologically associated with reproduction and explanations of their emotionality based on biological fluctuations related to the uterus [18]—is the emergence of a bodily awareness inextricably linked to feminized pain and pathologizing discourses. It is common to find women suffering from multiple painful conditions without an organic cause to justify them. Following Távora [19], symptoms related to the body reflects what remains unperceived: the body becomes a vehicle for expressing needs and conflicts, falling ill as a way of resisting imperatives and channeling dissatisfaction, bemoaning as a means of discovering alternative paths.

Beyond the bodily consideration of women's suffering, the treatment of their distress has also been biased by their exclusion from public spaces, once again relegating them to the private and invisible sphere of institutionalization. Authors such as Phyllis Chesler [20] and Sandra Caponi [21] reveal through historical and sociocultural analysis, the psychiatric institutionalization and medicalization of women's suffering and identities. First-person narratives from institutionalized women also bear witness to this, as seen in notable works like *The Looney-Bin Trip* [22] by influential feminist thinker Kate Millett, and *My Life in the Madhouse* [23] by pioneering Spanish journalist Ángeles Villarta. Also in Spain, psychiatrists Ana Conseglieri and Celia García Díaz contribute a vast body of research on the historical experiences of women in psychiatric institutions, analyzing subjective discourse within clinical histories.

12.4 Toward a Feminist Psychotherapeutic Approach

In her book *Women and Madness*, Phyllis Chesler [20] reflects on how much of what we take for granted today was unthinkable 50 or 60 years ago. She points out that "during the 1950s and 1960s, doctors were still taught that women suffered from penis envy, were morally inferior to men, and were innately masochistic, dependent, passive, heterosexual, and monogamous."

Along the same lines, it was asserted that "mothers were responsible for neuroses and psychoses," disregarding the multifactorial nature of psychological suffering, which is widely accepted today. Chesler continues, stating that "none of my professors ever said that women or men suffered from oppression or that oppression causes trauma, especially when those who experience it are blamed for their own misfortune and it is diagnosed as a pathology."

These excerpts highlight the thesis that this section aims to propose. Today, gender perspectives influence all areas of knowledge, and healthcare systems and traditional therapies are no exception. In light of the considerations mentioned, integrating a gender perspective into psychotherapeutic approaches is essential. It is even necessary to propose alternative models to traditional therapy, which has frequently relegated women's distress to an individual level, isolating it from social and environmental factors and masking the structural imbalances of society [24–26].

Historically, in psychiatry, women have been treated as passive objects of study, and patriarchal culture has shaped the way psychopathological knowledge has been developed. In the words of Theidon [17], the intrapsychic and individual treatment approach "systematically neglects the importance of contextual factors. It erases the sociopolitical and moral dimensions of suffering. It obscures the level of meaning, reducing it to a list of symptoms without considering what these symptoms seek to communicate" [pp. 42]. Without delving further into this point, studies have shown that gender biases affect the very definitions of mental disorders, their evaluation tools, and therapeutic approaches. In contrast, feminist psychotherapy considers the sociocultural structure in which we are situated and fosters critical awareness of how patriarchy pervasively impacts women's psychological suffering [27].

12.5 Integrative Psychotherapy

One of the proposals for developing a feminist psychotherapy is the integrative model. This psychotherapeutic approach advocates for a flexible and personalized philosophy to address suffering, integrating elements from different psychological approaches in a way that is adapted to everyone. It is a philosophical approach rather than a purely technical one [28, 29].

It is based on the client-centered approach, which emphasizes personal uniqueness and a horizontal, collaborative therapeutic relationship [29]. Combined with a gender perspective, this model seeks to co-construct a therapeutic space that is containing and non-judgmental, validating patients' experiences while recognizing the importance of structural determinants and promoting individuals' own resources within a capacity-based relationship.

Within this integrative psychotherapy model, literature has identified certain common elements or factors that facilitate the therapeutic change process. Systematic reviews and meta-analyses, such as those conducted by Laska, Gurman, and Wampold [30] and, more recently, by Norcross and Lambert [31], have highlighted that these factors are critical to the effectiveness of psychotherapy and have emphasized the need to consider them in daily clinical practice. As Wampold [32] argues in *The Great Psychotherapy Debate*, most therapeutic benefits derive from these shared elements rather than from isolated technical interventions.

Thus, these factors become transversal axes that, when enhanced, can significantly contribute to treatment effectiveness. Based on current reviews, the following have been identified: adaptability and flexibility in intervention; therapist empathy and authenticity, understood as the ability to genuinely connect, actively listen, and validate the patient's experiences; expectations and beliefs about change, which act as a driving force enhancing the intervention's effects; and finally, the therapeutic alliance.

Given its relevance to the central topic of this discussion, it is important to explore this last factor, the therapeutic bond, in greater depth. Numerous studies confirm that the quality of the relationship between therapist and patient is one of the strongest predictors of success in psychotherapy. An alliance based on empathy, authenticity, and collaboration fosters patient openness and the development of significant changes.

Considering the above, gender-sensitive psychotherapy, acknowledging the socio-cultural context of a patriarchal structure, offers a different way of conceptualizing this therapeutic bond. From this perspective, the essential goal is to create a therapeutic relationship that is not only based on emotional support and understanding but also on deconstructing power dynamics and patriarchal influences that have shaped women's lives.

To this end, various authors have suggested fundamental principles for achieving a more beneficial therapeutic alliance for female patients. Brown [33] emphasizes the importance of understanding the social, cultural, and historical context that shapes women's experiences recognizing power imbalances and the oppression many women encounter, particularly in relation to patriarchy, gender norms, and societal structures. On the other hand, Krantz [34] proposes a more horizontal and collaborative approach, where the therapist is not seen as a distant "expert" but as a co-creator of the therapeutic process, helping women feel empowered in their own healing journey and challenging traditional power dynamics that have historically normalized women's subordination.

Similarly, validation and empowerment are central to constructing the therapeutic relationship [35]. Women have historically been devalued and denied access to certain resources, particularly in the domain of mental health. Gender-informed therapists must foster a relationship where patients feel heard, their experiences are validated, and they are given space to reclaim their voice and autonomy, dismantling the internalized narratives of worthlessness that often accompany women's experiences. Finally, the therapeutic bond must serve as a medium for fostering critique of the patriarchal system. Women have been socialized to accept patriarchal norms, internalizing limiting standards, expectations, and beliefs about themselves. Psychotherapy must provide a safe space where these beliefs and norms can be questioned and redefined within the therapeutic relationship [36].

We can turn to the words of author Marta Suria [37], which perfectly illustrate the concepts discussed. Writing under a pseudonym, she narrates in *Ella soy yo* the abuse she suffered from childhood to early adulthood at the hands of her father. In her account, she describes key characteristics of her therapeutic process. She writes, "Not only in therapeutic listening but in the way of looking." She also speaks of the "white coat syndrome" and the transition from a hierarchical model to a more horizontal one, where emotional support, listening, and empathy is central to the therapeutic relationship.

Regarding her personal therapy experience, she writes about her therapist: "A feminist woman who approached me by sharing the pain of living. A woman who, instead of helping me open the door to leave the room, was willing to enter and observe it with me, despite the vertigo. Only when one truly feels can they approach another's place. And only at that moment are there no judgments, no recommendations, no prescriptions, no unbearable paternalism. Only shared pain and understanding."

Before discussing contributions from other psychotherapeutic models, it is important to highlight a fundamental aspect of the feminist approach to the therapist–patient relationship: the understanding of intersectionality. As emphasized in the literature, this concept involves recognizing how a person's multiple identities—such as gender, social class, ethnicity, sexual orientation, and more—interact to create distinct experiences of oppression or privilege. This recognition is crucial for addressing the needs of women who face multiple forms of discrimination, and it requires sensitivity to the diverse forms of suffering and resilience that patients experience, shaped by their complex social and political contexts [38].

Finally, we must highlight classic contributions such as Carl Rogers' *Person-Centered Therapy* [39], which bases change on self-concept and attitudes through self-directed behavior. This perspective's core pillars include the therapist's empathy, authenticity, and congruence. The rejection of the therapist's directive role, unconditional acceptance, and radical trust provide a favorable psychological climate for women to explore their own resources and feel empowered. These notions are also reflected in Erickson's contributions [40]. His therapy's horizontal structure, grounded in curiosity, flexibility, and each person's uniqueness, emphasizes solution-seeking through personal resources and creative potential.

In conclusion, gender-sensitive psychotherapy acknowledges how patriarchy influences women's mental health, perpetuating diagnostic biases, obscuring the impact of violence, and relegating their suffering to an individual level. A feminist perspective proposes an integrative therapeutic model that validates experiences, dismantles power dynamics, and fosters awareness of oppressive structures.

References

1. Lindqvist A, Sendén MG, Renström EA. What is gender, anyway: a review of the options for operationalising gender. Psychol Sex. 2021;12(4):332–44.
2. Bernabé F. Androcentrismo, ciencia y filosofía de la ciencia. Rev Humanid Valparaíso. 2019;14:287–313.
3. Cabanillas-Montferrer T, Giménez-Bonafé P. El sesgo de género en la asistencia sanitaria: definición, causas y consecuencias en los pacientes. MUSAS Rev Investig Mujer Salud Soc. 2022;7(1):106–29.
4. Lagro-Janssen T, Lo Fo Wong S, van den Muijsenbergh M. The importance of gender in health problems. Eur J Gen Pract. 2008;14(1):33–7.
5. Mauvais-Jarvis F, Merz NB, Barnes PJ, Brinton RD, Carrero JJ, DeMeo DL, et al. Sex and gender: modifiers of health, disease, and medicine. Lancet. 2020;396(10250):565–82.
6. Merone L. Exploring androcentricity in medicine, medical research and education, and the impacts on the experiences of female patients. Doctoral dissertation, James Cook University. 2022.
7. Toribio S. Psicopatología y género: determinantes socioculturales de los trastornos psicológicos en las mujeres. Doctoral dissertation, Universidad Complutense de Madrid. 2021.
8. Herman JL. Trauma and recovery. New York: Basic Books; 1992.
9. Burstow B. A critique of posttraumatic stress disorder and the DSM. J Humanist Psychol. 2005;45(4):429–45.
10. Li L, Shen X, Zeng G, Huang H, Chen Z, Yang J, et al. Sexual violence against women remains problematic and highly prevalent around the world. BMC Womens Health. 2023;23(1):196.
11. Chen LP, Murad MH, Paras ML, Colbenson KM, Sattler AL, Goranson EN, et al. Sexual abuse and lifetime diagnosis of psychiatric disorders: systematic review and meta-analysis. Mayo Clin Proc. 2010;85(7):618–29.
12. Jacobsen SA, Frostholm L, Buhmann CB, Petersen MW, Ørnbøl E, Dantoft TM, et al. Are sexual assaults related to functional somatic disorders? A cross-sectional study. Int J Environ Res Public Health. 2023;20(20):6947.
13. Fuentenebro F. El trabajo histórico conceptual de Germán E. Berríos. Una crítica del razonamiento psicopatológico. Rev Neuropsiquiatr. 1997;60(1):14–23.
14. De la Hermosa M, Polo C. Sexualidad, violencia sexual y salud mental. Rev Asoc Esp Neuropsiquiatr. 2018;38(134):349–56.
15. Despentes V. King Kong theory. New York: The Feminist Press at CUNY; 2010.
16. Yapp E. The double-edged sword trauma, mental health, and sexual violence testimony in England and Wales. Doctoral dissertation, University of Bristol. 2024.
17. Theidon K. Entre Prójimos: El conflicto armado interno y la política de la reconciliación en el Perú. Lima: Instituto de Estudios Peruanos; 2004.
18. Peñaloza MR, Ubach TC, Fuentealba PSG. ¿Feminización de la psicopatología o psicopatologización de lo femenino?: construcciones discursivas de cuerpos vulnerables. Athenea Digit. 2019;19(2):e2249.
19. Távora A. El cuerpo como lugar de expresión de los conflictos. In: Cuerpos de mujeres: miradas, representaciones e identidades. Universidad de Granada; 2007. p. 143–62.
20. Chesler P. Women and madness. Chicago: Chicago Review Press; 2018.
21. Caponi S. Política, psicofármacos y vida cotidiana. Xoroi Edicions; 2023.
22. Millett K. The loony-bin trip. Urbana: University of Illinois Press; 2000.
23. Villarta Á. Mi vida en el manicomio. Madrid: Self-edited; 1953.

24. Worell J, Remer P. Feminist perspectives in therapy: empowering diverse women. New York: Wiley; 2002.
25. Enns CZ. Feminist theories and feminist psychotherapies: origins, themes, and variations. 2nd ed. New York: Haworth Press; 2004.
26. Ballou M, Brown LS, editors. Rethinking mental health and disorder: feminist perspectives. New York: Guilford Press; 2002.
27. Brown LS. Subversive dialogues: theory in feminist therapy. New York: Basic Books; 1994.
28. Norcross JC, Goldfried MR. Handbook of psychotherapy integration. Oxford: Oxford University Press; 2005.
29. Castonguay LG, Beutler LE. Principles of therapeutic change that work. Oxford: Oxford University Press; 2006.
30. Laska KM, Gurman AS, Wampold BE. Expanding the lens of evidence-based practice in psychotherapy: a common factors perspective. Psychotherapy. 2014;51(4):467–81.
31. Norcross JC, Lambert MJ. Psychotherapy relationships that work III. Psychotherapy. 2019;56(4):423–30.
32. Wampold BE. The great psychotherapy debate: the evidence for what makes psychotherapy work. 2nd ed. New York: Routledge; 2015.
33. Brown LM. Betrayal and betrayed: feminist perspectives on therapy and power. Fem Psychol. 2002;12(3):369–92.
34. Krantz L. The feminist approach to psychotherapy: empowering women in therapy. New York: Springer; 1998.
35. Gergen KJ, McNamee S, Barrett FJ. Toward transformative dialogue. Int J Public Adm. 2001;24(7–8):679–705.
36. Walkerdine V, Lucey H. Democracy in the kitchen: regulating mothers and socializing daughters. Gend Psychol. 1989;3(3):309–30.
37. Suria M. Ella soy yo. Madrid: Círculo de Tiza; 2019.
38. Crenshaw K. Demarginalizing the intersection of race and sex: a black feminist critique of antidiscrimination doctrine, feminist theory and antiracist politics. Univ Chic Leg Forum. 1989;1989(1):140–67.
39. Rogers CR. On becoming a person: a therapist's view of psychotherapy. Boston: Houghton Mifflin; 1964.
40. O'Hanlon B. Taproots: underlying principles of Milton Erickson's therapy and hypnosis. New York: W. W. Norton & Company; 1987.

CBT and Gender

13

Marina Carretero-Gómez

13.1 Cognitive-Behavioral Therapy (CBT)

Cognitive-behavioral therapy (CBT) is a psychotherapeutic approach that focuses on the relationship between thoughts, emotions, and behaviors. The basic premise of CBT is that distorted or negative thoughts can lead to problematic emotions and behaviors. Through CBT, patients learn to identify, challenge, and modify the dysfunctional thinking and behavior patterns that cause and maintain emotional distress [1].

CBT is one of the most widely used models in contemporary psychotherapy for treating a wide range of emotional and psychological problems. It is a structured, practical, and goal-oriented therapy.

Traditional behavioral therapy was limited to working only with behaviors that could be objectively defined and measured [2]. Its scope expanded to include thought processes—internal processes—when Aaron Beck introduced cognitive therapy in 1976 in his book, *Cognitive Therapy and The Emotional Disorders.* In it, it is assumed that problematic patterns of thinking and behavior are learned under the same learning principles as any other human thought and behavior. Dysfunctional patterns can, therefore, be unlearned just as they are learned [3].

Cognitive therapy provides a way to assess and change interpretations of our experience that are dysfunctional and cause negative emotional repercussions. It's a way to rethink how we perceive the world.

Our perception of ourselves and our ideas on the world are formed in the context of meaningful interpersonal relationships. We learn who we are through our relationships with others, their responses to us, and our responses to them. As a result of the meanings we create from these experiences, we develop core beliefs or

M. Carretero-Gómez (✉)
Infanta Sofia Hospital, Madrid, Spain

M. López-Atanes, M. Sáenz-Herrero (eds.), *Applying the Gender Perspective in Psychiatry and Psychotherapy*, https://doi.org/10.1007/978-3-032-17883-1_13

thoughts that determine how we perceive the world and ourselves. Our behavior, what we do and how we feel, are profoundly impacted by the way we think about ourselves and about the world, as well as the meaning we give to our experiences. Negative experiences can produce core beliefs such as "I am incompetent," "I am unlovable." Often, we are not even aware of these automatic core beliefs that are triggered when we try to give meaning to experiences. The assumptions we use to give meaning to everyday experiences are closely related to these core beliefs.

The initial phase of cognitive-behavioral therapy is the assessment of problematic thoughts and behaviors: *what, when, where,* and *how often* [1]. Although the focus is on the present, the individual's history is important to understand how the problems have been developed. Core beliefs are often developed from childhood, in the family environment, and are subsequently influenced by other significant relationships and experiences throughout our lives. A woman, for example, who has experienced significant rejection or criticism in her early interpersonal relationships may develop the belief that she is not enough or worthy, thus believing that being valued by others is unlikely.

In Cognitive Therapy, an important part of changing automatic thoughts is identifying the cognitive distortions they contain. Through *cognitive restructuring*, we identify and correct erroneous thinking patterns; challenging core, automatic, and long-held beliefs.

Habitually, the majority of core beliefs have been learned in the family environment and from significant relationships. An important question to ask when automatic thoughts arise is: *Whose voice is this?* [4] In relation to this question, traditional cognitive-behavioral therapy has been criticized for failing to adequately consider the cultural and gender factors that influence individuals' lives, especially women's. Cognitive behavioral therapy with a feminist perspective (CBTFP) has emerged as an inclusive and transformative alternative.

13.2 Cognitive-Behavioral Therapy with Feminist Perspective (CBTFP)

Cognitive-behavioral therapy with feminist perspective (CBTFP) is an adaptation of traditional cognitive-behavioral therapy (CBT) that integrates the principles of feminism into the therapeutic process.

The feminist perspective assumes that gender, culture, power relations, and social norms influence people's mental and emotional health, as well as the automatic cognitive processes and dominant core beliefs, through which we interpret experiences and give meaning to interpersonal relationships and everyday events [5]. Cognitive-behavioral therapy with feminist perspective not only addresses cognitive distortions or dysfunctional behaviors of individuals from a microsystem perspective—their specific developmental experiences—but also considers other factors such as discrimination, violence, and oppression as elements that affect women's well-being.

By adopting this feminist approach, therapists incorporate a critique of the patriarchal system and its effects on women's core beliefs and behaviors, promoting a safe space where women can identify, explore, question, challenge, and redefine the roles and expectations imposed by society.

CBTFP uses various techniques for the identification and change processes, such as cognitive restructuring. As with traditional cognitive-behavioral therapy, cognitive restructuring is a fundamental procedure for identifying and modifying dysfunctional thoughts [1]. From a gender perspective, however, it explores how negative thoughts about oneself ("I am not enough," "I don't deserve respect," "I have to be perfect") can be directly influenced by the expectations of a patriarchal society. By identifying and questioning these beliefs and patriarchal societal norms, women can challenge them, adapting them to their unique development and experience, and thus developing healthier and more empowering behaviors [5].

That is, when it comes to cognitive restructuring from a feminist perspective, not only are individual thoughts addressed, but the political and sociocultural context that largely determines the development of these thoughts and their impact on behavior, which is also taken into account. The goal of CBT is to transform an individual's relationship with themselves and their environment through a critical understanding of power dynamics and gender norms, and by learning how all of these influence our behaviors and emotions, based on fundamental beliefs that have become automated.

The feminist approach to Cognitive Behavioral Therapy (CBT) has emerged relatively recently, yet it has garnered considerable attention and acceptance in recent decades. This perspective acknowledges the impact of power structures and gender norms on individuals' core beliefs. These, from a gendered perspective, can be understood through experiences of oppression, discrimination, or gender inequality.

Gender-influenced core beliefs are widely spread in patriarchal society, in which expectation of what is considered womanly behavior abides to a submissive, aesthetically pleasing, calm and demure disposition, paired with the need of external validation and high expectations and an ideal unachievable perfection. These beliefs may be internalized due to gender socialization and cultural messages about what it means to be a man or a woman.

Studies have found that these limiting beliefs can contribute to anxiety, depression, and low self-esteem, especially in women who experience conflicting social pressures and expectations.

A landmark study explored how women internalize experiences of being "good wives" or "good mothers" and how these beliefs generate guilt or anxiety when they fall short or fail to meet the internalized standard [6]. Cognitive restructuring in this context works to challenge these norms and redefine the concept of "wife," "mother," "woman," or "success" outside of patriarchal expectations.

Other studies have focused on how women's beliefs about their personal worth can be closely and directly linked to their role within the family.

Cognitive-behavioral therapy with feminist perspective aims to change thoughts and behaviors by recognizing, first of all, the influence of power structures:

women's experiences are directly influenced and shaped by systemic oppression and social expectations that shape how they perceive themselves and others. CBT works on identifying how internalized core beliefs on women's roles or gender stereotypes can influence thoughts, emotions, and behaviors. This approach encourages patients to critically examine the societal norms they have internalized during their development, which are influenced by patriarchal structures. By doing so, patients are less likely to passively accept these norms, which can directly contribute to dysfunctional behaviors. This promotes a critical understanding of how gender expectations can limit personal freedom.

By identifying automatic thoughts and beliefs developed from the patriarchal structure, one can challenge what has been learned, fostering self-knowledge and autonomy, empowering oneself.

The work validates and recognizes women's experiences of violence and victimization. It primarily aims to assist individuals in reframing their narratives and preventing them from becoming entrenched in victimization, fostering empowerment and a sense of agency.

Through cognitive restructuring, this approach enables the development of a new frame of reference. By encouraging the formation of healthier and more liberating beliefs, individuals are empowered to challenge imposed norms and live according to their own values, free from the constraints of traditional gender expectations.

Intersectionality is a key concept when assessing and measuring cognitions, beliefs, and behaviors: the feminist approach also considers other dimensions of identity (race, sexual orientation, social class) when assessing and identifying how cognitions, beliefs, and thoughts are experienced, as well as their impact [5]. These core beliefs usually lead to behaviors and interactions, to which we give meaning that impact our emotional well-being. It is important to assess and identify how the multiple layers of identity can influence the experience of discrimination and the core beliefs that develop from the vulnerability of childhood and determine the meaning given to significant relationships and experiences.

Racialized women, for example, may hold core beliefs that combine the effects of gender oppression with experiences of racism, creating more complex and sometimes more damaging thought patterns.

Studies have suggested [6] that therapeutic approaches that do not consider these intersections may overlook key aspects of people's subjective experience.

Although the literature on CBTFP is limited, several case studies have begun to explore how it improves outcomes in various contexts, for example:

- Cognitive-behavioral therapy for women victims of violence: in contexts where women have experienced gender-based violence, feminist CBT has proven effective in identifying core beliefs related to victimization and restoring personal autonomy [7–9].
- Treatment of depression in women: research has suggested that an approach combining CBT with feminist perspective has better results in addressing not only negative thoughts but also social pressures that contribute to low self-esteem and hopelessness in women [6, 10].

By identifying limiting core beliefs—such as those of worthlessness or failing in meeting other's expectations—in the treatment of anxiety and mood disorders, women can be helped to develop a more positive and autonomous self-image.

Ultimately, cognitive-behavioral therapy with feminist perspective offers a more holistic and inclusive approach to addressing women's mental health issues. By integrating a critique of patriarchy and recognizing the influence of social structures on emotional health, it provides a powerful method for women seeking not only to heal but also to challenge the norms that limit their thoughts, cognitions, beliefs, behaviors, and their well-being and potential.

References

1. Labrador Encinas FJ. Técnicas de modificación de conducta. Ed. Pirámide; 2008.
2. Martorell JL. Psicoterapias. Ed Pirámide; 2004.
3. Beck AT. Cognitive therapy and the emotional disorders. International Universities Press (New York); 1976.
4. Slater L, Daniel JH, Banks AE. The complete guide to mental health for women; 2003. p. 307–14.
5. Brown L. Feminist therapy 2nd ed. American Psychologist Association; 2010.
6. Sánchez AM. La terapia cognitivo conductual desde una perspectiva feminista en la intervención psicológica con mujeres; 2015.
7. Nielsen BB. Gender, power, and social justice: feminist approaches to cognitive-behavioral therapy; 2006.
8. Hara M, Brown L. The impact of cognitive behavioral therapy for women victims of domestic violence; 1999.
9. Yllö K, Bograd M (Eds). Brograd feminist perspectives on wife abuse: an introduction. Newbury Park: Sage; 1988. p. 11–26.
10. Worell J, Remer P. Feminist perspectives in therapy. Empowering diverse women. 2nd ed; 2002.

Systemic Therapy and Gender 14

Magdalena Marino Campos and Carolina Garcia

14.1 Introduction

Family systemic therapy, grounded in the principles of systems theory, understands family problems not as individual dysfunctions but as manifestations of dysfunctional relational patterns within the family system. This approach focuses on how interactions among family members influence the well-being and behavior of individuals. The therapeutic intervention, in this model, aims to modify these patterns of interaction and communication, facilitating new ways of relating that promote balance and conflict resolution within the system.

A key aspect that influences family dynamics is gender, whose structures and social expectations play a crucial role in shaping roles, power relations, and the distribution of responsibilities within the family. Culturally imposed gender norms influence family interactions, affecting how members communicate, resolve conflicts, and assume roles within the household. Hence, there is a need to integrate a critical gender perspective into the analysis and therapeutic intervention.

The gender perspective in family systemic therapy should not only consider traditional male and female roles but also incorporate an inclusive approach that addresses diverse gender identities, including non-binary and transgender identities. This is where the concept of gender-affirmative therapy comes into play, which focuses on validating and supporting the experiences of people with diverse gender identities, ensuring their identity is respected, and promoting an environment of acceptance both within and outside the family system. This approach also seeks to

M. M. Campos (✉)
NYC H+H | Roberto Clemente Center, New York, NY, USA

C. Garcia
Complejo Hospitalario Universitario Insular Materno-Infantil,
Las Palmas de Gran Canaria, Spain

M. López-Atanes, M. Sáenz-Herrero (eds.), *Applying the Gender Perspective in Psychiatry and Psychotherapy*, https://doi.org/10.1007/978-3-032-17883-1_14

reconfigure family patterns in ways that foster equity and justice for all members of the system, regardless of their gender identity.

Integrating a gender-affirmative approach into family systemic therapy involves recognizing the influences of socially constructed gender norms and how they affect interactions within the family system. It also seeks to transform family dynamics that may be based on rigid, hierarchical gender norms, instead fostering more inclusive, equitable, and respectful interactions of gender diversity. The therapeutic intervention must be sensitive to the experiences of discrimination and marginalization that family members may face due to their gender identity, which is key to promoting positive change in family relationships.

14.2 Evolution of Gender Perspective in the Systemic Therapy: A Transformative Journey

Systemic therapy emerged in the 1950s drawing mostly from the general systems theory proposed by Bertalanffy and the cybernetics of Bateson and his team [1, 2]. Systemic therapy defied the predominant model at the time, the Psychoanalysis, and changed the paradigm for the analysis of problems from the individual to the relational system. The emphasis was on the family as an interconnected system where each member influences and is influenced by the others. They operated under the idea that changes in one part of the system affect the whole system, and effective communication was a central focus [3]. Early systemic therapists, such as Murray Bowen, Salvador Minuchin or Jay Haley, focused on family systems, communication patterns, and relational dynamics. However, these initial models were gender blind, largely overlooking gender as a significant factor. The field operated under the assumption that family systems were neutral, failing to critically examine how patriarchal structures and gendered power dynamics shaped family roles and interactions (ref: Burke and Daniel). More problematic, these initial models often reinforced traditional gender roles (e.g., the mother as the primary caregiver, the father as the authority figure) that perpetuated inequality [4, 5].

In the 1970s, the second-wave feminist movement broadened the scope of feminist activism, bringing attention to gender inequality in all areas of society, including psychotherapy. Feminist theorists argued that systemic therapy, like other therapeutic approaches, was complicit in maintaining patriarchal norms [6]. Rachel Hare-Mustin (1978), a pioneer in integrating feminist theory into family therapy, critiqued the field for its "gender neutrality," which she argued masked the perpetuation of gender inequality, and introduced the concept of gender-sensitive therapy, urging therapists to examine how gender roles and power dynamics influence family systems [7]. Feminist therapists emphasized the need to deconstruct traditional gender binaries and explore how gendered expectations shape relationships and identities, highlighting issues like domestic violence and power imbalances within families [8]. This shift in perspective led to a more explicit recognition of gender as a central organizing principle in families and societies. More movements of systemic therapy began to include gender-sensitive approaches addressing the gender inequalities and power differentials within family systems.

During the late 1980s and throughout the 1990s, feminist systemic therapy expanded, emphasizing that gender is not merely a biological characteristic but a socio-cultural construct deeply influencing individuals' identity formation, emotional experiences, and interaction patterns. Feminist-informed systemic therapy aimed to promote women's empowerment, equality, and critical reflection on traditional family hierarchies and relational expectations [5, 6].

In 1989, Kimberlé Crenshaw published a black feminist critique that introduces the concept of intersectionality to understand how various forms of social identities (e.g., race, gender, class) intersect and interact to shape individuals' experiences of oppression and privilege. The intersectional framework has been instrumental in shaping contemporary understandings of how systemic inequalities operate and has provided a valuable tool for both scholars and activists in their efforts to promote social justice. Crenshaw's work has also profoundly influenced systemic therapy [9]. Therapists began to consider how gender intersects with other social categories, such as race, class, sexuality, and culture, to shape individuals' experiences and identities. Intersectionality also emphasized the importance of examining power dynamics within families and social systems, prompting systemic therapists to explore how power imbalances and systemic inequalities affect relationships and individual well-being [8, 10]. This broadened perspective allowed therapists to address the unique challenges faced by individuals and families more comprehensively. The field moved toward a more holistic approach that considered the broader social context and promoted a culturally informed practice, recognizing that gender norms and roles vary across cultures and contexts.

During the 1990s and 2000s, systemic therapy increasingly embraced postmodern theories and social constructionist ideas. From these perspectives, there was a conscious effort on deconstructing gender that came to be seen as a fluid and context-dependent construct rather than a fixed binary. This perspective opened the door for exploring diverse gender identities and expressions. Therapists began to challenge the male/female binary, recognizing the limitations of traditional gender categories and the need to affirm non-binary and transgender identities. Narrative therapy (White & Epston, 1980) also emphasized the importance of deconstructing dominant cultural narratives, including those related to gender. Narrative therapists help clients explore how societal expectations about gender have shaped their identities and relationships, empowering them to rewrite their own stories [11, 12].

Since the 2000s, systemic therapy has embraced contemporary developments that emphasize inclusivity. The integration of *queer theory* into systemic therapy has expanded the understanding of gender by challenging normative assumptions about gender and sexuality, emphasizing fluidity, diversity, and the performative nature of gender. Systemic therapists now work to create affirming spaces for LGBTQ+ clients, addressing issues such as coming out, family rejection, and societal discrimination [13, 14]. The field has increasingly recognized the importance of affirming transgender and non-binary identities, with therapists trained to use inclusive language, understand the complexities of gender transition, and support clients in navigating gender-related challenges.

Today, gender perspectives are integral to family therapy. Modern systemic therapists actively incorporate gender analysis into clinical practice, emphasizing cultural sensitivity, social justice, and advocacy for marginalized populations. Contemporary systemic therapy also incorporates intersectional and decolonial perspectives, examining how systems of oppression (e.g., racism, sexism, colonialism) intersect to shape clients' experiences and challenging Eurocentric and heteronormative assumptions in therapy. There is a growing emphasis on understanding gender within diverse cultural contexts, prompting therapists to engage with clients' cultural beliefs and practices related to gender, avoiding ethnocentric or universalizing assumptions. These advancements have enriched systemic therapeutic practices, resulting in more inclusive, socially aware, and ethically responsible interventions [15–18].

14.3 Systemic Interventions

14.3.1 Interventions with Gender Perspective

Systemic therapy interventions with a gender perspective aim to address family, relational, and individual dynamics by explicitly recognizing and challenging gender norms, stereotypes, societal expectations, and power imbalances. The goal is not only reducing conflict and improving relational well-being but also supporting individual empowerment by actively addressing the ways gender norms can impact human potential within a systemic context. Some essential elements and interventions:

14.3.1.1 Creating Gender-Awareness

Identifies explicit and implicit gender roles within the family or couple, understands transgenerational transmission of these roles and biases, explores relational dynamics influenced by gendered expectations.

- *Gender Genograms*: Construct a genogram that highlights the gender norms and expectations passed down through generations. Discuss how these inherited patterns shape current family interactions and individual decisions. Ask family members or couples to map out responsibilities, behaviors, decision-making roles, and emotional expressions based on gender, reflecting on how these roles influence relationships and individual well-being. Monica McGoldrick emphasizes the importance of understanding and addressing power and gender dynamics within therapeutic contexts, advocating for a culturally competent approach that considers broader social and political influences on individuals and families Reflections on Our Efforts to Help Mental Health Agencies Become More "Culturally Competent" [19].

- *Circular questioning*: Use questions that reveal how individuals perceive the gender roles and behaviors of others. These questions help family members see interactions from multiple perspectives, which can destabilize linear, causal narratives that often perpetuate issues, introducing the gender perspective and behaviors of others, such as "Who is expected to be strong in difficult situations?" or "What would change if your roles were reversed?"
- This approach, initially developed in the Milan School, has incorporated considerations of how power dynamics and gender roles influence family relationships, using principles of hypothesizing, circularity, and curiosity to guide the therapeutic process [20–23].

When working on creating gender awareness, it is key to analyze everyday language to understand how it reflects and promotes the interests of dominant groups, including gender assumptions. From this approach, working on developing gender genograms and using circular questions can help to understand the discourse that reinforce or alter traditional gender roles on the ecological system of the persons [24–26]. Many authors highlight how gender power dynamics and social gender processes can act as barriers to achieving reciprocity in couples therapy [25–28]. By focusing on these dynamics, therapists can use circular questioning to shift from an individual orientation to a relational one, promoting more equitable interactions. Furthermore, therapists can understand and bring to the therapeutic space clear examples of how language and power dynamics intersect, offering perspectives to promote gender equity in the family.

14.3.1.2 Deconstructing Gender Roles

Unpack societal expectations about masculinity and femininity that shape family interactions and individual behaviors.

- Invite family members to share stories that highlight gendered expectations (e.g., caregiving roles, emotional expression, decision-making power), analyze their origins, and discuss alternative narratives that empower each member equally.
- Explore how rigid gender norms affect family dynamics.
- Sexuality & Desire: Address how gendered expectations shape intimacy (e.g., the "male initiator" stereotype).

14.3.1.3 Reframing Power Dynamics

Identify and challenge gender-based power imbalances.

- Power Analysis: Examining how gender-based power imbalances influence decision-making, conflict resolution, and emotional labor in relationships.
- Highlight moments of imbalance, such as when one partner makes unilateral decisions due to gendered assumptions and reframe these interactions to encourage balanced, equitable decision-making
- Emotional Labor Discussions: Making invisible labor (often shouldered by women) visible and redistributing it fairly.

- Non-Hierarchical Relationships: Moving away from traditional dominance/submission dynamics.
- Psychoeducation on gender equality, equity, and rights to promote understanding and reduce conflict. Provide resources, facilitate discussions, and offer practical strategies to dismantle traditional gender roles within the family context.
- Role-Playing & Rehearsal: Practicing new ways of interacting outside traditional gender norms.

14.3.1.4 Empowering Marginalized Voices

Elevate voices historically marginalized by traditional gender roles.

- Actively facilitate discussions where historically silenced or marginalized individuals (women or LGBTQ+ family members) are explicitly encouraged to speak about their experiences and perspectives, assert their needs, and challenge oppressive structures in the family and society.
- Encourage equitable communication styles free of gender stereotypes. Model and facilitate dialogue promoting equality, validating emotional expression across genders, and fostering balanced participation.

14.3.1.5 Rewriting Family Narrative

Support family members to rewrite gendered stories that constrain individual and relational development.

- Use externalization techniques to separate individuals from restrictive gender expectations.
- Help family members to re-author their stories in empowering ways outside restrictive gender scripts.

Rewriting family narratives in systemic therapy, particularly in the context of gender, involves understanding and addressing the social constructs and power dynamics that influence family interactions and individual identities.Family therapists are increasingly adopting post-structural and postmodern perspectives, which view reality as constructed through social interactions rather than something fixed and universal, and gender as a social construct rather than inherent. Discourse analysis is especially important in this context, helping therapists identify and question the language and power dynamics that perpetuate gender inequalities within families [4, 11, 27, 29].

14.3.2 Gender-Affirmative Practice

Gender-affirmative interventions in family therapy are designed to support and validate individuals' gender identities, particularly for transgender, non-binary, and gender-diverse individuals. It involves assessing family dynamics and working with family members to better support the young person's gender identity and expression. Strategies include addressing common challenges faced by families and exploring options for gender expression and transition [30]. Overall, affirmative gender systemic therapy requires mental health professionals to have knowledge of transgender and gender-diverse issues, provide a validating and supportive environment, and incorporate interdisciplinary approaches to address their needs [29].

14.3.2.1 Creating a Safe and Affirming Space

- Ensure that the individual's chosen name and pronouns are consistently used and respected by all family members and the therapist.
- Foster a nonjudgmental attitude to create an environment where the individuals feel safe to express their gender identity without fear of judgment or rejection.

14.3.2.2 Exploring Family Dynamics

- Assess Family Reactions: Understand the range of reactions within the family, from acceptance to resistance or confusion.
- Facilitate Open Communication: Encourage family members to express their feelings and concerns in a respectful manner.

14.3.2.3 Addressing Family Concerns

- Normalize Emotional Responses: recognize that family members may experience a range of emotions, including grief, fear, or confusion, and provide a space to process these feelings.
- Educate the Family: Provide information about gender diversity, the difference between gender identity and biological sex, and the importance of affirmation for mental health.
- Address Myths and Misconceptions: Clarify common misconceptions about gender identity and transition processes.
- Challenge Transphobic Beliefs: Gently challenge and reframe any transphobic or binary gender beliefs within the family.

14.3.2.4 Supporting the Gender-Diverse Individual

- Acknowledge the individual's experiences and challenges related to their gender identity.
- Support them in making decisions about their gender expression and transition.
- Empower them to challenge oppressive gender norms and create more equitable relationships.
- Assert "chosen families" recognizing that support systems may extend beyond biological ties.

14.3.2.5 Cultural Sensitivity

- Be aware of and be sensitive to the cultural, religious, and social contexts that may influence the family's understanding and acceptance of gender diversity.
- Be prepared to adapt therapeutic interventions as the individual's needs and family dynamics evolve.

14.3.2.6 Advocacy and Allyship

- Model gender-affirmative behavior in your interactions with the family and the individual.
- Facilitate access to resources for gender-affirming care as support groups or medical professionals.
- Support the individual and family in navigating systems (e.g., schools, healthcare) to ensure their rights are respected.

14.3.2.7 Self-Reflection and Supervision

Therapists need to regularly engage in self-reflection to examine their own biases and assumptions about gender, ensuring they provide gender-affirmative therapy. Seeking supervision or consultation with colleagues who specialize in gender-affirmative practices can further enhance their approach. Additionally, utilizing reflecting teams with a gender perspective can expand awareness of gender biases through multiple viewpoints. These teams observe therapy sessions and provide feedback on gendered patterns in interactions, helping families gain insight into unnoticed gender dynamics.

14.4 Challenges

While the systemic models have made significant strides in promoting equity and intersectionality understanding, including developing more specific interventions to address the whole complexity of gender, there are still several challenges that need to be counted for and addressed from our discipline:

14.4.1 Cultural and Societal Resistance

Many societies still adhere to rigid gender norms, making it difficult for clients and even therapists to challenge or deconstruct these beliefs. Traditional gender norms can perpetuate stereotypes and limit the acceptance of diverse gender identities and expressions. Additionally, discussing gender-related issues, especially in conservative or patriarchal settings, can be met with resistance or stigma, which can limit open dialogue and hinder therapeutic progress [31]. This stigma can discourage clients from sharing their experiences and seeking support, while also creating barriers for therapists attempting to foster inclusive and affirming environments. Overcoming these cultural and societal resistances requires persistent efforts to promote awareness, education, and acceptance of gender diversity within therapeutic practices and broader communities [32].

14.4.2 Cultural Variations

Gender perspectives differ significantly across cultures, necessitating that therapists adapt their approaches to be culturally sensitive and relevant. Working with diverse populations requires therapists to be knowledgeable about various cultural norms and values related to gender to provide effective therapy. Additionally, legal and policy contexts in some regions may pose challenges to the application of gender-sensitive systemic therapy, particularly in cases involving LGBTQ+ rights or gender-based violence.

14.4.3 Evolving Gender Concepts

As the understanding of gender evolves to include non-binary and fluid identities, therapists must continuously update their knowledge and practices to remain inclusive. This ongoing education is crucial for providing effective support and validation to clients with diverse gender experiences. Keeping up with changing language and terminology around gender can be challenging, but it is essential for effective communication and ensuring that clients feel understood and respected. By staying informed about the latest developments in gender concepts, therapists can create a more inclusive and affirming therapeutic environment that acknowledges and celebrates the diversity of gender identities.

14.4.4 Therapist's Bias and Stereotyping

Despite progress, biases and stereotypes about gender roles still exist within therapy practices, posing challenges to equitable care. Therapists must continually work to recognize and address their own biases to provide effective and inclusive support. A lack of awareness or training in gender-sensitive approaches can lead to the unintentional reinforcement of gender stereotypes, which may affect the therapeutic process. Additionally, therapists' personal biases or blind spots regarding gender can influence their practice, potentially undermining the effectiveness of therapy. It is crucial for therapists to engage in ongoing education and self-reflection to ensure they are providing the best possible care for all clients, regardless of gender.

14.4.5 Intersectionality

Integrating an intersectional approach that considers multiple identities, such as race, class, and sexual orientation, alongside gender remains a challenge in therapy. Therapists need to understand how these intersecting identities impact family dynamics, recognizing that gender does not exist in isolation but intersects with other identities such as race, class, sexuality, and disability. Addressing these intersections in therapy requires nuanced understanding and skills to ensure that the unique experiences of each individual are acknowledged and validated. There is also a risk of overgeneralizing gender experiences without considering how other factors shape an individual's life, which can lead to incomplete or ineffective therapeutic interventions. Therefore, therapists must be vigilant in their efforts to integrate intersectionality into their practice, ensuring a comprehensive and inclusive approach to understanding and supporting their clients.

14.4.6 Power Dynamics in Therapy

Therapists inherently hold a position of authority, which can inadvertently replicate societal power dynamics if gender issues are not consciously addressed. This imbalance can affect the therapeutic relationship and the client's willingness to share openly. Ensuring client empowerment is essential, as it allows clients to voice their experiences and challenges related to gender. However, this can be difficult, especially in cases of systemic oppression where clients may feel marginalized or silenced [33]. Therapists must be mindful of these dynamics and strive to create a safe, inclusive environment that encourages clients to express themselves fully and authentically.

14.4.7 Family and Relationship Dynamics

Family members may resist changes in gender dynamics, particularly if they benefit from traditional roles. This resistance can create tension and conflict within the family unit, making it challenging for individuals to navigate their personal growth and identity [34, 35]. Therapists play a crucial role in addressing these dynamics, as they must balance the individual needs of their clients with the broader systemic context of their relationships and families. This delicate balance requires therapists to be sensitive to the complexities of family interactions while supporting their clients in achieving their personal goals and fostering healthier, more equitable relationships.

14.4.8 Systemic Barriers

Systemic barriers significantly impact access to mental health care for marginalized genders, including women, non-binary, and transgender individuals. These groups often face financial constraints and discrimination, which can hinder their ability to obtain necessary care. Additionally, institutional resistance poses a challenge, as organizations may lack the understanding or resources to integrate gender perspectives into systemic therapy practices. This resistance can stem from entrenched biases or a reluctance to change established protocols, further complicating efforts to provide inclusive and effective mental health support. Addressing these barriers requires a concerted effort to promote equity and inclusivity within mental healthcare systems.

14.4.9 Research and Evidence Base

There is a need for more research on the effectiveness of gender-sensitive systemic therapy, especially in diverse cultural contexts. This includes exploring how gender-sensitive approaches can be adapted to various populations and integrated with other therapeutic modalities like trauma-informed care and cognitive-behavioral therapy. Balancing evidence-based practices with gender-sensitive approaches can be challenging, as some interventions may not fully address gender and power dynamics. Therapists must adapt these perspectives to provide holistic and inclusive care, ensuring all aspects of clients' experiences are considered. Additionally, measuring the effectiveness of gender-sensitive systemic therapy requires innovative methods to capture nuanced changes in gender dynamics and empowerment and to assess the long-term impact on clients' relationships and societal gender roles [36].

14.5 Future Directions

Integrating and further developing a gender perspective in systemic therapy is crucial for addressing the complexities of gender roles, identities, and inequalities in therapeutic practice.

14.5.1 Gender Sensitivity Training and Education

It is essential to incorporate comprehensive gender-sensitivity training into systemic therapy education programs, not only to recognize and address gender biases and stereotypes but also to understand and apply intersectional frameworks [37]. For example, being culturally sensitive and relevant is crucial when adapting interventions, recognizing the diverse ways in which gender is understood and experienced across different cultures.

14.5.2 Supervision and Peer Support

Gender-focused supervision specifically addresses gender issues in therapy, giving therapists a space to reflect on their own biases and challenges. Establishing peer support networks for therapists can also be beneficial, allowing them to share experiences, strategies, and resources related to integrating gender perspectives.

14.5.3 Research and Evidence-Based Practices

Prioritize gender research that specifically examines the impact of gender perspectives in systemic therapy and evaluates the effectiveness of gender-sensitive interventions. Expand gender inclusivity exploring non-binary and transgender experiences in family contexts and develop interventions that address the complexities of gender in diverse cultural settings [38]. Create gender-inclusive metrics to create and validate assessment tools that capture changes in gender dynamics.

Research and evidence-based practices in systemic therapy and gender have evolved significantly, particularly in addressing the needs of sexual and gender minority populations. Recent efforts in psychological science have focused on developing evidence-based affirmative treatments for individuals, including identifying clear treatment goals, conducting efficacy studies, and reducing the stigma that hinders the development of affirmative treatments [39].

Gender-affirming psychotherapy has been developed to address the mental health needs of transgender youth, incorporating principles and skills designed to improve treatment engagement and outcomes. This is crucial given the high rates of discrimination and victimization faced by transgender youth, which contribute to disparities in mental health [40].

Additionally, the American Academy of Child and Adolescent Psychiatry emphasizes the importance of cultural competence, including gender identity, in behavioral health care. This involves adapting therapeutic approaches to be culturally sensitive and inclusive regarding diverse gender identities [41].

Systemic therapy approaches also highlight the importance of understanding and incorporating systems of power, such as gender, into psychotherapy. This includes recognizing the impact of gender-based power systems, oppression, and privilege on clients' mental health.

Overall, integrating affirmative and gender-inclusive practices into systemic therapy is essential for addressing the unique mental health needs and improving therapeutic outcomes.

14.5.4 Interdisciplinary Collaboration

Developing integrated care models that address both mental health and gender-related issues is essential for providing holistic support to clients. For that, it is necessary to integrate other disciplines such as sociology, gender studies, and public health that can enrich the understanding and application of gender perspectives in systemic therapy.

14.5.5 Policy and Institutional Support

It is necessary, especially in these challenging socio-political times, to advocate for institutional policies that defend and support the integration and implementation of gender perspectives, including anti-discrimination policies and gender-affirming care standards.

14.5.6 Advocacy and Social Change

Therapists are increasingly recognizing the importance of engaging in advocacy efforts to promote social justice and gender equity, addressing systemic inequalities that impact clients' mental health and well-being. This includes challenging oppressive structures and promoting policies that support gender equality. Launching public awareness campaigns to challenge gender stereotypes and promote the importance of gender-sensitive mental health care is also crucial in fostering a more inclusive and supportive society.

14.6 Conclusion

The integration of a gender perspective into systemic therapy has been a transformative journey, marked by critical reflection, theoretical innovation, and a commitment to social justice. This journey highlights the profound impact of feminist and postmodern critiques, the importance of intersectionality, and the ongoing need for inclusivity and cultural competence in systemic therapy. This continuous evolution reflects the field's responsiveness to social movements, and as it continues to grow, it must remain vigilant in challenging its own assumptions and recognize the diverse and dynamic realities of gender. It is the ultimate goal to continue evolving to become more inclusive, equitable, and effective in addressing the diverse and complex ways in which gender impacts individuals, relationships, and families.

References

1. Guerin PJ. Family therapy: theory and practice. New York: Gardner Press; 1976.
2. Beels CC. Notes for a cultural history of family therapy. Fam Process. 2002;41(1):67–82. https://doi.org/10.1111/j.1545-5300.2002.40102000067.x. PMID: 11924091.
3. Combrinck-Graham L. Being a family systems thinker: a psychiatrist's personal odyssey. Fam Process. 2014;53(3):476–88. https://doi.org/10.1111/famp.12090. PMID: 25074645.
4. Hare-Mustin RT. A feminist approach to family therapy. aaaaFam Process. 1978;17(2):181–94. https://doi.org/10.1111/j.1545-5300.1978.00181.
5. Burck C, Daniel G. Gender and family therapy. London: Karnac Books; 1994.
6. Walters M, Carter B, Papp P, Silverstein O. The invisible web: gender patterns in family relationships. New York: Guilford Press; 1988.
7. Hare-Mustin RT. A feminist approach to family therapy. Fam Process. 1978;17(2):181–94. https://doi.org/10.1111/j.1545-5300.1978.00181.
8. Knudson-Martin C, Mahoney AR, editors. Couples, gender, and power: creating change in intimate relationships. New York: Springer Publishing Company; 2009.
9. Crenshaw K. Demarginalizing the intersection of race and sex: a black feminist critique of antidiscrimination doctrine, feminist theory, and antiracist politics. Univ Chic Leg Forum. 1989;1:139–67.

10. Silverstein LB, Goodrich TJ, editors. Feminist family therapy: empowerment in social context. Washington, DC: American Psychological Association; 2003. https://doi.org/10.1037/10615-000.
11. Dickerson V. Patriarchy, power, and privilege: a narrative/poststructural view of work with couples. Fam Process. 2013;52(1):102–14. https://doi.org/10.1111/famp.12018.
12. Gómez AM, Cerezo A, Ajayi BC. Deconstructing meta-narratives: utilizing narrative therapy to promote resilience following sexual violence among women survivors of color. J Sex Marital Ther. 2020;46(3):282–95. https://doi.org/10.1080/0092623X.2019.1677836.
13. Allen KR, Henderson AC. Family theories today: a critical intersectional approach. San Diego: Cognella Academic Publishing; 2022.
14. Addison SM, Coolhart D. Expanding the therapy paradigm with queer couples: a relational intersectional lens. Fam Process. 2015;54(3):435–53. https://doi.org/10.1111/famp.12171.
15. Sutherland O, LaMarre A, Rice C, Hardt L, Le Couteur A. New sexism in couple therapy: a discursive analysis. Fam Process. 2017;56(3):686–700. https://doi.org/10.1111/famp.12292.
16. Knudson-Martin C, Huenergardt D, Lafontant K, et al. J Marital Fam Ther. 2015;41(2):205–20. https://doi.org/10.1111/jmft.12068.
17. Bryant T. Lessons from decolonial and liberation psychologies for the field of trauma psychology. Am Psychol. 2024;79(5):683–96. https://doi.org/10.1037/amp0001393.
18. Dunlop BJ, Lea J. It's not just in my head: an intersectional, social and systems-based framework in gender and sexuality diversity. Psychol Psychother. 2023;96(1):1–15. https://doi.org/10.1111/papt.12438.
19. McGoldrick M, Hines PM, García Preto N, Petry S. Reflections on our efforts to help mental health agencies become more "culturally competent". Fam Process. 2021;60(3):1016–32. https://doi.org/10.1111/famp.12704.
20. Esmiol DE, Knudson-Martin C, Delgado S. Developing contextual awareness: learning to address gender, social power, and culture in clinical practice. J Marital Fam Ther. 2012;38(4):573–88. https://doi.org/10.1111/j.1752-0606.2011.00232.
21. Knudson-Martin C. Gender policy in family therapy. J Marital Fam Ther. 1997;23(4):421–37, 439–44. https://doi.org/10.1111/j.1752-0606.1997.tb01054.
22. Telfener U, de Bustis E, Cazzaniga E, et al. The Milan approach today. Fam Process. 2025;64(1):e13075. https://doi.org/10.1111/famp.13075.
23. Diorinou M, Tseliou E. Studying circular questioning "in situ": discourse analysis of a first systemic family therapy session. J Marital Fam Ther. 2014;40(1):106–21. https://doi.org/10.1111/jmft.12005.
24. Dozier RM, Hicks MW, Cornille TA, Peterson GW. The effect of Tomm's therapeutic questioning styles on therapeutic alliance: a clinical analog study. Fam Process. 1998;37(2):189–200. https://doi.org/10.1111/j.1545-5300.1998.00189.
25. Ryan D, Carr A. A study of the differential effects of Tomm's questioning styles on therapeutic alliance. Fam Process. 2001;40(1):67–77. https://doi.org/10.1111/j.1545-5300.2001.4010100067.
26. Sutherland O, LaMarre A, Rice C. The primacy of discourse in the study of gender in family therapy. Fam Process. 2017;56(3):669–85. https://doi.org/10.1111/famp.12294.
27. D'Arrigo-Patrick E, Samman SK, Knudson-Martin C. Moving from "I" to "we": a grounded theory analysis of couple therapy with liver patients and their partners. Fam Process. 2020;59(4):1517–29. https://doi.org/10.1111/famp.12528.
28. Coolhart D, Shipman DL. Working toward family attunement: family therapy with transgender and gender-nonconforming children and adolescents. Psychiatr Clin North Am. 2017;40(1):113–25. https://doi.org/10.1016/j.psc.2016.10.002.
29. Spencer KG, Berg DR, Bradford NJ, et al. The gender-affirmative life span approach: a developmental model for clinical work with transgender and gender-diverse children, adolescents, and adults. Psychotherapy (Chicago). 2021;58(1):37–49. https://doi.org/10.1037/pst0000363.
30. Silverstein L, Wong YJ, Wester SR. Feminist masculinities: the end of gender as we know it. In: Wong YJ, Wester SR, editors. APA handbook of men and masculinities. Washington, DC: American Psychological Association; 2016. p. 145–72. https://doi.org/10.1037/14594-007.

31. Knudson-Martin C, Laughlin MJ. Gender and sexual orientation in family therapy: toward a postgender approach. Fam Process. 2004;43(4):467–83. https://doi.org/10.1111/j.0197-6664.2005.00009.
32. Young B, Seedall RB. Power dynamics in couple relationships: a review and applications for systemic family therapists. Fam Process. 2024;63(4):1703–20. https://doi.org/10.1111/famp.13008.
33. Lebow J, Snyder DK. Couple therapy in the 2020s: current status and emerging developments. Fam Process. 2022;61(4):1183–99. https://doi.org/10.1111/famp.12824.
34. Haddock SA, Zimmerman TS, MacPhee D. The power equity guide: attending to gender in family therapy. J Marital Fam Ther. 2000;26(2):153–70. https://doi.org/10.1111/j.1752-0606.2000.tb00286.
35. Hare-Mustin RT. The problem of gender in family therapy theory. Fam Process. 1987;26(1):15–27. https://doi.org/10.1111/j.1545-5300.1987.00015.
36. Fish JN, Russell ST. Queering methodologies to understand queer families. Fam Relat. 2018;67(1):12–25. https://doi.org/10.1111/fare.12297. Epub 2018 Feb 21. PMID: 30739971; PMCID: PMC6364998.
37. Singh S. Dismantling amatonormative biases and expanding Queer-affirmative psychotherapy: the role of trainers. Psychotherapy (Chicago, Ill.). 2025;62(1):98–104. https://doi.org/10.1037/pst0000558.
38. Pachankis JE. The scientific pursuit of sexual and gender minority mental health treatments: toward evidence-based affirmative practice. Am Psychol. 2018;73(9):1207–19. https://doi.org/10.1037/amp0000357.
39. Price MA, Rakhilin M, Johansen K, et al. Gender-Affirming Psychotherapy (GAP): core principles and skills to reduce the mental health care "GAP" for transgender youths. Psychiatr Serv. 2024;75(11):1075–83. https://doi.org/10.1176/appi.ps.20230460.
40. American Academy of Child and Adolescent Psychiatry (AACAP) Committee on Community-Based Systems of Care, AACAP Committee on Quality Issues. Clinical update: child and adolescent behavioral health care in community systems of care. J Am Acad Child Adolesc Psychiatry. 2023;62(4):367–84. https://doi.org/10.1016/j.jaac.2022.06.001.
41. Budge SL, Moradi B. Attending gender in psychotherapy: understanding and incorporating systems of power. J Clin Psychol. 2018;74(11):2014–27. https://doi.org/10.1002/jclp.22686.

Integrative Humanistic Psychotherapy and Gender. A Feminist Perspective

15

Ianire Estébanez

15.1 Therapeutic Relationship: Security, Power and Gender

The therapeutic relationship is not impervious to power relations between people, and to the oppressions and privileges that each one holds. Maintaining a gender perspective in therapeutic accompaniment means analyzing and identifying how people who come to psychotherapy perceive us.

In this sense, the fact of being a man or a woman as a therapist will have an obvious influence on the relationship established with the person who comes, taking into account that in the process of psychotherapy, the history of how this person relates to women, to men, and the relational experiences that he/she may have lived will be put into action. In this sense, the therapist as such is not an abstract and theoretical figure, but a human figure, and will be read by the person he/she accompanies as safe or not, depending on different factors. A clear example of this influence is shown by how some women who have experienced gender or sexual violence by a man express their discomfort in the presence of a male psychotherapist.

In fact, on the occasions when a person searches directly for a professional therapist, he or she may choose a professional with the objective of obtaining a similarity in experiences. In this sense, there are women who prefer to be accompanied by women, or who look for a therapist with a similar age to their own, or those who have been mothers seek to be accompanied by therapists who have also been mothers, people may try to find a therapist with the same sexual orientation, or those who are migrants may wish to find therapists who have also experienced a migratory process. In these personal searches, people would be prioritizing the confirmation of having a **shared experience** with their therapist, with respect to knowledge or

I. Estébanez (✉)
Bilbao, Spain

M. López-Atanes, M. Sáenz-Herrero (eds.), *Applying the Gender Perspective in Psychiatry and Psychotherapy*, https://doi.org/10.1007/978-3-032-17883-1_15

academic experience at the professional level, this choice being essential for the establishment of a safe therapeutic relationship.

In this sense, it is relevant to identify that, from a humanistic vision, the *supposed neutrality of the figure of the therapist cannot exist.* People will see and feel the relationship with other people from the social position that each professional represents in relation to gender, race, age, sexual orientation.

Working from a **situated** position and **knowledge** [1] could be, therefore, an important element in the establishment of a helping relationship in a feminist key, in a society that irremediably places us in differentiated positions of power, from which violence is exercised. Thus, perhaps we need to question not only the supposed neutrality of the therapist, but also the conceptualization of neutrality from which we analyze human psychology. In this sense, it is worth recognizing that psychology and psychiatry have studied, analyzed, researched and produced knowledge from the idea that the patient is a single neutral subject from which results can be generalized to the entire population, but the reality of the accompaniment in consultation shows that the gender of people is a differential factor in how, why, to what extent and in what ways people experience emotional discomfort. Sometimes gender is even the reason why people experience violence or exclusion in their lives, and it is this experience of violence that generates mental health problems.

Perhaps the neutrality of the therapist that we presuppose in psychotherapy is nothing more than *the stereotype of an upper class white male therapist* on which the different psychological theories in the history of our discipline have been based, since it is also this type of therapist who has had the privilege in the history of our discipline to publish, write, decide and teach how psychotherapy is practiced.

Practice tells us that when people see us as therapists, they also identify our gender or our life experience as an important element in emotional security. *Being security a central element to take care of in the therapeutic relationship.*

From a humanistic point of view, it is important to admit and accept that we all live in a system of **power hierarchies**. And the position we have as therapists accompanying people in a situation of suffering or discomfort is also a power relationship. When a person comes to a therapeutic service, he/she does it in a *position of vulnerability*, and he/she does it looking for an *answer of help*. From this position, it is impossible not to be in a power relationship, so it is important to keep this in mind. The prejudices and preconceived ideas that we have and the way we treat the person will be fundamental for the person to feel welcomed, listened to, understood and accompanied, or, on the contrary, to feel that our criteria are imposed on theirs, or they may feel pressured to act in a certain way that they would not have chosen.

However, the fact that being therapists places us in a position of power does not necessarily mean that we decide to use this power to impose our professional judgment. This position of power can be used consciously to accompany the person *to see and recognize his or her own power* and to accompany him or her respectfully to make good decisions for him or herself.

Therefore, for me it is important that at least as professionals, we are **aware of our position of power** and keep it in mind *to recognize and validate that person's* *vulnerability along with my own and put awareness into creating a relationship that can be healing, egalitarian, and where good treatment and equality are materializing in practice.*

Working in therapy as a feminist psychologist means for me to *work from the search for* ***horizontality****,* ***naming and making visible the violence*** *and social oppressions that are at the* ***base*** *of emotional discomfort and putting* ***care at the center of*** *the therapeutic relationship.*

15.2 Feminism as a Practice to be Implemented in the Therapeutic Relationship

Feminism is a critical theory of power, a theory of visibilization of women, of recognition of the situation of social oppression based on gender and of valuing care as an essential sustenance for survival. It is also a vision of criticism of capitalist productivity, and it is a collective and social movement. For me, therefore, feminist therapy has to include these elements in its own practice, since a feminist therapy **seeks the emancipation and interdependence** of the women we accompany, so that they can develop lives free of violence and approach experiences of health and wellbeing.

Taking into account feminist theories, but considering that feminisms are built collectively, I would like to share some of the questions I ask myself about how to bring to my own therapeutic relationship and practice all that feminism teaches us [2].

15.2.1 Diagnosis as a Power Tool

The diagnosis itself can sometimes become an abuse of power for therapists. Phyllis Chesler, in her book *Women and Madness* [3], relates how diagnostic labels have been used to categorize as pathological behaviors of women who did not conform to the **social norms** of the time. Wanting to separate, to show rage, or to establish certain sexual behaviors, thus, were punished from the labeling in a mental illness, instead of questioning the social beliefs that were behind those prejudices. Throughout the history of our discipline, the labeling of certain diagnoses in women has been able to serve, throughout history, to make invisible a structural and systematic violence that has been exercised against women.

It is much easier to place a pathological diagnosis on the victim than to fight collectively for a necessary change in the structure, the family or the institution that is perpetrating violence.

As Foucault theorizes, the possession **of Truth** is related to a status of power, and power enjoys a kind of self-sustaining development [4]. From the possession of Truth, traditional Psychiatry may consider as mental disorder a set of symptoms that have no biological explanation but are treated as such by prescribing psychotropic drugs. Traditional psychotherapy has assumed the biomedical postulates and the scientific method to explain human reality, including the androcentric postulates that are reflected in the diagnosis from which psychological treatment is proposed, or the objectives.

As feminist therapists, therefore, one element to review in the therapeutic relationship is always to keep in mind the critique of social norms that are taken as truth, because we can really do a lot of harm when we establish a diagnosis based on a norm from which we value and question a social behavior.

Therefore, to think of working in therapy by placing ourselves as *the one who knows the truth, the one who diagnoses, the one who decides the treatment* can be an exercise of power.

A feminist psychologist

- Can you impose your way of working without listening to what women ask for?
- Can you calm a symptom so that the person stays in a relationship that is oppressing him or her?
- Do you want to generate changes in a person to adapt to an imposed social norm?
- Would a feminist psychologist hide behind a diagnosis of depression so as not to inquire into issues of lived violence?
- Would you diagnose women's anger or rage as something to be controlled or silenced?

15.2.2 Bio-psycho-social Perspective and Power Structures

There is no doubt that human experience cannot be understood from a single variable of analysis. However, although there is evidence and professional agreement on the bio-psycho-social explanation of human experience, in recent years we have found psychological theories that integrate the biological and psychological perspectives (such as the polyvagal theory, or trauma-based theories), but the social perspective continues to be undervalued in research.

Thus, integrating **a social perspective in the psychopathological distress** experienced by people would imply analyzing the different oppressions and violence that people experience and have an impact on their mental health. In this sense, it is essential to rescue the figure of Judit Herman [5] in the recognition of how the experience of violence generates trauma, and how to repair these experiences implies the establishment of a healing relationship between therapist and survivor.

Sometimes, what is somehow present at the basis of different pathologies are power structures that are often unnoticed in an individualized account of distress. When we listen to a person in an individualized context, it is easy to focus only on those elements that the person is finding problematic or on those elements that have to do with the symptomatology that is becoming present in isolation. Therefore, perhaps sometimes we assume that it is not necessary to investigate further, and we forget that in our diagnosis, we could also make a premeditated analysis that we pay attention to in order to analyze how it has influenced that person:

- The dichotomous system of experience in which we are born, grow and learn, which criticizes and violates the feminine versus the masculine, the emotional versus the rational, the vulnerable versus the strong, the strange versus the normal, the margins versus the center.
- The social system that mistreats, violates and devalues women.
- Hierarchical and non-caregiving work structures that distress and pressure us.
- Symbolic violence towards non-normative bodies is internalized in the form of self-criticism and insecurity.
- Sexual norms that impose models of attraction, models of relationship and even models of identity.
- The inequality of power that justifies the violence exercised by people with privilege, or a socialization that imposes an expansive and dominating masculinity against a femininity that blames and over-care for the other.

15.2.3 The Power of the Therapist's Role

On the other hand, analyzing the power that our position as therapists gives us, we should also consider whether we are using this power for the **emancipation of the person or whether we are using this power to reproduce dependencies**. If as therapists we consider thar we hace ther truth and the knowledge, we could influence people's decisions and place in their history our labels, prejudices, diagnoses, ways of doing and routines because we have been doing it that way for a long time.

On the other hand, *as therapists we can also accompany that person to discover herself and to give light to what she brings.* And only this, in my opinion, could be called feminist and emancipatory.

In relation to power, I think it is worthwhile to inquire to what extent in our daily therapeutic practices:

- I am always the one who has **the criterion and the knowledge,** and I impose it on the person, or on the other hand, that criterion and that knowledge is shared and contrasted.
- Whether I make the diagnosis of the person exclusively or whether I build with that person an analysis of his or her situation.
- Analyze and review what the **space** I work in is like and how I set it up so that it is perceived as welcoming and safe, or if I use elements behind which to stand at a distance, such as a table behind which I stand as an expert.
- Identify when it might be relevant to **show something personal about myself as a person**, or if I place myself behind the figure of the invulnerable therapist who cannot be known about.
- Ask ourselves how we use **time**: who tends to use the last words and who is using more space and time in the therapeutic session.
- Question whether the **rules** I set for the process are flexible or do not take into account each person's situation.

- To be aware of **my own labels and prejudices** by doing a personal work of analysis my oppressions and my privileges.

From the power that our role gives us, placing ourselves in a therapeutic relationship in a superior position can also cause us to **lose sight of** *the personal resources that the person has*, which can generate a lot of dependence but also overprotection.

Sometimes in psychotherapy, we can harm our patients if we are not able to see what they need from the therapeutic relationship. It is important to be aware of this in order to repair it and to be able to review ourselves in spaces of supervision with other professionals. Calling ourselves invulnerable, neutral and believing that we are always right is one of the reasons why we may be doing harm without realizing it.

We have a huge responsibility, we have people in our hands in a vulnerable situation, and therefore, we have the **responsibility to also question our beliefs and our ways of acting in therapy.**

15.2.4 The Therapeutic Model and Methodology

Keeping in mind the therapeutic model from which we work or the contract we establish with people can also be interesting to analyze, to assess whether it is being a tool that is helping us or may be an imposition. It is usual for psychotherapy professionals to have a specific **working model** from which we read reality and establish the treatment. However, we can establish a certain flexibility in the way we work, integrating into our frameworks of analysis the work with different models, or working in relation with other professionals from **other therapeutic models**, which in some way could help us to intervene with people assuming the diversity of their needs and preferences.

Therapeutic models that do not include a feminist gender perspective in their development can serve us as a general framework of support, thinking about a general subject, that general subject from which we theorize. But perhaps it may be important to be able to identify when our model does not fit the needs or demands of people, or that we can include in our continuing education **less androcentric and colonial visions** that allow us to broaden our frameworks of analysis.

On the other hand, with regard to the **therapeutic contract**, we could ask ourselves whether ours takes into account the social situation of the people, or whether it is only taking into account our organizational needs. In that sense, it may be interesting to evaluate whether we have a standard contract that we give to everyone to sign in the same way, as it could be making invisible difficulties that I am not perceiving or we cannot know if this agreement respects their rhythms, their decisions, and their objectives.

In relation to methodology, it is important to understand how the language we use in how we conceptualize the therapeutic relationship also influences our thinking and our way of intervening:

- Perhaps if I see people as "patients," I can only see their disease and it prevents me from seeing aspects of their person that differ from their disease.
- Perhaps if I consider them "clients," we only understand the therapeutic relationship as professionals providing a service but forget to empathize with their basic needs as individuals.

In this sense, when I was training in psychotherapy, I did not feel comfortable with either the word patient or the word client. I decided to use the concept of **person**, so as not to forget that each person has multiple aspects, beyond the problematic ones. Likewise, in the case of talking about the therapy contract, I felt more comfortable talking about **an agreement**, because a contract comes pre-written, and an agreement is built and defined together. Finally, I wondered whether I wanted to carry out a standardized and protocolized practice with all the people or to personalize it in each case, deciding to call my work an **accompaniment,** which fluctuates and moves according to the needs of each person.

~~Patient/client~~—**PERSON**
~~Contract~~—**AGREEMENT**
~~Treat/intervene~~—**FOLLOW-UPs**

15.2.5 Referral and Professional Network

Often we, the professionals who accompany in psychotherapy, feel lonely. We are educated to keep in mind the therapeutic relationship at the individual level, but this can make us forget that being part of a network of professionals, in which each one can have different resources, skills and specialties, can help us to elaborate a more complete intervention plan. Knowing that a feminist therapist does not have to solve problems with a social base from solitude is also important at the level of self-care. A feminist therapist cannot work in consultation without sharing her analysis with other colleagues, without participating in *inter-vision* spaces or without referring other colleagues.

Society harms us collectively, so there are many **psychological** and psychiatric **ailments** that are based on that **social structure** that harms us. In these cases, no individual therapy will be able to repair absolutely everything, if there is no social and collective tool added. Perhaps as psychologists we do not only need to work in the consulting room, but to be able to build dialogues and alliances between professionals and to be able to disseminate information about the social situations that the people we accompany are experiencing in order to generate social change.

15.2.6 Autonomy as an Objective

When we consider the objectives of a therapeutic process, it is essential to take into account the improvement of women's autonomy. This autonomy (or agency) is important to identify from the idea that **autonomy is not independence**. From feminist knowledge, we recognize that all *people are interdependent.* We all need care, sometimes we care, sometimes we receive care, and sometimes we share care.

The idea of interdependence and mutual care helps us to be more aware of our position so as not to reproduce dependent therapeutic relationships in which the other person will always need the presence of the therapist to solve her problems. It is essential to rejoice in the steps women are taking towards autonomy and towards establishing support networks with other women. A feminist therapist

- Would you be able to pay attention to the relationship so as not to foster dependency?
- Could you take care of the relationship until the person recognizes your power and wants closure?
- Would you be happy when the person acquires an improvement, and no longer needs to attend therapy?
- Would it foster their collective and social empowerment?

15.2.7 Horizontality and Care

Finally, another aspect in which I consider important to be aware of is horizontality and daily care, understanding that the therapeutic relationship should be a relationship that prioritizes the care of the person, but in which daily care is valued.

To do this, a feminist therapist can name the **things we do to care for the relationship**: to take her into account, to remember her, to know her likes and dislikes, and to apologize if I have kept her waiting. We have a responsibility towards the wellbeing and care of people, so we can consider that the practice of this care is done during the time that women are coming to therapy, so that this learning can be generalized to their daily lives.

We have a great responsibility in the relationship with the people we accompany and a great responsibility implies a great awareness. If we are feminists, recognizing what we do to **care for that relationship** and making it visible will be essential, but also assessing how she is feeling and making the necessary changes to respond to the rhythm and needs of the specific person I am accompanying. **Evaluating the relationship with each person will be essential in order not to start from a pre-written (and normative) idea.**

But also from our position of power, we are also referents and we have a privileged opportunity to show the women we accompany how we take care of ourselves. How we set limits, how we stop to rest, and how we prevent stress. Being a good model of care, in a practical way, teaches more than theory.

Regarding **horizontality,** this concept has to do with the analysis of understanding ourselves as a person equal to the other person. Having a therapeutic relationship that seeks horizontality would lead us not to try to be saviors of women and tell them what to do, but to consider ourselves as partners and allies in the process of change.

15.3 A Feminist Look Beyond Individualism

In closing, I think it is also important to reflect on the idea of the therapist as omnipresent in any therapeutic process. It may be important that we recognize and give value to all forms of help that can achieve mental health gains.

A feminist therapist:

- Would you be able to refer a person when you perceive that another professional or resource can better accompany them?
- Would you take it upon yourself to learn about all the community resources available around you?

The experiences of **mutual aid groups**, the processes of **feminist self-knowledge**, belonging to a **social** support **network**, or what **reading** and discovering experiences of identification among peers means for many people show us the importance of community psychology in developing **the art of deciding when not to intervene as professionals**. Identifying that therapists do not have to be present at every change or improvement that a person experiences is important in order to find **other resources** for support.

For me, a basic element of power and hierarchy within psychology is held by individual and health psychology as opposed to **social and community psychology**. Perhaps it is necessary to begin to put interest in investigating the interventions that are carried out from collective spaces to take care of mental health problems.

Support groups, in which no professional is involved, can have an enormous therapeutic element for individuals. But from an individualistic scientific point of view, not enough attention is being paid to investigate them. *Feminism, sharing with peers and understanding that many of the problems we experience are not individual, but can be shared, can be enormously therapeutic. And validating and recognizing those experiences as therapeutic is necessary.*

As feminist psychologists, therefore, we must also recognize how peer support is healing and restorative. And we don't always have to be in the middle for that to happen.

References

1. Haraway D. Situated knowledges: the science question in feminism and the privilege of partial perspective. Fem Stud. 1988;14(3):575–99.
2. Estébanez I. Therapeutic relationship and professional helping relationship. I Summer Course of the University of the Basque Country UPV-EHU Mental health with a gender perspective. Towards a feminist professional practice. [Internet]. 2021. www.ianireestebanez.com.
3. Chesler P. Women and madness. Orlando: Houghton Mifflin Harcourt P; 1989.
4. Foucault M. Historia de la sexualidad, 1: La voluntad de saber. Siglo XXI Ediciones; 1990.
5. Herman JL. Trauma and recovery: the aftermath of violence—from domestic abuse to political terror. New York: Basic Books; 2019.

Creativity and Art Outside of PSY 16

Olatz Napal Fernández, Julia Mercedes Ontiyuelo Castellano, Teresa García-Carpintero García, and Eider Cordero Sánchez

There is no gate, no lock, no bolt that you can set upon the freedom of my mind. Virginia Woolf.

According to Winnicott, creativity is a human attribute, a capacity to be developed by anyone in any act or situation in their daily life. Creations are not only works of art, but also any task that goes beyond a simple adaptation or mechanical attitude of routine life, that is done in an original manner, an innovation. Creativity is an attitude, an approach to reality, a way of living life satisfactorily. The creative drive is universal [1].

Creativity plays a fundamental role in fostering resilience and psychological well-being, offering individuals a means to process emotions, navigate challenges, and regain a sense of control over their experiences. Engaging in creative practices allows for the externalization of thoughts and feelings that might otherwise remain unexpressed, facilitating both self-exploration and emotional regulation. The act of creating provides a structured yet flexible space where individuals can transform difficult emotions into tangible forms, making them more manageable and understandable [2]. Art is presence of the world; it draws from it and gives the world a new form that it did not have before. It is presence of subjectivity: *of oneself* (as it provides access to one's way of being and existence), *from the self to others*, and *from others to the self*. It is born from the sense of human transcendence.

According to Louise Bourgeois, art was always a form of therapy that also prevents the artist from going mad, from becoming a criminal. "To be an artist is a guarantee to your fellow humans that the wear and tear of living will not let you

O. N. Fernández (✉) · J. M. O. Castellano · T. G.-C. García · E. C. Sánchez
Cruces University Hospital, University of the Basque Country, Bizkaia, Spain
e-mail: Olatz.napalfernandez@osakidetza.eus

M. López-Atanes, M. Sáenz-Herrero (eds.), *Applying the Gender Perspective in Psychiatry and Psychotherapy*, https://doi.org/10.1007/978-3-032-17883-1_16

become a murderer, and the way to avoid it is to become a murderer in your work. In my art, I am the murderer." If in life Bourgeois can sometimes be seen as vulnerable, in art she regains control by selecting her victim [3].

Spanish philosopher María Zambrano relates creativity to metamorphosis: "Metamorphosis is the way in which all living beings avoid suffering. And all those intoxicated with life, eager to be something other than mere human beings, have dreamed of traversing the world by metamorphosing, a desire that is the key to all urges for escape, even the legitimate one that is called art" [4]. Beyond emotional processing, creativity supports cognitive flexibility, encouraging individuals to approach problems from new perspectives and adapt to changing circumstances. This adaptive quality is relevant in the context of resilience, as it enables people to reframe adversity, imagine alternative possibilities, and reconstruct their sense of self beyond moments of crisis [2].

For Siri Hustvedt, the secret to creativity lies not in the higher cognitive processes but in dreamlike reconfigurations of emotional meanings that take place unconsciously. She insists on the importance of remembering that emotions can never be *unreal*, even when triggered by fiction. She highlights the discrepancy between *what happens* in a story and *how it is told. What happens* "feels to me as if it is already there in me, a part of the subliminal self that must either be dredged to the surface." And, *how to tell it?* "It happens that parts of books or poems are written in trances. The underground pushes upward and becomes a poem" [3].

Entering the world of creativity is, at its core, a restorative adventure. Creation itself holds a function of internal reconstruction, self-repair, self-creation, and integration into the world coming from a dissociated and fragmented self, which, in the case of female authors, also fights gender related conflicts. It is not uncommon that this constant observation of inner fragmentation exposes the creator to anguish and imbalance, as Lispector notes: "I'm afraid to write. It's so dangerous. Anyone who's tried, knows. The danger of stirring up hidden things – and the world is not on the surface, it's hidden in its roots submerged in the depths of the sea. In order to write I must place myself in the void. In this void is where I exist intuitively. I write as if I were going to save someone's life, probably my own life" [5].

16.1 Creativity and Gender

Being a woman places you in a specific position where you can observe and create, even if the fruits of that work have been rendered invisible throughout history. When we analyze art in museums and public spaces, we see that men seem to have been the only creators. Hernando explains that women have grown up in environments with defined freedom of movement and were educated to develop relational identities, whereas men were encouraged to develop their individuality beyond the confines of the family circle. Thus, while men constructed an external self through their professional achievements and projection into the public sphere, gender pressure directed female creativity toward motherhood and creation of pleasant environments for others—that is, care (such as the small details that surround us and are also creations: a bouquet of flowers, a collage to celebrate a birthday, a colorful wool scarf, photographs strategically placed on the wall… the so-called *art of caresses*). Women have sought ways outside the public sphere to channel their creative drive, and in the realm of the arts, one of the most accessible from the beginning was creation of stories [6].

The creative process also generates distress and, in the case of female creators, difficulties in reconciliation between their desires and the possibilities offered by the world, self-understanding and socially assigned labels, as can occur when transitioning from object-muse to subject-creator. The concept of muse implies that the true source of creation is women, while the artist is merely the channel. However, history reflects how the secondary role was not meant to be male, leaving women as enshrined muses and men as geniuses—a distribution of roles that has been projected into the universal collective imagination, replicating itself time and again. There are no male muses [7].

A recently published meta-analysis [8] suggests that men and women tend to express their creativity in different ways: men are more inclined to take risks, while women harness their empathic skills. Creativity is often portrayed as a trait associated with independence, risk-taking, and self-confidence, qualities more aligned with traditional masculine gender roles. Previous studies have shown that people tend to perceive men as more creative than women, even when the ideas presented are identical. This perception may come from an overestimation of novelty as defining characteristic of creativity, underestimating the role of utility. Researchers sought to challenge this one-sided view by exploring whether creativity can also arise from communal behaviors, such as empathy, which align more closely with traditional feminine gender roles. Notably, the study demonstrates that empathy can be a more powerful boost of creativity than risk-taking, especially when the utility of ideas is considered.

López Mondéjar identifies artist block and suicide, whether symbolic or real, are the symptomatology of failure when sublimation is not achieved. The reasons that have driven female artists down these dead-end paths are at times linked to the difficulties they encounter in developing their work and establishing their own identity as authors. Expectations derived from the condition of being a woman combined with the internal contradictions they experience can lead them either to rebel or to succumb. Taking these factors into account helps us understand some of the issues related to the mental health of female artists [9].

Within creativity, artistic self-references are a performative act that constitutes a subjectivity in which identity, agency, memory, experience, and embodiment converge. In cases of trauma, processes that involve temporal organization, such as writing, comics, and theater, are especially revealing, as they allow pain to be narrated and structured, so that it can first be endured and then integrated. The ways in which an artist can express themselves include text, image, voice, body, performance, sculpture, and photography. Photographer Francesca Woodman, whose work is a constant exploration of herself, a journey inward, remarked, "Am I in the picture? Am I getting in or out of it? I could be a ghost, an animal or a dead body, not just this girl standing on the corner?" [10].

16.2 Creativity Made into Text

A word after a word after a word is power.—Margaret Atwood

Some authors [11] suggest that writing about traumatic, stressful, or emotional events improves physical and psychological health in both clinical and non-clinical populations. Writing about neutral events does not produce these benefits. Although the immediate effect of writing about distressing experiences may result in a temporarily *negative* emotional and physical state, long-term comparisons with control groups show improvement of the immune function, lower blood pressure, enhanced liver function, and better mood. Researchers describe four mechanisms that may explain these positive effects of writing: (1) catharsis (emotional release) after inhibition (intense crying or hitting the wall are examples), (2) facing previously inhibited emotion, (3) cognitive processing, seeking a coherent narrative that helps reorganize traumatic memories, leading to more adaptive internal schemas, and (4) repeated exposure that may result in the extinction of negative emotional responses to traumatic memories.

Writing is a perceived transition from within to without, creating space for dialogue. We write with a receiver in mind, even diaries are intended for another, even if that other is just another version of ourselves, the person who returns years later to those words and finds a past self. Writing pulls us out of ourselves and jumping into putting words on paper, stimulates self-reflection, the examination of the self as another. Writing is not simply a translation of thought into words but a process of discovery, "it is the subject's taking up a position in the world of its meanings" (Merlau-Ponty) [12]. Hustvedt describes writing "as a movement from one place to another, a form of traveling, and once the journey is over, the resulting text may help organize a person's view of her subjectivity as she regards it now from the outside, instead of from the inside. This externalized self on paper can become a lifeline, a more organized mirror image that makes it possible to go on" [3]. Sontag distinguishes between the "I" who writes and the "I" who lives [13]. In this sense, Anne Sexton stated, "Some think I have been cured, but I have only become a poet."

Virginia Woolf (United Kingdom, 1882–1941) a renowned twentieth-century writer, stated, "A woman must have money and a room of her own if she is to write fiction." She faced significant mental health challenges throughout her life, including episodes of depression and bipolar disorder. From an early age, Woolf suffered profound losses, such as the death of her mother when she was 13, which triggered her first depressive episode. Throughout her life, she alternated between periods of intense literary productivity and phases of withdrawal and depression. Despite these struggles, her creativity remained a constant, allowing her to transform pain into art and introspection. In her novels, Woolf explored the complexity of the human mind and the Sontag subtleties of subjective experience. Works like *Mrs. Dalloway* and *To the Lighthouse* showcase her ability to delve into the psyche of her characters, addressing themes such as time perception, memory, and identity [14].

In confessional poetry, melancholy serves as the driving force behind raw, narrative, and often unsettling texts. Sylvia Plath and Anne Sexton carved out a space for themselves writing about their personal experiences and emotions, allowing an intimate connection with their readers by addressing taboo subjects with unflinching honesty, challenging gender conventions and emphasizing female subjectivity in a deeply personal and courageous way.

Anne Sexton (USA, 1928–1974) transitioned from a housewife to one of the most influential poets in the USA in just over a decade, winning the Pulitzer Prize. “Until I was twenty-eight, I had a kind of buried self who didn’t know she could do anything but make white sauce and diaper babies. I didn’t know I had any creative depths. I was a victim of the American Dream, the middle-class dream. All I wanted was a little piece of life, to be married, to have children. I thought the nightmares and the demons would go away if there was enough love to put them down.” When Sexton turned 28, “I had a psychotic break and tried to kill myself.” She was diagnosed with bipolar disorder. Even though she had written poetry in her teenage years, she had abandoned the practice long ago at that time. Her therapist encouraged her to take it up again, “Maybe your poems will mean something to someone else one day.” This notion “gave me a sense of purpose” (Paris Review, 1968).

Sylvia Plath (USA, 1932–1963), first winner of the Pulitzer Prize posthumously as a poet and author of *The Bell Jar*, an iconic feminist novel whose title serves as a metaphor for depression. Plath’s poetry and journals reveal an obsessive fascination with the dualities of life and death, joy and despair, beauty and decay. Her verses capture the constant struggle between a desire to live fully and the lure of self-destruction. Recurring themes in her work include death and rebirth, as well as the figure of the absent yet oppressive father, both a source of protection and constraint, frequent theme in her work. Plath’s autobiographical work openly addresses her experiences with depression and psychiatric hospitalizations, including electroconvulsive therapy. As she once wrote, “And I a smiling woman. And like the cat I have nine times to die.”

Plath and Sexton became friends in a creative writing workshop. They shared an interest in poetry that emerged from personal experience and used language to illuminate their inner darkness, becoming close in their life and their writing. Suicide was a shared secret between them; they frequently discussed it and contemplated the idea together. From an early age, they both struggled with depression and other mood disorders, and at some point, they each felt they could no longer endure it. Their deaths have similarities, inhaling carbon monoxide (Plath at the age of 30, inhaling gas from her oven in her home, after ensuring that breakfast was prepared for her children, and 11 years later, Sexton, inside her car in the garage).

16.3 As Readers

Reading, unlike watching a movie, a portrait, or a photograph, requires the transformation of abstract symbols into vivid mental images. Once we learn to read and write, this conversion is almost instantaneous. The relationship we establish with the characters in a novel is a unique form of intersubjectivity, one that develops through imagination.

Zambrano emphasizes that poetry serves to ensure that what is not said, the unspoken is not left in solitude. This helps shortening distances and making us feel less isolated [15]. An article published in *Psychology Today* [16] suggests that the abstract nature of poetry facilitates the observation of painful experiences that might otherwise feel too overwhelming to confront. The poetry's power to provide comfort lies in its ability to expand perspective; poems soften our emotional response to certain experiences and reshape our perception of them, offering new angles to face our concerns in a more creative way. We, the authors of this text, believe that poetry brings solace also because it allows us to connect through a shared human experience, fostering a sense of companionship. At times, people stop reading poetry out of fear of their own vulnerability, as engaging with it requires being open to a feeling of defenselessness that accompanies the silence of facing a poem alone. Anne Sexton paraphrased Kafka describing her vision of poetry by "A poem must be the axe for the frozen sea within us."

16.4 Creativity Turned into Music

Music plays a role in reviving the past, even the simplest tune can "transport each person back into their own history" [17]. Langer writes that the true power of music lies in its ability to remain *faithful* to the life of emotions in a way that language cannot, as its forms possess an *ambiguity* that words cannot achieve. Musical meanings reach below consciousness´ threshold (and) undoubtedly beyond the limits of discursive thought [18].

Musician and composer Tori Amos (USA, 1963) is known for her unique combination of virtuosic piano playing, poetic and confessional lyrics, and a versatile voice that ranges from delicate whispers to powerful high notes. Her music explores themes such as religion, female empowerment, sexuality, pornography, homophobia, misogyny, and trauma, combining the personal with the universal. She is one of the pioneers of the 1990s alternative rock and one of the first female artists to openly challenge the patriarchal norms of the music industry. In 1991, she released *Me and a gun*, where she tells when she was sexually assaulted and performs it a cappella in her concerts. She explained, "I really do feel as though I was psychologically mutilated that night and now I'm trying to put the pieces back together again. Through love, not hatred. And through my music. My strength has been to open again, to life, and my victory is the fact that, despite it all, I kept alive my vulnerability" [19]. In the lyrics Amos speaks about survival: "It was me and a gun. And a man on my back. But I haven't seen Barbados. So I must get out of this."

Within collective creative processes, the Riot Grrrl cultural and musical movement stands out in the early 1990s in the USA. It is a subgenre of punk rock characterized by its feminist perspective and its focus in raw and direct emotional expression and confrontation of issues such as sexual abuse, gender-based violence, and inequality. The movement arose as a way for women to claim their space in a male-dominated music scene and to address gender, sexuality, and abuse through artistic expression. It started with punk bands seeking a safe and autonomous environment where women could express themselves without being judged based on their gender. In addition to punk music, fanzines played a central role in the movement. Kathleen Hanna was the singer of the band Bikini Kill, whose concerts often began with the rallying cry "Girls to the front!", a call encouraging women to move closer to the stage. It was common to pass around a microphone to the audience, giving women a platform to share their experiences of discrimination. Another famous motto of the movement was: *We didn't come here to fuck the band; we are the band.* Role of women were no longer as *groupies* or mere admirers of male musicians; instead, they took the center stage, setting an example that inspired others to do the same. Music became a powerful vehicle for messages that reinforced self-esteem, challenged sexism, and encouraged women to take an active role in their own lives [20].

16.5 Creativity Turned into Images

Camille Claudel (France, 1864–1943) dedicates herself to sculpture. She became romantically involved with Rodin, 24 years older, a regarded artist of the time who was already in a long-term relationship with another woman. Camille Claudel's work *L'Âge Mûr* (1899) portrays the love triangle they experienced. Camille Claudel's emotional suffering escalated alongside Rodin's increasing violence, who dismissed her artistic talent and abused her as a partner. Isolated at home for years, she fell into a deep depression and destroyed many of her own works, diagnosed with delusions of grandeur and persecutory mania, Camille Claudel was institutionalized in a psychiatric hospital for 30 years despite doctor's reluctance, who tried to convince her family that she did not need prolonged hospitalization. Nevertheless, her brother, Paul Claudel, and another physician signed the hospital admission order. Years later, the abuse and manipulation that Camille Claudel suffered at the hands of the men in her life were documented in letters that not only demonstrated her mental clarity but also expressed her desperate longing for freedom and her desire to return home to work. At the turn of the twentieth century, women who departed from the traditional roles of daughter, mother, or wife were quickly labeled as hysterical and subjected to psychiatric confinement. Camille Claudel met all the criteria: she lived alone, refused male guardianship, and pursued a profession that belonged almost exclusively to men. In her sculptures Camille Claudel sculpt naked women cowered or devoted (sometimes desperate), never static or indifferent. "There is always something missing that torments me," she once said. Perhaps finding it fueled the creation of the nearly 90 pieces that we preserved of her [21].

Yayoi Kusama, the renowned Japanese artist, has used her creativity as a therapeutic tool to cope with her mental health challenges. Since childhood, Kusama has experienced hallucinations and obsessive-compulsive disorders, conditions she has channeled into her art as a way to mitigate her symptoms. In *Infinity Mirror Rooms*, using immersive spaces, covered in mirrors and lights, she creates the illusion of infinite space, reflecting her internal perception and allowing her to share her world with the audience. Kusama has used repetitive patterns, such as polka dots and nets, in her paintings and sculptures, transforming her obsessions into artistic expressions. Throughout her career, Kusama has turned her personal experiences into works showing how creativity can be a catalyst for healing and emotional well-being [22].

16.6 Creativity Turned into Body: Performance and Dance

In performance the artist's body is both the medium and the message, the fundamental element to experiment, explore, question, and transform. Body becomes both tool and product. Artists seek a definition for their physical presence and their way of existing in the world. By incorporating elements of everyday life into their work, performance allows them to explore personal, political, economic, and social issues. They establish a complex relationship between artist and audience and make the spectator an active participant. Performance allows to experience the moment, an instant immediacy gain meaning in this art form.

One of the pioneers in this field is Serbian artist Marina Abramovic, *the grandmother of performance art* for many. In 1974, she staged a six-hour performance called *Rhythm 0*, during this time she remained passive while the audience could use her body and operate on it using any of the objects that were placed on a table—ranging from flowers and lipstick to knives, razor blades, an axe, and even a loaded gun that a member of the audience eventually placed against her throat. Abramovic has said that pain and suffering can be transformed while stabbing a knife between her fingers repeatedly recording the scene.

Ana Mendieta (Cuba, 1948–USA, 1985) was a Cuban-American artist who developed body art throughout the 1970s and 1980s. She was deeply troubled by her identity conflict as an exile, a fragmented (borderline) identity disclosed in her work. She tries to open a dialogue between the Cuban-Caribbean culture she grew up in and the identity introduced by her arrival to the USA at the age of 12 as part of *Operation Peter Pan*. She was a survivor, a nomad, and used her own body as an experimentation area, her own *border identity* as a channel for artistic expression. In *Silueta* series, created in Mexico, she carved and shaped her figure into the earth, merging with mud and water, covering her form with leaves and flowers [23]. Blood is another recurring element in her work, it serves to give bodies carnality and presence leaving traces and vestiges, it is both origin and death. Mendieta denounced gender violence and all forms of violence in general: political, verbal, acoustic, perpetuated through socialized mechanisms, the media… Her life came to a sudden and violent end in 1985 when she fell from the 34th floor of her apartment in New York after an argument with her husband, the artist Carl Andre. He was tried for murder but acquitted after his lawyer argued that Mendieta suffered from a fragile mental state, describing her as extreme with suicidal tendencies. This verdict sparked outrage among feminist collectives such as Guerrilla Girls and the Women's Action Coalition [24].

Angelica Liddell (Spain, 1966) is a playwright and psychology graduate. Her works are structured around tensions between opposing poles: spiritual/corporeal, purity/scatology, beauty/pain, innocence/guilt, abstract/concrete. It defines what is aberrant, monstrous, or inhuman, constant obsessions in her artistic universe. In *Anfaegtelse*, Liddell inflicted cuts on her legs, letting her blood flow freely.

> "Blood has an extraordinary aesthetic power, it's beautiful: I use it pictorially. To reveal what's within, I begin in the surface, I make public what is private. When you choose force, blood, and selfconfession, at its core, you are speaking of your fragility. Using a blade is declaring war, and exposing oneself is exposing the other, stripping them bare. That is my intention; then, everything depends on the relationship with the audience and the power dynamic" [25].

The art of Regina José Galindo (Guatemala1974) is constructed through the body and its relationship with the environment, highlighting the sociopolitical context in which she and other women live. Her work reflects the ongoing struggle for women's rights. She began her career with the piece *Pain in a Handkerchief* (1999) in which, while lying on bed with her hands and feet tied with handkerchiefs and blindfolded, her body became a projection screen for newspaper clippings of women who had been abused, murdered, and raped. Her works allude to different representations of women: the victim, the raped, the survivor, the heroine, and the standard bearer (bearer of hope). All of her projects take place within patriarchal contexts, pushing further the struggle for equality and women's empowerment with the intention of making an impact on the public by exposing the systemic violation of women's rights, by sexism and dictatorial policies [26].

Isadora Duncan (USA, 1877–France, 1927), the pioneer of modern dance, one that goes beyond the classical formalism of ballet based on natural movements of the human body, breathing, and fluid gestures. She chose dance elements and movements that had never been considered before: imbalance, falling, and pendular motion. She was a strong advocate for women's bodily *freedom*, representing the desire of women at the time to *break free* from their traditional roles as mothers or wives, as well as the pursuit of sexual freedom and personal fulfillment beyond social clichés. In her performances, she sought for both herself and the audience to experience emotional catharsis, a release through movement. Throughout her life, she faced personal tragedies that profoundly affected her mental health (the death of her two children in a car accident among others) and by dancing, she seemed to seek a way to understand and manage her emotions, especially pain, loss, and suffering. "If I could tell you what it meant, there would be no point in dancing it."

Pina Bausch (Germany 1940–2009), based in her childhood memories, speaks about the tragedies she experienced (World War II) and other daily dramas. In her works, such as *Café Müller*, she collectively constructs a co-biography with her dancers, expressing universal emotions such as despair and anguish, not in a rationalized way, but embodied in a form of synchronized, shared catharsis emerging from bodily experience. Her dance seeks connection with the world and support from others as a means to soothe suffering and heal trauma. Bausch universalizes human drama, and what happens in her pieces connects us all. From the idea that movement is also thought, emotion, action, and expression, and every act is a form of dance, she became the creator of the Dance-Theater. Her choreographies portray human beings with all their flaws and virtues, focusing on *what drives people rather than movement itself*. Bausch uses the dancers' own fears, desires, insecurities, their vulnerabilities to create a raw and vivid humanity, forcing the audience to confront these issues. Her preferred themes are love and death, male-female relationships, violence against women, and the dynamics between the individual and the group. "Sometimes, we can only clarify something by confronting ourselves with what we don't know. And sometimes, the questions we have bring us back to experiences that are much older," she said. "Dance, dance, because otherwise we are lost" [27].

References

1. Winnicott DW. Playing and reality. London: Tavistock Publications; 1971.
2. Firestone S. Art as a catalyst for resilience: women artists with life-threatening illness. 2013 [cited 2025 Mar 20]. Available from: https://digitalcommons.lesley.edu/expressive_dissertations.
3. Hustvedt S. La mujer que mira a los hombres que miran a las mujeres: ensayos sobre feminismo, arte y ciencia. 2017;446.
4. Cerezo AC. María Zambrano. "Obras Completas VI. Escritos autobiográficos. Delirios. Poemas (1928–1990). Delirio y destino (1952)". Barcelona: Galaxia Gutenberg; 2014. Available from: https://www.academia.edu/10420862/Mar%C3%ADa_Zambrano_Obras_Completas_VI_Escritos_autobiogr%C3%A1ficos_Delirios_Poemas_1928_1990_Delirio_y_destino_1952_Barcelona_Galaxia_Gutenberg_2014.
5. Lispector C. Un soplo de vida. Siruela; 2016.
6. Hernando Gonzalo A. La fantasía de la individualidad. Buenos Aires: Traficantes de sueños; 2012.
7. Montejo J. Todas esas chicas de zapatos rojos. Madrid: Huso Editorial; 2023.
8. Abdulla Alabbasi AM, Thompson TL, Runco MA, Alansari LA, Ayoub AEA. Gender differences in creative potential: a meta-analysis of mean differences and variability. Psychol Aesthet Creat Arts. 2025;19(1):87–100.
9. Borrego MJP. Literatura y psicoanálisis. Si digo agua ¿beberé?. 2022.
10. Baños Palacios G. El autorretrato fotográfico de Francesca Woodman: entre la fabulación y la metamorfosis. Anu Dep Hist Teor Arte. 2021;33:43–60.
11. Baikie KA, Wilhelm K. Emotional and physical health benefits of expressive writing. Adv Psychiatr Treat. 2005;11:338–46.
12. Merleau-Ponty M. Phenomenology of perception. Londres; 1997. p. 352–3.
13. Sontag S. Cuestión de énfasis. Debolsillo; 2010.
14. Figueroa CG. Virginia Woolf: enfermedad mental y creatividad artística. Rev Méd Chil. 2005;133(11):1381–8.
15. Zambrano M. Algunos lugares de la poesía. Madrid: Editorial Trotta SA; 2007.
16. Will a poem a day keep the doctor away? | Psychology Today [Internet]. [cited 2025 Mar 24]. Available from: https://www.psychologytoday.com/us/blog/minding-the-body/201101/will-poem-day-keep-the-doctor-away.
17. Barbara. Il était un piano noir. Mémoires interrompus. Paris: Le Livre de Poche; 1999.
18. Langer K. S. Nueva Clave De La Filosofía. Buenos Aires: Sur; 1958.
19. Jackson J. The Tori Amos Interview. Copyright: Joe Jackson [Internet]. Joe Jackson. 2020 [cited 2025 Mar 24]. Available from: https://www.joejacksoninterviewer.com/2020/04/07/the-joe-jackson-interview-tori-amos/.
20. Marcus S. Girls to the front: the true story of the Riot Grrrl revolution. Nueva York: Harper Perennial; 2010.
21. Delbée A. Camille Claudel (Biografía). Circe; 1989.

22. Kusama Y. The visionary who used art to deal with mental illness. Arts Help [Internet]. 2022 [cited 2025 Mar 24]. Available from: https://www.artshelp.com/yayoi-kusama/.
23. Blocker J. Where is Ana Mendieta? Duke University Press; 1999.
24. Roulet L. Ana mendieta as cultural connector with Cuba. Am Art [Internet]. 2012 [cited 2025 Mar 20]; 26(2):21–7. Available from: https://www.researchgate.net/publication/275296986_Ana_Mendieta_as_Cultural_Connector_with_Cuba.
25. Liddell A. La casa de la fuerza: Te haré invencible con mi derrota. La Uña Rota; 2011.
26. Vista de Arte, feminismo y cuerpo político. Estrategias de lucha activista en la performance de Regina José Galindo [Internet]. [cited 2025 Mar 20]. Available from: https://turia.uv.es/index.php/ITAMAR/article/view/29148/pdf.
27. Biography @ ORLAN OFFICIAL WEBSITE/SITE OFFICIEL D'ORLAN [Internet]. [cited 2025 Mar 20]. Available from: http://www.orlan.eu/bibliography/biography/.

Part V

Gendered Interventions in Specific Psychiatric Disorders

17 Gender Differences in Depressive Disorder

Saioa López-Zurbano

17.1 Introduction

In this chapter, we will focus mostly on the gender differences on major depressive disorder (MDD) and related diseases such as persistent depressive disorder (previously known as dysthymia), premenstrual dysphoric disorder, depressive symptoms and subsyndromic symptoms, since bipolar disorder will be described elsewhere is this book).

Major depressive disorder (MDD) is a common mental disorder which can affect all aspects of life, including relationships with family, friends and community, school or work.

According to the *Diagnostic and Statistical Manual of Mental Disorders*, fifth edition [1], a major depressive disorder implies to suffer from depressed mood or loss of interest and pleasure in activities, associating a feeling of sadness, dejection, irritability, hopelessness, loss of interest or pleasure. It also appears with biological or neurovegetative symptoms, such as impairment in sleep, libido, appetite, energy level, psychomotor activity and cognitive signs; impairment in concentration, increased distractibility and guilt and death thought. All these symptoms cause a great change from previous functioning in the patient [2, 3], affecting their physical health, their ability to think or move, but also their work, leisure activities, family economy or social relationships. That is the reason why unipolar major depression is the main source of disease-related disability for females all over the world [2–4].

Sex differences in the prevalence of MDD are observed since the 1970s [5]. Women are twice more likely to experience depression than men in clinical and

S. López-Zurbano (✉)
Araba University Hospital, OSI Araba, Vitoria-Gasteiz, Spain

Neuroscience Department, University of Basque Country, Leioa, Spain
e-mail: saioa.lopezzurbano@osakidetza.eus

M. López-Atanes, M. Sáenz-Herrero (eds.), *Applying the Gender Perspective in Psychiatry and Psychotherapy*, https://doi.org/10.1007/978-3-032-17883-1_17

non-clinical samples [6, 7]. This difference begins as early as at 12 years old [6, 8]. There are also symptomatology differences, where depressed women suffer more "atypical" symptoms (sleep and appetite disturbances, fatigue), more somatic symptoms and more suicide attempts [6, 9]. Women, characteristically, have more anxiety comorbidities [9].

The response to treatment is also different in pharmacokinetics, pharmacodynamics and in side effects [5].

All these differences occur because MDD is a multifactorial disorder with a wide range of biological, psychological and social risk factors [4, 9, 10].

Biological factors include genetic and epigenetic factors, brain function and neural correlates, hormonal factors, stress response and immune system response, metabolism and fat distribution. The cognitive factors involve negative cognitive style (neuroticism), objectified body consciousness and rumination. The sociocultural factors include trauma exposure, more commonly child sexual abuse, but also partner maltreatment or sexual harassment and structural gender inequality and patriarchal culture.

17.2 Epidemiology

17.2.1 Prevalence

Depression is a major public health problem, affecting around 280 million people in the world [11] and been one of the primary causes of disability and poor quality of life [2, 3, 12].

Even though there are differences between countries, the 12-month worldwide MDD prevalence is estimated to be 5.8% in females and 3.5% in males. This gender disparity is also reflected in lifetime prevalence, which ranges from 6% to 25% for women and 5% to 12% for men [2–4, 12, 13]. Epidemiological studies consistently show that women are more likely to experience depression, with the female-to-male ratio for MDD ranging from 1.2 to 2.7, depending on the region. Even though the rates are different among countries, the gender gap keeps similar for high-income countries and low-income countries [14].

The race and sexual orientation may be a risk factor for MDD. A study carried in the US [15], with data between years 2012 and 2020, showed that the groups with greatest prevalence of MDD were multiracial bisexual women (past year: 19.7%; lifetime: 35.1%), White bisexual women (past year: 19.1%; lifetime: 36.5%), Multiracial bisexual men (past year: 14.0%; lifetime: 22.6%) and White bisexual men (past year: 13.1%; lifetime: 26.0%). Groups with lowest MDE prevalence were Asian heterosexual men (past year: 1.9%; lifetime: 5.1%), Black heterosexual men (past year: 2.2%; lifetime: 4.5%) and Hispanic/Latino heterosexual men (past year: 2.3%; lifetime: 5.3%).

Furthermore, the hormonal importance as a risk factor is confirmed by the fact that worldwide more than 10% of pregnant women and women who have just given birth experience depression [16].

These differences are not limited to major depression but also extend to dysthymia and subclinical depression. Dysthymia has a lifetime prevalence of 4.6%, but when a lifetime MDD happens, it can raise to a 29.4%. Subclinical depression symptoms are also more common in women [9, 17]. According to an epidemiological study carried in China, prevalence of any depressive disorders is higher in women than in men with lifetime prevalence odds ratio (OR) 1.44 and a 12-month prevalence OR of 1.41 [18]. Research is needed to inform about the magnitude of this difference in subthreshold symptoms because they also can determinate significant impairment [8, 19] and a future risk of developing an MDD or committing or attempting suicide [8].

Age predicts a variability in the effect size [8, 17]. Major depression is rare in preschool-aged children (0.3% in general population) and there is no gender gap at this age [20]. Differences emerge around the age of 12 (OR = 2.7) and peak during adolescence (age 13–15, OR = 3.02). This gender gap narrows afterwards and remains stable thereafter (OR = 1.72 for ages 20–29 and OR = 1.57 for ages 60–69) [8, 20]. However, the risk of recurrence and chronicity is bigger in female patients. Women with MDD background have a significantly higher risk of relapse, particularly when arriving to menopause, where the risk is 4–6 times higher than in men of the same age [21–23].

Referring to dysthymia, which is a risk factor for MDD itself, the onset age is usually at early adulthood and the prevalence ranges between 1% and 6% [18, 24].

When MDD becomes a persistent depression, the prevalence is around 33–50% of patients with depressive disorders. The rate of chronic depression is nearly twice in women than in men [24].

The global variability in depression rates, particularly the gender gap, suggests that cultural and socioeconomic factors play a critical role. Countries with higher levels of gender equity and economic development tend to exhibit a narrower gender gap in depression prevalence, indicating that societal factors, such as gender roles and access to mental health care, may influence the rates at which men and women experience depression [25]. In addition, as we have seen, studies from the United States [15] have highlighted that sexual orientation is an important factor driving disparities in depression prevalence, with bisexual women and men showing significantly higher rates of depression compared to their heterosexual counterparts. These findings point to the complex interplay between gender, sexual orientation and mental health, with marginalized groups facing unique vulnerabilities.

Moreover, the COVID-19 pandemic has exacerbated the global mental health crisis, with an increase of 27.6% in global MDD prevalence in 2020 [26]. This has particularly affected women, young people and gender diverse people due to social isolation, economic uncertainty and health-related fears [26, 27].

17.2.2 Clinical Features and Course

The clinical presentation of the depression symptomatology varies according to gender. It is not just the age of onset, which is earlier in women as we have seen, but also the type of symptoms, the severity and the risk of chronicity and recurrence.

Epidemiological data reveals that while depression rates are similar between the sexes during childhood, the prevalence in females doubles the rates of men during adolescence [18, 20].

Women suffering from MDD tend to exhibit more "atypical" depressive symptoms, with a frequency more than twice higher comparing to men. Atypical symptoms are described as: excessive fatigue, increased appetite, weight gain, hypersomnia, interpersonal sensitivity and gastrointestinal symptoms. These symptoms are often associated with younger age of onset, greater depression severity and more overall comorbidity (social anxiety and specific phobia and more severity, disability and suicide attempts), and because of that women are also more likely to report comorbid anxiety.

Apart from atypical symptoms, women more often suffer from anxiety, anger, somatic symptoms and psychomotor retardation. It is also more common that female patients report symptoms, particularly in self-ratings; report antecedent stressful events; and display increased comorbidity of anxiety and eating disorders, thyroid disease and migraine headaches, as well as lower lifetime prevalence of substance abuse and dependence [6, 21]. Women suffer more commonly from sleep disturbances [7] which have a bidirectional relation with depression; it can be a risk factor for developing MDD and it can also be a common symptom of the disease [28].

Women with clinical depression may tend to experience a greater severity of depressive symptoms, and their depression is often associated with a greater functional impairment [9].

Gender differences are especially prominent in the self-reported severity of depressive symptoms as compared to interview-based measures of depression severity, which implies that women express more their psychic distress [6].

When females suffer from subthreshold depressive symptoms it has also been reported to endorse a greater overall number of depressive symptoms in comparison to men.

Also, the duration of the depressive episodes is larger in female patients [6, 20]. However, findings from longitudinal studies do not show conclusive sex differences in remission, recurrence or chronicity [9, 29–31].

Even though, there are two gender-related course moderating factors in depression. First, the incidence of suicide, which is higher among men [9, 32]. Suicide rates vary between regions, beinge a rare event in psychiatry and not all suicide deaths are due to MDD. Second, the excess mortality in depressed patients compared to general population is higher in male patients. It can partially be explained because of the deaths by suicide, the increased somatic comorbidity or the substance abuse in men [9]. Even though men are more likely to make a lethal attempt, women make more suicide attempts [9, 32].

The hormonal cycle also seems to influence the symptom severity: in the premenstrual phase the severity of depressive symptoms is bigger, even if the antidepressants have been previously effective. Premenstrual worsening of depression symptoms has been associated to faster relapses [33].

Comorbidity is also different in men and women. Anxiety disorders are much more frequent in women, in both clinical and population samples [29, 30]. Anxiety disorders, beginning in childhood and puberty, can develop a chronic course and if that happens it can end in a depressive episode [29, 34]. Research also shows that the presence of previous anxiety disorders is a risk for developing depression in both sexes, but since women have higher lifetime prevalence, the risk is increased in them [9, 29].

17.3 Why Is There a Gender Gap in Depression?

As we have seen, the prevalence of depression is higher in women when the adolescence is reached (12–14 years old), while the gender gap is non-existing during childhood [7]. Many theories have been formulated to explain this situation. Nowadays, there is a consensus that the preponderance of MDD in women underlays in a multifactorial aetiology: including biological factors, affective and cognitive factors, and psychosocial factors [6, 7, 9].

17.3.1 Biological Factors/Vulnerability

17.3.1.1 Genetics

The heritability of major depressive disorder is estimated at 30–40% [35], which has been confirmed not only by twin studies, but also by national register and electronic health records (EHR) studies [36–38]. The largest twin studies for MDD to date found that the heritability of MD was bigger in women [39] and genetic risk factors for MDD were not identical between the sexes [9, 40].

The evidence to establish a greater genetic risk for women than for men is still weak [9]. In fact, the different genetic studies trying to identify genetic markers of MDD until today have not been very fortunate. It is likely that this is due to the heterogeneity, the great extent of the risk factors, and the sample in most of the published genome-wide association studies (GWAS) is of European descent [41].

Transcriptome analysis works by analysing RNA of groups of cells, in this case neurons, and tries to identify differences in the expression of genes between healthy and "depressed" cells or brain tissues. Transcripts of the brain rely on the identification of differences in the regulation and expression of genes between normal tissues of numerous brain regions or between normal tissues and diseased tissues [7, 42]. Gender differences have been found in gene expression and RNA transcripts that take part in the susceptibility for stress and depression [42]. Labonté et al. [43] demonstrated that both male and female MDD patients showed different transcriptional profiles with minimum overlap across cortical and subcortical brain areas [42, 43]. Other studies show that gene expression may be in opposite direction in depressed women and men [42, 44].

The largest studies to find sex-differences in depression have been carried by the genome-wide association approach (GWAS), which are similar to transcriptome studies. A meta-analysis identified 44 independent and significant loci associated to MDD [6, 9]. Surprisingly, no 5-HTTLPR gene or genes on X or Y chromosomes were among those 44 loci. This same study confirmed that genetic risk for depression is not categorical but, instead, is continuous, with numerous genes participating [6].

Another GWAS study [45] for neuroticismn identified high genetic correlation between MDD and a similar single-nucleotide polymorphism (SNP)-based heritability for both female and male, concluding that gender differences in neuroticism are attributable to non-genetic factors [9, 45].

Postmortem investigations showed that women have more alterations in gene expression of serotonin and glutamate receptors [42]. Investigation in men showed variations in the expression of brain-derived neurotrophic factor (BDNF) genes and its receptor TrkB [42]. Another study by Seney et al. [46] performed gene-ontology analyses and determined that synapse-related genes are upregulated in MDD female patients and downregulated in males, while the reverse relation happened to the microglia- and oligodendrocyte-related genes [46].

A GWAS that incorporated a genome-wide environment interaction approach (GWEIS) was conducted on a population of Han Chinese women with recurrent major depression and considered the exposure to adverse events [40]. They found that genes that contribute to depression may not be the same in those who experienced major negative life events and in those who have not [47].

Despite the importance of investigating with large sample sizes, GWAS often fail to replicate.

Epigenetic processes have been theorized as possible collaborating factors to MDD, that is why gene–environment (G*E) studies are carried out. Sex differences have been found [48] suggesting that DNA methylation and other epigenetic mechanisms are important processes for the brain feminization and establishment of women and men behaviour [42, 48]. Furthermore, the transgenerational transmission of stress susceptibility may be hereditable [42]. Female children of depressed mothers have bigger likelihood to develop depression [42].

There is a serotonin transporter-linked polymorphic region (5-HTTLPR), which correlates with a long (L) and a short (S) allele variant. The short allele variant diminishes the transcriptional efficiency of the 5-HTT gene promoter, decreasing 5-HTT function [9]. Researchers observed that carriers of the short allele are more vulnerable to suffer from depression in response to environmental stress [9, 49, 50]. Other studies associate the S allele, in the presence of environmental stress, to a higher risk of depression and anxiety in women and with more externalizing behaviour in men [51, 52].

Other known genetic polymorphisms in depression associates with FKBP5, a gene locus involved in the stress response. It is associated with vulnerability, in the presence of stressful life events, to develop different mental health problems, such as; depression, psychosis or aggressive behaviour [51]. Women carrying the minor allele of FKBP5 SNP rs1360780 showed more depressive symptoms under high peer stress but fewer symptoms under low peer stress [52].

The corticotropin-releasing hormone receptor 1 (CRHR1) gene also has variants associated with vulnerability to MDD when exposed to childhood trauma [53]. However, these results have been difficult to replicate [9, 53].

17.3.1.2 Brain Structure and Function

Sex differences in brain anatomy and function have been progressively documented in imaging studies. These structural differences may contribute to sex-specific susceptibilities to neuropsychiatric conditions [9, 41].

In healthy controls, structural differences show that men have 8–13% larger total brain volumes compared to women, even once corrected by total body mass [54]. Historically, it has been said that men have higher grey-white matter rate than females. However, it was demonstrated that these differences are due to the brain's size. That is, the larger the brain is, the bigger the grey-white matter ratio will be, no matter the sex [55].

A meta-analysis of sex differences in human brain structure determined that sex differences on size are more notable in the intracranial volume and cerebrum volumes. Large effects are also found for total brain volume, grey matter, white matter, cerebrospinal fluid and cerebellum volumes [56]. For specific brain tissue density, it was found that males on average have larger volumes and higher tissue densities in the left amygdala, hippocampus, insular cortex, and putamen, higher densities in the right VI lobe of the cerebellum and in the left claustrum, and larger volumes in the bilateral anterior parahippocampal gyri, posterior cingulate gyri, precuneus, temporal poles and cerebellum, areas in the left posterior and anterior cingulate gyri, and in right amygdala, hippocampus and putamen. Females have higher density in the left frontal pole; and larger volumes in the right frontal pole, inferior and middle frontal gyri, pars triangularis, planum temporale/parietal operculum, anterior cingulate gyrus, insular cortex and Heschl's gyrus; bilateral thalami and precuneus; the left parahippocampal gyrus and lateral occipital cortex [56].

On depressed patients we can find that in male patients there is an increased volume in the left cerebellum and reduction in the right superior/middle temporal gyrus, left middle temporal gyrus and ventro-medial prefrontal cortex; while a grey matter volume reduction in the left lingual gyrus and dorsomedial prefrontal cortex occurred selectively in female patients [57].

Hippocampus In healthy controls there are no sex differences in this brain region [58]. In first depression episodes, men appear to exhibit a smaller hippocampal volume than healthy male controls. This volume difference was not found between female patients and controls [59]. However, newer researches seem to correlate the hippocampal smaller volume in MDD compared to controls just on patients whose illness length was longer than 2 years or who had more than one MDD episode, regardless of sex [60].

Cortical morphometry differences Studies have shown that females with MDD show reduced surface area in the left ventrolateral prefrontal cortex (vlPFC) and right rostromedial prefrontal cortex (mPFC), along with increased local gyrification index (LGI) in the left visual cortex compared to healthy controls [57, 61].

Meanwhile, males with MDD show an increased surface area in the left cerebellum and decreased grey matter volume in the right superior/middle temporal gyrus, left middle temporal gyrus, grey matter volume in the right superior/middle temporal gyrus, left middle temporal gyrus and ventromedial prefrontal cortex [7].

Amygdla Volume Differences Research indicates that depressed women tend to have a smaller amygdala compared to healthy females. Depressed men exhibit a positive association between depression history and lower grey matter volumes in the amygdala [62].

Corpus Callosum and Internal Capsule Alterations While depressed women show focal abnormalities in the genu of the corpus callosum, depressed men tend to have alterations in the anterior limb of the internal capsule [63].

Functional Connectivity Functional MRI research has demonstrated that resting-state functional connectivity in brain network in depressed women is altered, particularly in emotion regulation and self-referential processing. On the contrary, depressed men exhibit different patterns of functional connectivity, specifically in cognitive control and reward processing [64].

Observations so far have been very heterogeneous, showing the complexity of MDD and the difficulty of carrying out brain exams.

A further difficulty is that the brain and neural correlate in healthy and depressed females is influenced by the hormonal situation, which varies with the age, the reproductivity life stages and the moment of the menstrual cycle. All these factors make it challenging to find epidemiological and brain differences between sexes.

17.3.1.3 Hormonal Influences

Since the gender difference emerges during puberty (by the age of 12–14), it is very likely that the hormonal change that happens at this age may be involved in the development of MDD in young girls. The hormonal factor is also supported by the decompensations and relapses happening during peripartum and menopause [9, 20]. However, this hormonal influence on depression risk is complex and interacts with genetic factors, particularly those related to neurotransmitter systems.

One of the biggest biological differences between sexes in mammary species are the sexual hormones. Oestrogens are a group of ovarian hormones that include three subtypes, viz. estrone, estradiol and estriol. Even if they are a family of hormones, they are often referred as estrogens to the three of them. The most potent one, according to its affinity for oestrogen receptors in rodents and humans, is 17β- estradiol [65]. Other sex hormone cyclically produced in the ovary is progesterone. It is also produced by the placenta during pregnancy, the adrenal glands and again by cells in the central nervous system where it's formed by steroidogenesis from cholesterol in both males and females [66]. Both oestrogens and progesterone act as neuromodulators and are involved in several brain actions such as, mood regulation, stress response or neuroplasticity.

Oestrogens

Oestrogen is a potent neuromodulator that influences many of the brain neurotransmitter systems, such as serotonergic, noradrenergic, dopaminergic, glutamatergic and GABAergic [67, 68]. This is why, among other processes, this sexual hormone can impact on emotion reward processing, cognition and mood [68].

Research shows that oestrogen has a protective role against depression in women: it improves serotonin activity by promoting serotonin receptor density and enhancing spine formation and synaptic plasticity [41].

The functional studies demonstrate a positive correlation between estradiol concentrations and hippocampal grey matter volume, white matter integrity and activity during affective processing [67–70]. Oestrogen also regulates the prefrontal cortex. Hippocampus and prefrontal cortex are both regions associated with mood regulation [70].

As Albert et al. demonstrate, women with high estradiol levels showed significantly less deactivation in limbic regions and less subjective distress during psychosocial stress compared to women with low estradiol levels [70]. This means that the normal cycling high estradiol levels in premenopausal women attenuate the brain activation changes and the negative mood response to psychosocial stress.

Oestrogen can enhance the expression of the serotonin transporter gene, increasing serotonin signalling in the brain. In women, particularly those in premenstrual or postmenopausal states, hormonal fluctuations may impact the SLC6A4 gene expression, potentially making them more susceptible to depression [68]. The SLC6A4 gene codes for the serotonin transporter protein. Variations in the short allele of the SLC6A4 gene are known to increase depression risk, particularly in the context of stress. Recent studies have suggested that oestrogen may interact with this gene to modulate its expression [68].

Oestrogens increase the expression of serotonin receptors and the release of serotonin in the brain, contributing to mood stabilization. Oestrogen promotes the growth of dendritic spines (which are involved in synaptic plasticity) in the hippocampus, a region critical for memory and emotion regulation. Fluctuations in oestrogen levels, especially during the menstrual cycle or menopause, can result in cognitive and emotional instability [41, 65].

Oestrogen also enhances the expression of BDNF, which supports the growth and survival of neurons. Lower BDNF levels have been implicated in major depressive disorder (MDD), with research showing that oestrogen's effects on BDNF may be one reason women are more susceptible to depression during periods of hormonal decline [71].

All women that were pharmacologically treated with a gonadotropin-releasing hormone agonist developed depressive symptoms [72].

Lipophilic oestrogens go through cell membrane and attach to intracellular oestrogen receptors (ER) alpha (ERα) and beta (ERβ). These receptors operate as transcription factors. Both ERα and ERβ have been proposed to contribute to the pathophysiology of mood disorders and especially in depression [73]. Polymorphisms in the genes that encode both receptors, specifically rs2234693 single nucleotide polymorphism for ERα may have a role in the vulnerability to "reproductive depression subtypes" [74]. No ER polymorphism in men has been found to correlate with depression [6].

These findings highlight the bidirectional relationship between hormonal fluctuations and genetic predispositions in women [75].

Progesterone

Progesterone, same as estradiol, also has neuroprotective properties by potentiating the expression of different neurotrophins, like BDNF [66, 76]. Progesterone also activates neuronal proliferation signalling pathways [67, 68]. This hormone can impact in the GABAergic system, which is involved in inhibitory neurotransmission, by modulating GABA-A receptors [66, 76]. This way, low progesterone levels contribute to anxiety and depressive symptoms, especially during the luteal phase of the menstrual cycle and postpartum depression [67, 68, 77].

Pubertal Depression

We have already described how the gender gap raises dramatically at puberty, remaining stable across adulthood.

There are different explanations for it; the biopsychosocial perspective explains that adolescence may be more disadvantageous for girl than for boys. Girls find more peer pressure, premature sexual activity, peer sexual harassment and greater body dissatisfaction than boys [6, 7, 9].

From a biological perspective, puberty is a period where reproductive hormones suffer intense fluctuations, new functions and induce several body changes which are very different between sexes. Females suffer a rise in pituitary hormones, luteinizing hormone (LH) and follicle-stimulating hormone (FSH), inducing the ovarian maturation and hence a big release of oestrogen. In males, on the other hand, the rise of LH levels induce the testicles to produce more testosterone, and FSH induces the spermatogenesis [6, 9, 78].

Both sexes go through an increase in LH secretion similarly, but FSH increases greatly in girls across the peripubertal transition [79]. The hypothalamic-pituitary-gonadal (HPG) axis is regulated by negative feedback of gonadal steroids in both males and females. But girls have a second control mechanism. This second mechanism is the positive feedback correlated with the menstrual cycles [7]. So, if estradiol level gets higher than determinate values, it provokes a central release of LH and FSH, which lasts less than 2 days and induces ovulation.

The different feedback sex steroids induce on the regulation on the hypothalamic-pituitary-adrenal (HPA) axis have an influence in its modulation and reactivity [80]. In addition, not in women, but only in men, estradiol stimulates the production of corticosteroid-binding globulin, diminishing the quantity of free corticosterone. This very likely prevents men from the stimulative effects of estradiol on the HPA axis [80].

The higher excitability of HPA axis through HPG axis activity, associated with more exposition to stressful and traumatic experience, exposes the big role sexual hormones have in the risk and development of depression among female adolescents [7].

Premenstrual Dysphoric Disorder and Premenstrual Syndrome

A big proportion of women experiment physical, psychological and/or behavioural changes during the luteal phase of the menstrual cycle. This combination of changes is called premenstrual syndrome (PMS) [6, 77, 81, 82]. About 3–8% of females at reproductive age suffer from even more severe symptoms, that include: depressed mood, decreased interest in usually enjoyable activities, irritability, anxiety, lethargy, difficulties in concentration, appetite and sleep disturbance, which are the diagnostic criteria for premenstrual dysphoric disorder (PMDD) [81, 82]. Even though we can find these group on symptoms in MDD, the principal difference is that they tend to happen specifically during luteal phase, experiencing an improvement within a few days after the menstruation.

It is intuitive to assert that the biological mechanism of the disease must be related to the gonadal sex hormone changes that happen in the female body in the luteal phase. There is a quick drop in sexual hormone levels, both steroid levels and particularly progesterone. At the same time, pituitary gonadotropins, FSH and LH, remain low and stable [83].

As we have already asserted, estradiol and progesterone have neuroprotective roles [41, 67, 68, 76]; and their sudden decline has an impact in serotonin, γ-aminobutyric acid and dopamine neurotransmitter systems. This neurotransmitter fluctuations may be responsible for the psychological symptoms suffered by vulnerable females. Nevertheless, sexual hormonal levels are not significantly different between affected women and healthy controls, so there must be a further explanation [84]. However, we can assert that PMDD is characterized by an abnormal response to normal hormonal changes during the luteal phase of the menstrual cycle, as described by Kuehner et al. [85].

PMS seems to have a strong heritability, and genetic variations of the oestrogen receptor (ER) sequence have been thought to induce an abnormal response to hormonal fluctuations [81, 85], but this proposal needs yet to be confirmed.

The use of contraceptive hormones as a treatment for PMS or PMDD shows that the prescription of oral combined contraceptives does not specifically improve premenstrual depressive symptoms, but it does improve overall premenstrual symptomatology [81, 85].

There is also to be said that PMDD has not been included in DMS manual until 2013 because there is an ongoing debate about whether this categorization may medicalize a normal physiological process. On one hand, PMDD can be seen as the medicalization and pathologizing women's normal physiological processes, particularly those related to reproduction [84]. And on the other hand, PMDD can develop into a stigma due to its symptoms and because of social pressure for women to adapt to gender norms of femininity as caregiving, affectivity and emotional stability against irrationality or overemotionality [84, 86].

Perinatal Depression

Postpartum depression is one of the most frequent complications during childbirth. It can affect one in eight women [16], with deleterious effects for both the mother and the child. Unfortunately, suicide is one of the leading causes of mortality after giving birth [87].

We are not going to focus on peripartum disease, since there is going to be a specific chapter about it in this book.

Perimenopausal Depression

The perimenopause is another challenging period in a woman's life; it occurs around 42–52 years old. This period is described as "the period immediately prior to the menopause, when the endocrinological, biological, and clinical features of approaching menopause commence, and until at least the first year after the final menstrual period" by the World Health Organization [88]. This period can be as long as 3–9 years, and 80% of women report neuropsychiatric symptoms [21], such as vasomotor symptoms (commonly called hot flashes), sleep disturbances, vaginal dryness and loss of libido and cognitive impairment; 20% may suffer from depression symptoms [21, 22].

During perimenopause, women experience big hormonal changes, oestrogen and progesterone levels fall, influencing both dopamine and serotonin neurotransmitter systems [6, 9, 22]. These variations are associated with higher rates of depressive symptoms and mood swings. Research supports that hormonal changes during perimenopause are linked to both the frequency and severity of depressive symptoms [21–23].

Risk factors for perimenopausal depression are: a history of depression or a family history of mood disorders, high stress levels, lack of social support and prior traumatic experiences [22]. If a woman was experiencing an MDD, it is likely that during menopause the symptoms get worse [6, 21]. It is also a bidirectional process, because women who have experienced adverse childhood experiences also have more menopausal symptoms [23].

Men also experience andropause, it happens later in life (from 50 years old onwards) and with different and less pronounced biological, physical and psychological features: there is no hormonal level drop like in females, total testosterone levels keep more stable over the years [89]. Men can experience fatigue, sexual dysfunction, weakness, irritability, depression, insomnia, anxiety, memory impairment and reduced cognitive function [89]. Since the biological changes are less intense, the risk of depression also is milder [75].

As a conclusion, we may say that the relationship between perimenopause and depression is complex and multifactorial. While hormonal fluctuations during this transitional period undeniably play a significant role in mood disturbances, psychosocial factors and individual health history are also critical. Recognizing and addressing depression during perimenopause is essential for improving quality of life and ensuring women receive the care and support they need during this challenging time.

Testosterone and Depression

Although testosterone is primarily a male hormone, it plays a role in mood regulation for both sexes. Low circulating testosterone levels have also been associated with increased risk of developing anxiety- and stress-related disorders in males [90, 91].

Testosterone has a neuroprotective effect, helping to increase serotonin receptor binding in key brain regions. Decreased testosterone levels in older men have been associated with increased rates of depressive symptoms. Testosterone replacement therapy can serve as an adjunct treatment to improve mood and alleviate depressive symptoms [90, 91].

Testosterone in women has been shown to influence libido, mood and energy levels, and lower levels of testosterone may contribute to fatigue, irritability and depression [90].

17.3.1.4 Physiological Stress Response and HPA Axis

Depressive disorders associate with an abnormal stress-related HPA axis activation [6, 42, 92]. Research confirms depressed patients, due to this altered HPA axis activation, exhibit different levels and altered response to cortisol, although results are very heterogenous [42, 92].

Sex differences in HPA axis activation begin in puberty [6, 92, 93] and are none or small before adolescence and after menopause [94]. We must take into account that HPA axis is influenced and regulated in many different ways, particularly by sex hormones. As we have explained before, there is a complex HPA-HPG axis mutual interaction. Both androgens and estrogens influence the response to stress by regulating the cortisol receptor's activity [75, 94]. Testosterone inhibits the activation of HPA axis, while oestrogens and progesterone stimulate its function [92, 93] and diminish the sympathoadrenal response [95]. Female hormones regulate cortisol production and circulation as a result of the bigger cortisol levels during the follicular phase versus the luteal phase during women's menstrual cycle. This means that the cortisol-sex hormones correlation may play a part in premenstrual symptoms [42] and that the use of oral contraceptives and the hormone fluctuations (pregnancy, menopause or menstrual cycle) may influence women's cortisol response [6, 94].

There also seem to be sex differences in how neuropeptides such as oxytocin, arginine, vasopressin or corticosteroid-binding globulin concentrations activate the HPA axis [42, 94].

Men exhibit bigger physiological responses to a larger variety of psychosocial stressors than women [37, 92, 96]. This means a greater HPA axis activation, more elevated diastolic blood pressure, broader conditioned fear reactions and more negative and aggressive emotional answers [9, 42, 97]. This greater HPA axis response persists also when adjusting for depressive symptoms, which predict for a flatter cortisol response curve in females, compared to males [98, 99]. The nature of the stressor may also vary the stress response; males react more strongly to achievement challenges and females to social rejection and conflict [98, 100]. The nature of the stressor while being depressed have also shown to be different between genders: depressed women have bigger cortisol responses to negative events than depressed men [101]. The evolutionary hypothesis for women's attenuated stress response is that it may help protect the foetus from the deleterious effects of maternal stress [95]. Even if men have bigger HPA axis activation, women experience more stress vulnerability, subjectively suffer greater stress than men and describe more somatoform symptoms [7].

Studies of HPA axis dysregulation in MDD show inconsistent results, describing both hypercortisolism and hypocortisolism [99, 102, 103]. On one hand, the chronic activation of the HPA axis is associated with the development of depression. The presence of elevated cortisol levels and the persistent cortisol dysregulation—either if it is elevated morning cortisol or inhibited night cortisol—is a strong predictor of depression onset, especially in individuals with a genetic predisposition [41, 103, 104]. Hypercortisolemia in depression is thought to downregulate serotonin receptors, impair hippocampal function and increase vulnerability to stress. Elevated cortisol is particularly significant in chronic depression or treatment-resistant depression [102–104]. Depressed women often show higher cortisol levels than depressed men, particularly following stressful events [9, 33], higher early morning cortisol levels and greater cortisol reactivity to stress [33, 99]. On the other hand, hypoactivation of the HPA axis is seen in different stress-related disorders, including posttraumatic stress disorder, where stress-related HPA axis hypoactivation is correlated with higher premenstrual symptoms [105]. Hypocortisolemia can diminish negative affect and subjective stress, contributing to the normalization of emotional circuits after exposure to stressors.

Atypical depression, characterized by the inhibition of the HPA axis, and related symptomatology of profound fatigue and reversed neurovegetative symptoms, represents a more homogeneous phenotype, which is particularly common among women [106, 107]. But no sex correlation has been found between HPA axis and atypical features [99].

As Stadtler and Neigh explain [108]: "*Women disproportionally experience lasting physical effects of stress when compared to their male counterparts. Chronic stress can increase HPA axis dysregulation and disrupt glucocorticoid balance in women, which negatively impact neurobiology and cognition. Differences in neural plasticity fuelled by hormonal differences between women and men could contribute to increased susceptibility of women to stress*" [108].

Sex differences also influence the interaction between the immune system and the hypothalamic–pituitary–adrenal (HPA) axis [42], whose role in sex differences will be discussed in the following section.

17.3.1.5 Immune System Response

The immune system response has been a target when addressing the sex differences in mood and anxiety disorders [7, 9, 42]. There is a bidirectional correlation between inflammation/immune activation and neuropsychiatric diseases, as mood disorders, schizophrenia, neurodegenerative disorders or other medical illness. Based on this statement the neuroimmune theory of MDD was described [109]. Different researches have demonstrated that brain inflammatory cytokines have a key role in the development of depression and anxiety, proposing that persistent neuroimmune activation in adulthood impacts on brain's health and contributes to the appearance and maintenance of depression symptoms in women [109, 110]. Furthermore, depression also activates some inflammatory paths even though the ways this happens have not been fully explained yet [109, 111].

IN MDD there is an immune activation, which derives in increased levels of C-reactive protein (CRP), and peripheral interleukins (IL) and cytokines (IL-12, IL-1b, IL-8), and tumor necrosis factor alpha (TNF-α) [42, 108, 109, 112]. This induces the activation of microglia and higher monocyte traffic in to the brain [113]. The amelioration of depression is associated to a reduction in this pro-inflammatory interleukins [109, 114]. And we can find this in all ranges of patients, even in old-aged patients with cognitive impairment [115].

Male and female immune systems do not work the same way, situation that can easily be argued by the prevalence of autoimmune diseases among women [7], which independently is a risk factor for developing MDD. The sex differences in the immune system include divergence in immune cell number, ratio and activity. Women have a higher amount of some peripheral immune cells, such as B cells, Th2 cells and neutrophils, and show a stronger response to infections, with higher phagocytic capacity and synthesis of some cytokines [116]. In addition, research in mice shows that in the central nervous system, microglial cells' ("brain macrophages") number, morphology and functionality is sexually dimorphic, and influenced by the stage of development and the specific brain region [42, 117, 118].

Furthermore, the chromosome with the biggest proportion of immune-related genes is the X chromosome, including those coding for the CD40LG protein (expressed on T cells), the toll-like receptor 7 [119] and the CXCR3 chemokine receptor, defies X-inactivation mechanisms, with a double gene product in women [7, 117, 118, 120].

The same way, the inadequate function of immune system in depressed patients occurs in different ways in men and women patients. Depressed women have higher levels of IL-6, pro-inflammatory IL-8, interferon-γ and leptin and lower levels of the pro-inflammatory IL-5 and anti-inflammatory adiponectin [121]. And those depressive symptoms seem to be associated with higher CRP levels in women, but not in men [122].

When inflammatory activation is induced, for example by the administration of bacterial endotoxins, healthy women develop depressed mood and social disconnectedness, but not men. This effect is associated to the mediation of TNF-α and IL-6 levels [123].

17.3.2 Individual Difference Susceptibility: Psychological Factors

17.3.2.1 Affective Factors: Neuroticism, Negative Affect, Absence of Positive Affect

Some models of depression postulate temperament as a vulnerability factor for MDD [124, 125]. Children with elevated scores in the temperament dimension of negative emotionality (also known as negative affectivity or "difficult temperament") are at higher risk for depression later in life [124, 125].

As it is described in the reviews by Hyde and Mezulis [6, 126], negative emotionality can drive to depression through diverse pathways. First, negative emotionality may have a direct effect on depression; being itself a risk factor. Second, negative emotionality may contribute to the development of other vulnerability factors such as negative cognitive style, which in turn is a more proximal risk factor. Third, negative emotionality may induce a bigger reactivity to stress, and the social and hormonal changes that happen at adolescence may act as stressors to that exacerbated negative emotionality, leading to depression [6, 126].

In early childhood, girls are better at regulating attention and restraining impulses [9]. Boys, on the contrary, have more externalizing problems and score higher on surgency. This means that boys are a little more active and impulsive, and experience more pleasure from high-intensity stimuli [9, 127].

In early childhood can already be seen a small but consistent difference between boys and girls in personality traits of interpersonal orientation such as empathy and prosociality [97], warmth and agreeableness [128]. Empathy is usually associated with better mental health, but some models have linked it to internalizing problems in women, which starst at puberty [128, 129].

A meta-analysis of studies on gender differences in temperament, however, found a trivial gender difference for negative affect, $d = -0.06.27$ [127].

So in early childhood there is mixed evidence for gender gap in negative affectivity.

In the absence of a gender difference in negative emotionality, another possible mechanism is a temperament-stress interaction, with girls and women experiencing more stress than boys and men, beginning in early adolescence [6]. Gender differences in the experience of stressors are discussed later in this chapter. Several studies have found that temperament predicts depression differently for girls than for boys. A study [130] described that girls who were high in negative affectivity in infancy typically displayed more depressive symptoms in adolescence, whereas boys high in negative affectivity in infancy typically displayed initial higher levels of depressive symptoms and then decrease at adolescence [6, 9].

Even if there is mixed evidence for low extraversion correlated to depression [127], positive affectivity lack, a subfacet of extraversion, has been described as a risk factor for depression [131]. This changes in adolescence, when girls score higher for neuroticism and negative affectivity than boys, and these scores are kept over lifetime [128]. In puberty, negative affectivity correlates to anhedonic symptoms, especially if combined with low positive affectivity in both sexes [132].

Neuroticism is a known risk factor for MDD [131], but also for other internalizing and externalizing disorders [133]. The gender gap for neuroticism shows cross-cultural differences, pointing to culture-related gender stereotypes in modelling these traits [96, 128, 134, 135]. The biggest gender difference in neuroticism is usually found in developed countries [96, 128, 134, 135]. The explanation for this dissimilarity is attributed to the demands for gender role in different societies: while in more traditional societies gender roles are assumed as the "normality," the more progressive ones attribute this behaviour to trait characteristics [128].

Aside from this, the way adolescents, males and females, interact has been greatly changed by the use of social media. This use has raised the peer harassment [136] and the sexualization of women [137]. This way, the body consciousness and the isolation have grown during the last decades, and so have the internalizing problems in girls [138].

17.3.2.2 Cognitive Factors

Negative Cognitive Style It has been described for a long time the impact of cognitive vulnerability-stress models for the development of depression. This theory postulates [139] that certain cognitive styles make people more vulnerable to MDD when they suffer stressful events. The two most known of these theories are the hopelessness theory and the ruminative response styles theory [6, 140].

In hopelessness theory, negative cognitive style (also known as attributional style) describes the inclination when negative life events occur to jump to negative conclusions about the self, causality and consequences [6, 141]. Research demonstrates that both adults and adolescents, no matter the sex, with this negative cognitive style, when a new stressor appears are at higher risk of developing an MDD [142–144]. However, the gender differences in negative cognitive style are uncertain. There is mixed information for children, addressing no gap between genders or a more negative style in boys [145]. In adolescence, on the contrary, girls have more negative cognitive styles in response to stressors [146].

The fact that gender gap in depression appears before the gender gap in negative cognitive style indicates that this theory by itself is unlikely to describe the gender differences in MDD [147].

Objectified Body Consciousness Investigation shows that the cognitive vulnerability for depression should extend to the cognitions girls and women have about their body. As Hyde and Merzulis [6] describe it, objectified body consciousness which leads to a negative perspective of one's body include two mental processes: first, the self-surveillance, the habitual monitoring of body's outward appearance [148] so that it matches with specific standards; and second, the body shame, where individuals feel shame if their bodies do not meet those specific standards [149]. Objectified body consciousness, which correlates with the cultural and societal standards about the ideal appearance, is internalized by the individual. This is believed to impact more in women. A proof ot this is the sex gap observed in the prevalence and incidence A of eating disorders during adolescence [150, 151]. Longitudinal investigations show that sex differences in self-surveillance are seen at an age as young as 11 ($d = 0.49$) and it broadens with age ($d = 0.64$ at age 13; $d = 0.79$ at age 15) [149, 150, 152]. Investigations also show that adolescents and adult women experience more body shame [127]. Since this gender difference emerges so early, it is thought to contribute to the sex difference in the appearance of depression. In fact, self-surveillance at age 11 correlates to depressive symptoms at age 13 for girls but not for boys [150]. Gender differences in body shame and dissatisfaction precede those in depression, and may intervene in the association between gender and the increase in depression in adolescents [9, 153].

It is important to note that it has been demonstrated that self-surveillance mediates the effect of media exposure on depressive symptoms [6, 133].

Rumination Rumination is the inclination to repetitively, passively, and unproductively analyse problems and distress-generating negative emotions and no taking actions [6, 9]. This way of thinking anticipates depressive symptoms in life and the onset of MDD [154, 155]. It can also interact with stressful life events to predict depressive symptoms [131, 142, 154]. Rumination is associated with neuroticism, and it is even more correlated to depressive symptoms [131]. But rumination is not only associated with the development of depression, but also with internalizing and externalizing psychopathologies and their co-occurrence [6, 9].

Meta-analysis [156, 157] show that women tend more intensely to ruminate, especially in childhood and adolescence [156], but no so much in adulthood [157]. So rumination may play a role in the sex differences for depression [154]. Mood disorder patients scored higher than controls on rumination too [155, 158].

Co-rumination is the tendency to ruminate problems with another person. Girls score higher on co-rumination than boys in adolescence [6, 158] and this tendency to response to distress seems harmful for pubertal girls [159] and to correlate with depression rates.

17.3.3 Environmental Factors: Individual (Micro) Level

As Kuehner describes, "gender roles, social expectations, and cultural stressors disproportionately affect women, potentially heightening their genetic susceptibility to depression" [9].

The correlation between negative life events and the onset of depression and the higher depressive symptoms in lifetime is well known [160, 161]. It is also robustly demonstrated that girls have more stressors and are more vulnerable to those stressors than boys. Interpersonal stressors (peer events) make a bigger sex difference in adolescence, measured by the use of a daily diary in adolescents [17]. Another stressor described in adolescent girls is peer sexual harassment, that is more prevalent in girls than in boys (56% vs 40%) and include verbal, physical and electronic harassment. Girls are more affected, describing sleeping disorders and unwillingnes to go to school [6, 9]. Longitudinal research on peer sexual harassment in adolescence reports that victimization correlates with depressive symptoms in a reciprocal relation [162].

In adult samples, having a paid job correlated with a minor prevalence of depressive and anxiety disorders for both sexes, but for women, the protective role of having a job was limited to the ones without children [6, 9]. Different investigations have described gender-specific stressor associated with MDD: for men, being currently working and legal problems were the main factors, and for women, there were the perceived failure in interpersonal relationships and lack of social support [9, 37, 96, 135].

17.3.3.1 Violence Against Girls and Women

Violence against girls and women is a serious worldwide public health and human rights problem. It can appear in different forms, such as child sexual abuse, rape, intimate physical and sexual violence, sex trafficking and, in some regions, child or forced marriage, female genital mutilation or violence in the name of so-called honour [9, 163]. Gender-based violence has important consequences for physical, reproductive and mental health, and a huge economic impact [9, 163].

Sexual assault for adults is demonstrated to be a main stressor, with a much higher prevalence in women. US data shows that, 18% of women and 1.4% of men have ever been raped in their lives [6].

17.3.3.2 Childhood Sexual Abuse

Early adversity is established as a main non-specific risk factor for diverse somatic and mental disorders in childhood, adolescence and adulthood [9, 163, 164]. This causes dysfunctional development of the stress response and autoimmune processes, structural and functional brain variations and epigenetic effects [9, 164]. Boys and girls suffer similar rates of early adversity with one difference: the child sexual abuse (CSA) [9, 165]. Lifetime prevalence of CSA is about 18% in girls and 8% in boys [165]. CSA victims more commonly suffer from internalizing and externalizing symptomatology compared to victims of other maltreatment [9]. Results of epidemiological studies show that exposure to CSA reduces the gender gap in depression, internalizing and externalizing disorders [9, 164, 165].

To summarize, there is proof that the higher prevalence of MDD in women is partially because of the higher rate of CSA in girls. And this higher prevalence is not due to women's higher vulnerability to adversity [9, 164]. Nevertheless, victimization may have extended- or delayed-onset effects, causing an increased psychiatric risk in adolescents and adult women when exposed to early adversity. It is described that tough early adversity, as CSA is, provokes higher risks in pubertal transition, especially in girls, developing increased psychopathology later in life [9].

17.3.3.3 Other Forms of Interpersonal Violence

WHO assesses that 30% of women in the world have been victims of physical or sexual partner violence, and 7% have had non-partner sexual assaults [9, 163]. Being a woman increases the risk of multiple coercive, sexual and severe physical partner violence. Female violence victims are twice as likely to develop depression and substance-related disorders as non-affected women [9, 163].

Revictimization is also an important factor, because CSA victims are more prone to be adult sexual abuse victims, and this also develops into a higher risk of psychopathology in adulthood compared to CSA alone [9].

Intimate partner violence correlates with peripartal depression: women who suffered lifetime or during pregnancy partner violence have three times more odds of developing a postpartal depression, and 27–30% of peripartal depressed women had suffered domestic violence the previous year [166].

17.3.4 Sociocultural Factors: Macro Level

17.3.4.1 Structural Gender Inequality

Structural gender inequality is the differences in access to power, social status and resources between men and women, and it is well documented by United Nations Development Programme and the World Economic Forum. It includes various socio-economic factors as political participation, reproductive rights, economic autonomy or education, which are correlated with mental health [6, 9, 166]. The hypothesis is that gender inequality, in detriment of women, would drive to more depressive symptoms in women and consequently amplify the gender differences in depression.

Patriarchy has allowed men to sexually harass women, which connects to depression, anxiety and posttraumatic stress disorder (PTSD) [6]. Income inequality and the difficulty to leave an abusive heterosexual relationship, and the intimate partner violence contribute to depression [6, 163, 166].

Meta-analysis investigating gender differences in depression observed that, contrary to hypotheses, gender-equity indicators did not predict the magnitude of the gender difference or greater equality was positively associated with larger gender differences in depression [6, 20]. The explanation for this counterintuitive discovery is proposed to be the subjective nature of reports of depression symptoms, and in investigations for subjective self-ratings, gender differences are usually bigger in more progressive nations [6]. The more gender interaction in equitable nations may facilitate the girls to compare themselves with boys and see themselves as more depressed than boys. There is no way where we declare gender equality to be bad for women, it is just that social comparisons between genders are much less frequent in non-equitable nations [6]. However, these results do not correlate with findings in the US and Europe, where women in regions with lower gender equality report more depressive symptoms than those from regions with higher gender equality [9].

Data from the National Epidemiologic Survey on Alcohol and Related Conditions (NESARC) showed that gender discrimination in terms of gendered wage gap in the workforce explained a significant part of gender disparities in mood and anxiety disorders. This results were controlled by gender differences in individual-level productivity [6].

Results of an analysis of macro-level predictors including 56 surveys and 30 countries observed that gender-related structural factors such as male authority over women, gender discrimination in family law, lack of education or access to property or bank credit for women correlated with the prevalence of partner violence [6, 163].

17.3.4.2 Culture

Culture is described as the values, ideas and norms that shape human societies, and are transmitted to members of that specific society. It can have several components: art, technology, religion, traditions and the media. We will describe how media can determine the mental health of citizens.

There are two ways to relate to media; on one hand there is traditional media (movies, music, TV or magazines), which historically and still nowadays contains huge amount of sexual content that objectifies girls and women. On the other hand, social media acts differently, by encouraging the sexual engaging with others and punishing when sexual information is rebelled [6, 167].

Media consumption for adolescents and adults is correlated to depressive symptoms [167]. In girls and women, media consumption links self-objectification and body shame, which also predicts for depressive symptoms [9, 167]. For adolescent girls, opposite to adolescent boys, time spent on social media correlates significantly with depressive symptoms. By contrast, the same study observed that sports and exercise linked negatively with depressive symptoms for both girls and boys [6, 167]. On the contrary, data for minorities (black or lesbian women) and the use of social media correlated with wellbeing [6].

In summary, the media's effects depend on a variety of factors, which include individual factors (reasons for using media, ethnicity or sexual orientation) and media factors (sexualized portrayal of women and portrayal of the strong black ideal woman) [6].

17.4 Psychopharmacological Treatment

Knowledge about the physiologic differences between men and women is widening in the last decades. These differences provoke variations among the two sexes in pharmacokinetics, pharmacodynamics pharmacotoxicity and effectiveness [42, 168, 169]. However, the clinical prescription for men and women is usually at the very same dose [169, 170]. This is because in all the steps of pharmacological research the presence of female animals (rats, mice, humans or other mammals) has been and is historically underrepresented [42, 171]. Science has assumed that results in male and female individuals are equivalent, avoiding not only the presence of hormonal cycles, but also the possibility of pregnancy, childbirth or breastfeeding [172].

An estimated 15.9% of adult women in the US take antidepressants, compared to 7.7% of men [170].

The recognition of sex differences in the genetic susceptibility to depression has important implications for personalized medicine and treatment strategies. Recent findings have emphasized how biological differences, hormonal fluctuations, genetic predispositions and sociocultural factors all contribute to the distinct ways men and women experience and respond to depression treatments [42, 170]. Treatment of depression needs a multifaceted approach tailored to the individual patient's requirements. This means that it must associate, apart from the pharmacological treatment, psychoeducation and counselling/psychotherapy. When pharmacotherapy for depression is needed, the most commonly prescribed class of medications is the selective serotonin reuptake inhibitors (SSRI), followed by serotonin-noradrenaline reuptake inhibitors (SNRI), whereas tricyclic antidepressants and monoamine oxidase inhibitors have been progressively abandoned apart from some exceptions.

17.4.1 Sex Differences in Pharmacokinetics

Pharmacokinetics may be modified by sex differences in different levels, such as absorption, distribution, metabolism and drug excretion [173–175].

Gastric acid secretion and intestinal enzymatic activity are reduced in women and gastrointestinal motility is slower, which reduces the maximum concentration of medication in the blood [173]. In addition, drugs', and specifically antidepressants', bioavailability is bigger in women [42, 168]. Females have lower body weight and higher body fat mass, so the distribution of lipophilic structures, like antidepressants, is faster and broader, with lower redistribution rate and clearance [173–175]. The higher proportion of adipose tissue can lengthen the half-life of lipophilic drugs, such as trazodone and bupropion. Antidepressants' absorption and distribution are also influenced by hormonal fluctuations during menstrual cycles [176]. Furthermore, the free fraction of drug molecules is higher in women because antidepressants' binding to proteins is weakened [177].

P-glycoprotein (P-gp) is a drug transporter which plays a critical role in the absorption and distribution of antidepressants. It has been reported that a gender difference exists in the expression of P-gp so women express one-third to one-half of protein compared to men [178]. This is, in part, because the expression of multidrug resistance protein 1 (MDR1) gene expression is influenced by sex hormones, diminishing P-gp levels. This has several implications. We can find the P-gp inhibited by sex hormones in the gastrointestinal tract, increasing antidepressants absorption [179]. A higher absorption implies an increased blood concentration of the drug, and therefore a higher toxicity in women [179].

The P-glycoprotein (P-gp) transporter in the blood-brain barrier (BBB) is responsible for efflux of antidepressants, and consequently, for the effects of antidepressants in the brain [180]. Since women appear to express less P-gp protein, there are diminished brain levels of P-gp's substrates, such as venlafaxine, fluvoxamine or fluoxetine, among others [181].

The most important cytochromes (CYPs) in antidepressant metabolism are CYP2D6, CYP2C, CYP3A and CYP1A [180, 182], and it seems that there is a differential expression of CYPs among sexes [183]. CYP3A4's activity is increased in females, so its substrates, such as sertraline, citalopram, fluoxetine, escitalopram, amitriptyline, imipramine and clomipramine usually clear faster. On the contrary, cytochrome P450 2D6 (CYP2D6) clears faster in males for desipramine, and mirtazapine, the same as Cytochrome P450 1A2 (CYP1A2) for escitalopram to desmethylcitalopram and didesmethylcitalopram. Cytochrome P450 2B6 (CYP2B6) genotype and phenotype were only observed in women, and it is important for the metabolism of bupropion to its active metabolite hydroxybupropion. In the same way, CYP2C19 activity has also been evidenced to be diminished in women, and it has been also suggested that this may be a direct result of inhibition by oestrogen [184] and oral contraceptives [171, 185, 186].

Female sex hormones alter hepatic enzyme activity, which can result in decreased elimination and accumulation of some drugs. However, the way oestrogen and progesterone affect pharmacokinetics of drugs is hard to predict and assess, with studies yielding conflicting results [171, 174, 180]. Oestrogen is also a substrate for some of the same cytochrome P450 isozymes as antidepressants, and the presence of both can shift the metabolism for both. It seems that these differences may also be associated to genetic polymorphisms, comorbid illnesses, hormonal effects (including fluctuation during the menstrual cycle), interactions with other prescribed medications and epigenetic factors [42].

We can also find differences in medication excretion. The excretion depends on the molecule polarity: polar molecules are excreted through the kidneys and non-polar are metabolized in the liver. Both processes are affected by the decreased blood flow in females. This difference has been proposed to be the reason for the reduced metabolism of antidepressants in women [42]. Even though it is not regarded in guidelines it is well known that, at the same dose of antidepressant, women show higher blood levels of the drug.

17.4.2 Sex Differences in Pharmacodynamics

Pharmacodynamic differences are more difficult to evaluate, as pharmacological effects are difficult to measure.

Different researches have demonstrated that men have a better therapeutic response to tricyclic antidepressants (TCA) than women [42, 173]. For serotonine reuptake inhibitors (SSRI), monoamine oxidase inhibitors (MAOI) and serotonine/norepinephrine reuptake inhibitors (SNRI), are women who have a stronger antidepressant response than men [175]. The most used antidepressants, SSRI and SNRI, show that women were about 1.5 times more likely to accomplish remission than men [42]. However, the biggest antidepressant effect in women seems to be with SSRI.

The difference between genders is more common in the middle ages of life, before the menopause and out of the peripartum period. This is due to different factors, as we will see [187].

The genic (SLC6A4) expression of the serotonin transporter (5-HTTLPR) intensely influences the pharmacodynamics of SSRIs. There are three important allelic variants: the short one "S" was associated with a poorer response and non-remission to SSRI, particularly escitalopram, in men but not in women [188].

Hormones seem to have a role in the effectiveness of antidepressants: younger women (premenopausal) seem to be the ones that have the best response to antidepressants, specifically the serotoninergic ones. On the other hand, at post-menopausal period, when LH levels are high, women's response to antidepressants appears to be similar to what men show: they respond better to TCAs, such as imipramine, and less to fluvoxamine compared to younger female patients [189]. Furthermore, hormonal replacement therapy (HRT) (which decreases LH, FSH, and increases estradiol) or oestrogen replacement therapy (ERT) improve the response to SSRI antidepressants in postmenopausal women [190, 191]. This confirms the theory that administrating HRT or oestrogens (specifically 17-β estradiol) [189] in association with the antidepressant may be more efficacious than antidepressants alone and have a longer antidepressant effect. This synergic effect has also been confirmed with sertraline, fluoxetine and imipramine [42, 171, 188, 191].

Oestrogen treatment in perimenopausal and antidepressant naïve women demonstrated efficacy in depression. HRT of oestrogen in women at 40 years old with a recurrency in depression background was effective for depression [190]. LH levels correlate with the response to antidepressants in postmenopausal women, because lower LH levels correlate with higher serotonin levels at baseline [42].

Oestrogen promotes the growth of dendritic spines in neurons and the liberation of neurotrophic factors. It influences the synthesis of serotonin and the expression and binding of the molecule to transporter receptors which have a direct impact on SSRIs' efficacy [41, 65, 192]. This can be an explanation of why women in their reproductive period are more responsive to SSRIs and SNRIs. Additionally, women produce less cortisol and more tryptophan if exposed to SSRIs.

Another explanation may be that the subtype of depression can modify the response to antidepressant drugs [192]. As we have seen, the clinical presentation is different between genders, where women tend to exhibit more somatic and atypical symptoms, which seem to respond better to SSRIs, as women do [192].

Physiologically, patients with lower body weight, more frequent among women, respond better to fluoxetine [187]. Additionally, the magnitude of the effect of body weight on antidepressant activity seems to be related to gender. Obese men did not respond to any of the tested SSRIs better than a placebo, whereas obese women showed superior response [171, 192].

We can also find differences in augmentation strategies (drugs which primarily have other indications but are used to increase the effect of antidepressants). Apart from HRT and ERT, adding triiodothyronine (T3), lithium and stimulants seems to be more effective to increase the antidepressive effect of antidepressants in women compared to men [192]. Women also are more benefited by the use of folic acid and association with benzodizepines [171, 173].

On the other hand, men appear to have a better antidepressant response when testosterone is added to treatment [91].

17.4.3 Sex Differences in Side Effects of Antidepressants

Women experience more frequent and intense side effects than men, very likely in correlation with higher drug blood concentrations [42].

Weight gain is more common only in women (not men) who had been prescribed SSRI for at least 90 days. Women also suffer more nausea and reduced libido [192].

On the contrary, men are more prone to develop indigestion, sexual dysfunction and urinary tract disorders during antidepressant treatment.

Women show decreased tolerability of TCAs and tend to report side effects, such as nausea, constipation, dizziness, somnolence and abnormal vision [42].

Women are more likely to experience anticholinergic effects (such as dry mouth, constipation and blurred vision), while men may be more prone to orthostatic hypotension (a sudden drop in blood pressure upon standing) [42, 173].

Women suffering from dysthymia present more intense withdrawal symptoms after discontinuing paroxetine compared to men [193].

17.4.4 Sex Differences by Groups of Antidepressants

Tricyclic Antidepressants (TCA)

Pharmacokinetic studies report that TCA blood levels (imipramine, nortriptyline and desipramine) are reportedly higher in women [171, 192]. Probably because of that, females have increased rates of secondary effects and tolerate TCAs worst.

The receptor mechanism for TCAs is inhibiting the reuptake of noradrenaline and serotonin, but they also antagonize postsynaptic 1-adrenoceptors, histamine (H1) receptors, muscarinic cholinergic receptors and serotonin (5-HT2) receptors, resulting in a different side effect. Anticholinergic effects include sweating, dry mouth, constipation, tremor and sedation. It is described that these anticholinergic side effects are more acceptable in men than in women [42].

All these, the more side effects and the less acceptance of them in women, explain why women are nearly three times more likely to cease treatment with imipramine than with sertraline, whereas men showed similar cessation rates [75, 76].

Selective Serotonin Reuptake Inhibitors (SSRIs)

At the reproductive age women's response to SSRI is twice as high compared to men. The explanations proposed are several. First, Oestrogen modulates the synthesis of serotonin and the transcription and function of its transporter. Particularly in those with polymorphisms in the gene coding for serotonin transporter (SLC6A4), which are more likely to respond to SSRIs than men with similar genetic profiles [42, 175]. The short "S" allelic variant for 5-HTTLPR was associated with a poorer response and non-remission to SSRI [9]. This suggests that hormonal fluctuations, such as those experienced during the menstrual cycle, pregnancy or menopause, may modulate how women respond to SSRI treatment.

Second, SSRI may induce the activity of 3-alpha reductase, which synthesizes anxiolytic metabolites allopregnanolone (3-alpha, 5-alpha metabolite of progesterone) and the metabolites of androstanedione and dihydrotestosterone. These metabolites boost the improvement of depressive symptoms [175].

In case of chronic depression, recent studies have found that females respond more favourably to sertraline and to fluoxetine than men [175].

Females metabolize SSRIs slower than males, which apart from contributing to increased drug efficacy induces a higher risk of side effects, such as weight gain, sexual dysfunction and insomnia. Weight gain was observed only in women (not in men) who had received treatment for at least 90 days with SSRI [118, 119].

Serotonin-Norepinephrine Reuptake Inhibitors (SNRIs)

Serotonine/norepinephrine reuptake inhibitors (SNRIs) increase both serotonin and norepinephrine levels in the brain. Women respond more to SNRIs than men, but in a smaller magnitude than SSRI. Women also experience a more rapid symptom improvement compared to men [175]. It is proposed that women may have an increased sensitivity to norepinephrine because of oestrogen-associated changes.

The influence of sex on serum levels of venlafaxine and its metabolite has been determined and found that women have 30% higher levels of venlafaxine and its metabolite *O*-desmethylvenlafaxine than men. Despite these results, research has not found sex difference between women and men treated with venlafaxine [42].

Maybe because of the higher blood levels, SNRIs also have more pronounced side effects in women, such as nausea, fatigue and sexual dysfunction, which are often more intense than in men [175].

17.5 Psychotherapy: Gender-Specific Approaches and Effectiveness

Women tend to use psychotherapy more often than men. In addition, they ask for help and are committed to treatment with far less difficulty than men. The way feminine gender is thought to deal with emotions makes women more prone to attend psychotherapy.

Psychotherapy, therefore, must take into account the gender perspective and therapist should discuss and analyse their cultural burden when treating men, women or trans individuals.

Psychotherapy can be conducted alone or with associated psychopharmacological treatment. When antidepressants are prescribed with psychotherapy, the pharmacological response is bigger [175].

17.5.1 Cognitive Behavioural Therapy (CBT)

Cognitive behavioural therapy (CBT) is a widely used psychotherapy for depression. Research has demonstrated that both men and women benefit from CBT, but gender differences influence how they engage with and respond to the treatment. For CBT, educational, behavioural assignments and cognitive structures are the target, and these are highly correlated with psychosocial structures and gender bias.

Women's greater emotional expressiveness may influence their response to CBT; women tend to engage more actively with the cognitive restructuring component of CBT and are more likely to report improvements in emotion regulation and self-esteem. Socialized gender roles may contribute to this increased willingness to discuss emotions and internal conflicts during therapy [130].

For men, however, research suggests that the cognitive restructuring component of CBT may be less effective unless combined with more action-oriented strategies. Men respond better to a more structured, problem-solving approach that focuses on concrete goals and tasks rather than introspective emotional exploration. Male patients may find it difficult to engage in therapies that ask them to delve deeply into emotions, potentially due to societal expectations of masculinity, which discourage emotional vulnerability [123, 147].

In a more plausible analysis comparing cognitive behaviour therapy (CBT) with pharmacotherapy and comparing either CBT or pharmacotherapy with placebo, no sex-modulating effects on treatment were detected regardless of therapeutic intervention.

17.5.2 Interpersonal Therapy (IPT)

Interpersonal therapy (IPT) focuses on improving interpersonal relationships and social functioning and has demonstrated to be effective in acute treatment of depression. IPT directs its efforts to address interpersonal difficulties such as interpersonal loss or grieving, role transitions, interpersonal disputes and social deficits. Depressed women could benefit from IPT since they are often more affected by interpersonal stress such as relationship difficulties or caregiving stress [68, 87].

17.5.3 Mindfulness-Based Cognitive Therapy (MBCT)

Mindfulness-based cognitive therapy (MBCT) is another effective treatment for depression that combines cognitive therapy with mindfulness practices. Women seem to benefit more than men from MBCT [194]. The reason for it may be that women tend to have a more ruminative style of thinking and that is what MBCT specifically addresses.

In contrast, men may show lower adherence to mindfulness-based therapies, possibly due to cultural norms that discourage practices perceived as "soft" or "emotionally vulnerable." However, integrating structured action steps within MBCT may improve engagement and outcomes for men.

17.6 Transcranial Magnetic Stimulation (TMS)

Transcranial magnetic stimulation (TMS) is a non-invasive brain stimulation treatment that has shown effectiveness for depression. Women have better response to TMS than men, and Hanlon and McCalley [195] propose it may be due to three reasons: (1) closer proximity of the brain to the scalp at the prefrontal cortex, leading to larger TMS-induced electric fields especially at the medial prefrontal cortex, (2) greater grey matter density and gyrification in the prefrontal cortex and (3) high levels of estradiol which facilitate cortical excitability [195].

17.7 Conclusions

Epidemiological research has demonstrated important sex-related differences in the onset, prevalence and clinical symptomatology of depression. The reason for this imbalance is contributed by several factors. Biological factors are undeniable: the sexual differences include genetics, brain regions and functional hormones, stress response systems and the immune system. Psychological factors include both affective factors as neuroticism and cognitive factors, such as negative cognitive style, objectified body conscious and rumination. Environmental and sociocultural factors refer to the systematic violence against women and how it is suffered individually and collectively.

It is obvious that the factors described are interconnected in a multidirectional way that makes it very difficult to investigate. There are also differences in pharmacokinetics, pharmacodynamics and in side effects of antidepressant drugs.

Based on all this observed data, it is important that medicine and investigation teams develop researches that highlight the sex differences and the age differences by sex. Women are exposed to periods of particular vulnerability to MDD, associated with hormone alterations that cannot be found in men. All this taken into account, we should move towards a more inclusive and patient-dependent medicine.

References

1. American Psychiatric Association (APA). Diagnostic and statistical manual of mental disorders: DSM-5™. 5th ed. Arlington: American Psychiatric Publishing, Inc; 2013. xliv, 947 p.
2. Ferrari AJ, Santomauro DF, Aali A, Abate YH, Abbafati C, Abbastabar H, et al. Global incidence, prevalence, years lived with disability (YLDs), disability-adjusted life-years (DALYs), and healthy life expectancy (HALE) for 371 diseases and injuries in 204 countries and territories and 811 subnational locations, 1990–2021: a systematic analysis for the Global Burden of Disease Study 2021. Lancet. 2024;403(10440):2133–61.
3. GBD 2019 Mental Disorders Collaborators. Global, regional, and national burden of 12 mental disorders in 204 countries and territories, 1990–2019: a systematic analysis for the Global Burden of Disease Study 2019. Lancet Psychiatry. 2022;9(2):137–50.
4. Impact of major depressive disorder on comorbidities: a systematic literature review. Psychiatrist.com [Internet]. [cited 2025 Apr 2]. Available from: https://www.psychiatrist.com/jcp/impact-major-depressive-disorder-comorbidities-systematic-literature-review/.
5. Pavlidi P, Kokras N, Dalla C. Antidepressants' effects on testosterone and estrogens: what do we know? Eur J Pharmacol. 2021;899:173998.
6. Hyde JS, Mezulis AH. Gender differences in depression: biological, affective, cognitive, and sociocultural factors. Harv Rev Psychiatry. 2020;28(1):4–13.
7. Di Benedetto MG, Landi P, Mencacci C, Cattaneo A. Depression in women: potential biological and sociocultural factors driving the sex effect. Neuropsychobiology. 2024;83(1):2–16.
8. Klein DN, Shankman SA, Lewinsohn PM, Seeley JR. Subthreshold depressive disorder in adolescents: predictors of escalation to full-syndrome depressive disorders. J Am Acad Child Adolesc Psychiatry. 2009;48(7):703–10.
9. Kuehner C. Why is depression more common among women than among men? Lancet Psychiatry. 2017;4(2):146–58.
10. Flint J, Kendler KS. The genetics of major depression. Neuron. 2014;81(3):484–503.
11. Institute of Health Metrics and Evaluation. Global Health Data Exchange (GHDx) [Internet]. 2023. Available from: https://vizhub.healthdata.org/gbd-results/.
12. World Health Organization. Depression and other common mental disorders: global health estimates. Geneva: World Health Organization; 2017.
13. de la Torre JA, Vilagut G, Ronaldson A, Bakolis I, Dregan A, Martín V, et al. Prevalence and variability of depressive symptoms in Europe: update using representative data from the second and third waves of the European Health Interview Survey (EHIS-2 and EHIS-3). Lancet Public Health. 2023;8(11):e889–98.
14. Seedat S, Scott KM, Angermeyer MC, Berglund P, Bromet EJ, Brugha TS, et al. Cross-national associations between gender and mental disorders in the World Health Organization World Mental Health Surveys. Arch Gen Psychiatry. 2009;66(7):785–95.
15. McGuire FH, Beccia AL, Peoples JE, Williams MR, Schuler MS, Duncan AE. Depression at the intersection of race/ethnicity, sex/gender, and sexual orientation in a nationally representative sample of US adults: a design-weighted intersectional MAIHDA. Am J Epidemiol. 2024;193(12):1662–74.

16. Treatment and management of mental health conditions during pregnancy and postpartum: ACOG Clinical Practice Guideline No. 5. Obstet Gynecol. 2023;141(6):1262–88.
17. Hankin BL. Development of sex differences in depressive and co-occurring anxious symptoms during adolescence: descriptive trajectories and potential explanations in a multiwave prospective study. J Clin Child Adolesc Psychol. 2009;38(4):460–72.
18. Lu J, Xu X, Huang Y, Li T, Ma C, Xu G, et al. Prevalence of depressive disorders and treatment in China: a cross-sectional epidemiological study. Lancet Psychiatry. 2021;8(11):981–90.
19. Lewinsohn PM, Solomon A, Seeley JR, Zeiss A. Clinical implications of 'subthreshold' depressive symptoms. J Abnorm Psychol. 2000;109(2):345–51.
20. Salk RH, Hyde JS, Abramson LY. Gender differences in depression in representative national samples: meta-analyses of diagnoses and symptoms. Psychol Bull. 2017;143(8):783–822.
21. Kulkarni J. Perimenopausal depression – an under-recognised entity. Aust Prescr. 2018;41(6):183–5.
22. Turek J, Gąsior Ł. Estrogen fluctuations during the menopausal transition are a risk factor for depressive disorders. Pharmacol Rep. 2023;75(1):32–43.
23. Kapoor E, Okuno M, Miller VM, Rocca LG, Rocca WA, Kling JM, et al. Association of adverse childhood experiences with menopausal symptoms: results from the Data Registry on Experiences of Aging, Menopause and Sexuality (DREAMS). Maturitas. 2021;143:209–15.
24. Schramm E, Klein DN, Elsaesser M, Furukawa TA, Domschke K. Review of dysthymia and persistent depressive disorder: history, correlates, and clinical implications. Lancet Psychiatry. 2020;7(9):801–12.
25. Bromet E, Andrade LH, Hwang I, Sampson NA, Alonso J, de Girolamo G, et al. Cross-national epidemiology of DSM-IV major depressive episode. BMC Med. 2011;9:90.
26. COVID-19 Mental Disorders Collaborators. Global prevalence and burden of depressive and anxiety disorders in 204 countries and territories in 2020 due to the COVID-19 pandemic. Lancet. 2021;398(10312):1700–12.
27. Thompson EJ, Stafford J, Moltrecht B, Huggins CF, Kwong ASF, Shaw RJ, et al. Psychological distress, depression, anxiety, and life satisfaction following COVID-19 infection: evidence from 11 UK longitudinal population studies. Lancet Psychiatry. 2022;9(11):894–906.
28. Fang H, Tu S, Sheng J, Shao A. Depression in sleep disturbance: a review on a bidirectional relationship, mechanisms and treatment. J Cell Mol Med. 2019;23(4):2324–32.
29. Kuehner C. Gender differences in unipolar depression: an update of epidemiological findings and possible explanations. Acta Psychiatr Scand. 2003;108(3):163–74.
30. Mackenzie CS, El-Gabalawy R, Chou KL, Sareen J. Prevalence and predictors of persistent versus remitting mood, anxiety, and substance disorders in a national sample of older adults. Am J Geriatr Psychiatry. 2014;22(9):854–65.
31. Penninx BWJH, Nolen WA, Lamers F, Zitman FG, Smit JH, Spinhoven P, et al. Two-year course of depressive and anxiety disorders: results from the Netherlands Study of Depression and Anxiety (NESDA). J Affect Disord. 2011;133(1–2):76–85.
32. World Health Organization. Suicide worldwide in 2019: global health estimates. Geneva: World Health Organization; 2021.
33. Bangasser DA, Valentino RJ. Sex differences in stress-related psychiatric disorders: neurobiological perspectives. Front Neuroendocrinol. 2014;35(3):303–19.
34. Davies SJC, Pearson RM, Stapinski L, Bould H, Christmas DM, Button KS, et al. Symptoms of generalized anxiety disorder but not panic disorder at age 15 years increase the risk of depression at 18 years in the Avon Longitudinal Study of Parents and Children (ALSPAC) cohort study. Psychol Med. 2016;46(1):73–85.
35. Sullivan PF, Neale MC, Kendler KS. Genetic epidemiology of major depression: review and meta-analysis. Am J Psychiatry. 2000;157(10):1552–62.
36. Docherty AR, Mullins N, Ashley-Koch AE, Qin X, Coleman JRI, Shabalin A, et al. GWAS meta-analysis of suicide attempt: identification of 12 genome-wide significant loci and implication of genetic risks for specific health factors. Am J Psychiatry. 2023;180(10):723–38.
37. Kendler KS, Ohlsson H, Sundquist J, Sundquist K. Risk for mood, anxiety, and psychotic disorders in individuals at high and low genetic liability for bipolar disorder and major depression. JAMA Psychiatry. 2022;79(11):1102–9.

38. Wray NR, Ripke S, Mattheisen M, Trzaskowski M, Byrne EM, Abdellaoui A, et al. Genome-wide association analyses identify 44 risk variants and refine the genetic architecture of major depression. Nat Genet. 2018;50(5):668–81.
39. Flint J, Kendler KS. The genetics of major depression. Neuron. 2014;81(5):1214.
40. Peterson RE, Kuchenbaecker K, Walters RK, Chen CY, Popejoy AB, Periyasamy S, et al. Genome-wide association studies in ancestrally diverse populations: opportunities, methods, pitfalls, and recommendations. Cell. 2019;179(3):589–603.
41. Iqbal J, Huang GD, Xue YX, Yang M, Jia XJ. Role of estrogen in sex differences in memory, emotion and neuropsychiatric disorders. Mol Biol Rep. 2024;51(1):415.
42. Pavlidi P, Kokras N, Dalla C. Sex differences in depression and anxiety. In: Sex differences in brain function and dysfunction. Cham: Springer International Publishing; 2022. p. 103–32.
43. Labonté B, Engmann O, Purushothaman I, Menard C, Wang J, Tan C, et al. Sex-specific transcriptional signatures in human depression. Nat Med. 2017;23(9):1102–11.
44. Seney ML, Glausier J, Sibille E. Large-scale transcriptomics studies provide insight into sex differences in depression. Biol Psychiatry. 2022;91(1):14–24.
45. Kong X, Jin F, Tang G, Qin Y, Liu D, Sun J. Causality between neuroticism personality clusters and female reproductive diseases in European population: a two-sample bidirectional Mendelian randomization study. BMC Womens Health. 2024;24(1):507.
46. Seney ML, Huo Z, Cahill K, French L, Puralewski R, Zhang J, et al. Opposite molecular signatures of depression in men and women. Biol Psychiatry. 2018;84(1):18–27.
47. Peterson RE, Cai N, Dahl AW, Bigdeli TB, Edwards AC, Webb BT, et al. Molecular genetic analysis subdivided by adversity exposure suggests etiologic heterogeneity in major depression. Am J Psychiatry. 2018;175(6):545–54.
48. Hodes GE, Walker DM, Labonté B, Nestler EJ, Russo SJ. Understanding the epigenetic basis of sex differences in depression. J Neurosci Res. 2017;95(1–2):692–702.
49. Caspi A, Sugden K, Moffitt TE, Taylor A, Craig IW, Harrington H, et al. Influence of life stress on depression: moderation by a polymorphism in the 5-HTT gene. Science. 2003;301(5631):386–9.
50. Sharpley CF, Palanisamy SKA, Glyde NS, Dillingham PW, Agnew LL. An update on the interaction between the serotonin transporter promoter variant (5-HTTLPR), stress and depression, plus an exploration of non-confirming findings. Behav Brain Res. 2014;273:89–105.
51. Gressier F, Calati R, Serretti A. 5-HTTLPR and gender differences in affective disorders: a systematic review. J Affect Disord. 2016;190:193–207.
52. VanZomeren-Dohm AA, Pitula CE, Koss KJ, Thomas K, Gunnar MR. FKBP5 moderation of depressive symptoms in peer victimized, post-institutionalized children. Psychoneuroendocrinology. 2015;51:426–30.
53. Heim C, Bradley B, Mletzko TC, Deveau TC, Musselman DL, Nemeroff CB, et al. Effect of childhood trauma on adult depression and neuroendocrine function: sex-specific moderation by CRH receptor 1 gene. Front Behav Neurosci. 2009;3:41.
54. Eliot L, Ahmed A, Khan H, Patel J. Dump the 'dimorphism': comprehensive synthesis of human brain studies reveals few male-female differences beyond size. Neurosci Biobehav Rev. 2021;125:667–97.
55. de Jong LW, Vidal JS, Forsberg LE, Zijdenbos AP, Haight T, Alzheimer's Disease Neuroimaging Initiative, et al. Allometric scaling of brain regions to intra-cranial volume: an epidemiological MRI study. Hum Brain Mapp. 2017;38(1):151–64.
56. Ruigrok ANV, Salimi-Khorshidi G, Lai MC, Baron-Cohen S, Lombardo MV, Tait RJ, et al. A meta-analysis of sex differences in human brain structure. Neurosci Biobehav Rev. 2014;39:34–50.
57. Yang X, Peng Z, Ma X, Meng Y, Li M, Zhang J, et al. Sex differences in the clinical characteristics and brain gray matter volume alterations in unmedicated patients with major depressive disorder. Sci Rep. 2017;7(1):2515.
58. Tan A, Ma W, Vira A, Marwha D, Eliot L. The human hippocampus is not sexually-dimorphic: meta-analysis of structural MRI volumes. NeuroImage. 2016;124(Pt A):350–66.
59. Frodl T, Meisenzahl EM, Zetzsche T, Born C, Groll C, Jäger M, et al. Hippocampal changes in patients with a first episode of major depression. Am J Psychiatry. 2002;159(7):1112–8.

60. McKinnon MC, Yucel K, Nazarov A, MacQueen GM. A meta-analysis examining clinical predictors of hippocampal volume in patients with major depressive disorder. J Psychiatry Neurosci. 2009;34(1):41–54.
61. Hu X, Zhang L, Liang K, Cao L, Liu J, Li H, et al. Sex-specific alterations of cortical morphometry in treatment-naïve patients with major depressive disorder. Neuropsychopharmacology. 2022;47(11):2002–9.
62. Mohammadi S, Seyedmirzaei H, Salehi MA, Jahanshahi A, Zakavi SS, Dehghani Firouzabadi F, et al. Brain-based sex differences in depression: a systematic review of neuroimaging studies. Brain Imaging Behav. 2023;17(5):541–69.
63. Lyon M, Welton T, Varda A, Maller JJ, Broadhouse K, Korgaonkar MS, et al. Gender-specific structural abnormalities in major depressive disorder revealed by fixel-based analysis. Neuroimage Clin. 2019;21:101668.
64. Piani MC, Maggioni E, Delvecchio G, Ferro A, Gritti D, Pozzoli SM, et al. Sexual dimorphism in the brain correlates of adult-onset depression: a pilot structural and functional 3T MRI study. Front Psychiatry. 2021;12:683912.
65. Heldring N, Pike A, Andersson S, Matthews J, Cheng G, Hartman J, et al. Estrogen receptors: how do they signal and what are their targets. Physiol Rev. 2007;87(3):905–31.
66. González-Orozco JC, Camacho-Arroyo I. Progesterone actions during central nervous system development. Front Neurosci. 2019;13:503.
67. Barth C, Villringer A, Sacher J. Sex hormones affect neurotransmitters and shape the adult female brain during hormonal transition periods. Front Neurosci. 2015;9:37.
68. Kundakovic M, Rocks D. Sex hormone fluctuation and increased female risk for depression and anxiety disorders: from clinical evidence to molecular mechanisms. Front Neuroendocrinol. 2022;66:101010.
69. Dubol M, Epperson CN, Sacher J, Pletzer B, Derntl B, Lanzenberger R, et al. Neuroimaging the menstrual cycle: a multimodal systematic review. Front Neuroendocrinol. 2021;60:100878.
70. Albert K, Pruessner J, Newhouse P. Estradiol levels modulate brain activity and negative responses to psychosocial stress across the menstrual cycle. Psychoneuroendocrinology. 2015;59:14–24.
71. Chhibber A, Woody SK, Karim Rumi MA, Soares MJ, Zhao L. Estrogen receptor β deficiency impairs BDNF-5-HT2A signaling in the hippocampus of female brain: a possible mechanism for menopausal depression. Psychoneuroendocrinology. 2017;82:107–16.
72. Frokjaer VG, Pinborg A, Holst KK, Overgaard A, Henningsson S, Heede M, et al. Role of serotonin transporter changes in depressive responses to sex-steroid hormone manipulation: a positron emission tomography study. Biol Psychiatry. 2015;78(8):534–43.
73. Levey DF, Gelernter J, Polimanti R, Zhou H, Cheng Z, Aslan M, et al. Reproducible genetic risk loci for anxiety: results from ~200,000 participants in the million veteran program. Am J Psychiatry. 2020;177(3):223–32.
74. Li C, Xie M, Wang W, Liu Y, Liao D, Yin J, et al. Association between polymorphisms in estrogen receptor genes and depression in women: a meta-analysis. Front Genet. 2022;13:936296.
75. Borrow AP, Cameron NM. Estrogenic mediation of serotonergic and neurotrophic systems: implications for female mood disorders. Prog Neuro-Psychopharmacol Biol Psychiatry. 2014;54:13–25.
76. Singh M, Su C. Progesterone and neuroprotection. Horm Behav. 2013;63(2):284–90.
77. Hantsoo L, Payne JL. Towards understanding the biology of premenstrual dysphoric disorder: from genes to GABA. Neurosci Biobehav Rev. 2023;149:105168.
78. Fechner PY. Gender differences in puberty. J Adolesc Health. 2002;30(4 Suppl):44–8.
79. De Rose L, Wright AJ, Brooks-Gunn J. Does puberty account for the gender differential in depression. In: Women and depression: a handbook for the social, behavioral, and biomedical sciences. New York: Cambridge University Press; 2006. p. 89–128.
80. McCormick CM, Mathews IZ. HPA function in adolescence: role of sex hormones in its regulation and the enduring consequences of exposure to stressors. Pharmacol Biochem Behav. 2007;86(2):220–33.
81. Hofmeister S, Bodden S. Premenstrual syndrome and premenstrual dysphoric disorder. Am Fam Physician. 2016;94(3):236–40.

82. Dennerstein L, Lehert P, Heinemann K. Epidemiology of premenstrual symptoms and disorders. Menopause Int. 2012;18(2):48–51.
83. Reed BG, Carr BR. The normal menstrual cycle and the control of ovulation. In: Feingold KR, Ahmed SF, Anawalt B, Blackman MR, Boyce A, Chrousos G, et al., editors. Endotext [Internet]. South Dartmouth (MA): MDText.com, Inc.; 2000 [cited 2025 May 5]. Available from: http://www.ncbi.nlm.nih.gov/books/NBK279054/.
84. Beddig T, Reinhard I, Kuehner C. Stress, mood, and cortisol during daily life in women with Premenstrual Dysphoric Disorder (PMDD). Psychoneuroendocrinology. 2019;109:104372.
85. Kuehner C, Nayman S. Premenstrual exacerbations of mood disorders: findings and knowledge gaps. Curr Psychiatry Rep. 2021;23(11):78.
86. Beddig T, Reinhard I, Ebner-Priemer U, Kuehner C. Reciprocal effects between cognitive and affective states in women with Premenstrual Dysphoric Disorder: an Ecological Momentary Assessment study. Behav Res Ther. 2020;131:103613.
87. Ghaedrahmati M, Kazemi A, Kheirabadi G, Ebrahimi A, Bahrami M. Postpartum depression risk factors: a narrative review. J Educ Health Promot. 2017;6:60.
88. Research on the menopause in the 1990s. Report of a WHO Scientific Group – PubMed [Internet]. [cited 2025 May 5]. Available from: https://pubmed.ncbi.nlm.nih.gov/8942292/.
89. Lc S, Aa O. Andropause (male menopause): valid concepts, fables and controversies. Univ Lagos J Basic Med Sci [Internet]. 2022 [cited 2025 May 5];1(1). Available from: https://www.jbms.unilag.ng/index.php/jbms/article/view/113.
90. Maharjan DT, Syed AAS, Lin GN, Ying W. Testosterone in female depression: a meta-analysis and Mendelian randomization study. Biomolecules. 2021;11(3):409.
91. Walther A, Breidenstein J, Miller R. Association of testosterone treatment with alleviation of depressive symptoms in men: a systematic review and meta-analysis. JAMA Psychiatry. 2019;76(1):31–40.
92. Ceruso A, Martínez-Cengotitabengoa M, Peters-Corbett A, Diaz-Gutierrez MJ, Martínez-Cengotitabengoa M. Alterations of the HPA axis observed in patients with major depressive disorder and their relation to early life stress: a systematic review. Neuropsychobiology. 2020;79(6):417–27.
93. Oldehinkel AJ, Bouma EMC. Sensitivity to the depressogenic effect of stress and HPA-axis reactivity in adolescence: a review of gender differences. Neurosci Biobehav Rev. 2011;35(8):1757–70.
94. Kajantie E, Phillips DIW. The effects of sex and hormonal status on the physiological response to acute psychosocial stress. Psychoneuroendocrinology. 2006;31(2):151–78.
95. Hillerer KM, Slattery DA, Pletzer B. Neurobiological mechanisms underlying sex-related differences in stress-related disorders: effects of neuroactive steroids on the hippocampus. Front Neuroendocrinol. 2019;55:100796.
96. Kendler KS, Gardner CO. Sex differences in the pathways to major depression: a study of opposite-sex twin pairs. Am J Psychiatry. 2014;171(4):426–35.
97. Fattore L. Reward processing and drug addiction: does sex matter? Front Neurosci. 2015;9:329.
98. Powers SI, Laurent HK, Gunlicks-Stoessel M, Balaban S, Bent E. Depression and anxiety predict sex-specific cortisol responses to interpersonal stress. Psychoneuroendocrinology. 2016;69:172–9.
99. Young EA, Carlson NE, Brown MB. Twenty-four-hour ACTH and cortisol pulsatility in depressed women. Neuropsychopharmacology. 2001;25(2):267–76.
100. Stroud LR, Salovey P, Epel ES. Sex differences in stress responses: social rejection versus achievement stress. Biol Psychiatry. 2002;52(4):318–27.
101. Peeters F, Nicholson NA, Berkhof J. Cortisol responses to daily events in major depressive disorder. Psychosom Med. 2003;65(5):836–41.
102. McKay MS, Zakzanis KK. The impact of treatment on HPA axis activity in unipolar major depression. J Psychiatr Res. 2010;44(3):183–92.
103. Mikulska J, Juszczyk G, Gawrońska-Grzywacz M, Herbet M. HPA axis in the pathomechanism of depression and schizophrenia: new therapeutic strategies based on its participation. Brain Sci. 2021;11(10):1298.

104. Lei AA, Phang VWX, Lee YZ, Kow ASF, Tham CL, Ho YC, et al. Chronic stress-associated depressive disorders: the impact of HPA axis dysregulation and neuroinflammation on the hippocampus—a mini review. Int J Mol Sci. 2025;26(7):2940.
105. Huang Y, Zhou R, Wu M, Wang Q, Zhao Y. Premenstrual syndrome is associated with blunted cortisol reactivity to the TSST. Stress. 2015;18(2):160–8.
106. Blanco C, Vesga-López O, Stewart JW, Liu SM, Grant BF, Hasin DS. Epidemiology of major depression with atypical features: results from the National Epidemiologic Survey on Alcohol and Related Conditions (NESARC). J Clin Psychiatry. 2012;73(2):224–32.
107. Lamers F, Vogelzangs N, Merikangas KR, de Jonge P, Beekman ATF, Penninx BWJH. Evidence for a differential role of HPA-axis function, inflammation and metabolic syndrome in melancholic versus atypical depression. Mol Psychiatry. 2013;18(6):692–9.
108. Stadtler H, Neigh GN. Sex differences in the neurobiology of stress. Psychiatr Clin North Am. 2023;46(3):427–46.
109. Jeon SW, Kim YK. Neuroinflammation and cytokine abnormality in major depression: cause or consequence in that illness? World J Psychiatry. 2016;6(3):283–93.
110. Remus JL, Dantzer R. Inflammation models of depression in rodents: relevance to psychotropic drug discovery. Int J Neuropsychopharmacol. 2016;19(9):pyw028.
111. Miller AH, Raison CL. The role of inflammation in depression: from evolutionary imperative to modern treatment target. Nat Rev Immunol. 2016;16(1):22–34.
112. Ganguly P, Brenhouse HC. Broken or maladaptive? Altered trajectories in neuroinflammation and behavior after early life adversity. Dev Cogn Neurosci. 2015;11:18–30.
113. Ramirez K, Fornaguera-Trías J, Sheridan JF. Stress-induced microglia activation and monocyte trafficking to the brain underlie the development of anxiety and depression. Curr Top Behav Neurosci. 2017;31:155–72.
114. Osimo EF, Pillinger T, Rodriguez IM, Khandaker GM, Pariante CM, Howes OD. Inflammatory markers in depression: a meta-analysis of mean differences and variability in 5,166 patients and 5,083 controls. Brain Behav Immun. 2020;87:901–9.
115. Kokras N, Stamouli E, Sotiropoulos I, Katirtzoglou EA, Siarkos KT, Dalagiorgou G, et al. Acetyl cholinesterase inhibitors and cell-derived peripheral inflammatory cytokines in early stages of Alzheimer's disease. J Clin Psychopharmacol. 2018;38(2):138–43.
116. Rainville JR, Tsyglakova M, Hodes GE. Deciphering sex differences in the immune system and depression. Front Neuroendocrinol. 2018;50:67–90.
117. Yanguas-Casás N. Physiological sex differences in microglia and their relevance in neurological disorders. Neuroimmunol Neuroinflamm. 2020;7(1):13–22.
118. Han J, Fan Y, Zhou K, Blomgren K, Harris RA. Uncovering sex differences of rodent microglia. J Neuroinflammation. 2021;18(1):74.
119. Souyris M, Cenac C, Azar P, Daviaud D, Canivet A, Grunenwald S, et al. TLR7 escapes X chromosome inactivation in immune cells. Sci Immunol. 2018;3(19):eaap8855.
120. Villa A, Della Torre S, Maggi A. Sexual differentiation of microglia. Front Neuroendocrinol. 2019;52:156–64.
121. Birur B, Amrock EM, Shelton RC, Li L. Sex differences in the peripheral immune system in patients with depression. Front Psych. 2017;8:108.
122. Köhler-Forsberg O, Buttenschøn HN, Tansey KE, Maier W, Hauser J, Dernovsek MZ, et al. Association between C-reactive protein (CRP) with depression symptom severity and specific depressive symptoms in major depression. Brain Behav Immun. 2017;62:344–50.
123. Moieni M, Irwin MR, Jevtic I, Olmstead R, Breen EC, Eisenberger NI. Sex differences in depressive and socioemotional responses to an inflammatory challenge: implications for sex differences in depression. Neuropsychopharmacology. 2015;40(7):1709–16.
124. Lengua LJ, West SG, Sandler IN. Temperament as a predictor of symptomatology in children: addressing contamination of measures. Child Dev. 1998;69(1):164–81.
125. Sherman BJ, Vousoura E, Wickramaratne P, Warner V, Verdeli H. Temperament and major depression: how does difficult temperament affect frequency, severity, and duration of major depressive episodes among offspring of parents with or without depression? J Affect Disord. 2016;200:82–8.

126. Hyde JS, Mezulis AH, Abramson LY. The ABCs of depression: integrating affective, biological, and cognitive models to explain the emergence of the gender difference in depression. Psychol Rev. 2008;115(2):291–313.
127. Else-Quest NM, Hyde JS, Goldsmith HH, Van Hulle CA. Gender differences in temperament: a meta-analysis. Psychol Bull. 2006;132(1):33–72.
128. Costa PT, Terracciano A, McCrae RR. Gender differences in personality traits across cultures: robust and surprising findings. J Pers Soc Psychol. 2001;81(2):322–31.
129. Balzer BWR, Duke SA, Hawke CI, Steinbeck KS. The effects of estradiol on mood and behavior in human female adolescents: a systematic review. Eur J Pediatr. 2015;174(3):289–98.
130. Mezulis A, Salk RH, Hyde JS, Priess-Groben HA, Simonson JL. Affective, biological, and cognitive predictors of depressive symptom trajectories in adolescence. J Abnorm Child Psychol. 2014;42(4):539–50.
131. Klein DN, Kotov R, Bufferd SJ. Personality and depression: explanatory models and review of the evidence. Annu Rev Clin Psychol. 2011;7:269–95.
132. Wetter EK, Hankin BL. Mediational pathways through which positive and negative emotionality contribute to anhedonic symptoms of depression: a prospective study of adolescents. J Abnorm Child Psychol. 2009;37(4):507–20.
133. Caspi A, Houts RM, Belsky DW, Goldman-Mellor SJ, Harrington H, Israel S, et al. The p factor: one general psychopathology factor in the structure of psychiatric disorders? Clin Psychol Sci. 2014;2(2):119–37.
134. Hakulinen C, Elovainio M, Pulkki-Råback L, Virtanen M, Kivimäki M, Jokela M. Personality and depressive symptoms: individual participant meta-analysis of 10 cohort studies. Depress Anxiety. 2015;32(7):461–70.
135. Leach LS, Christensen H, Mackinnon AJ, Windsor TD, Butterworth P. Gender differences in depression and anxiety across the adult lifespan: the role of psychosocial mediators. Soc Psychiatry Psychiatr Epidemiol. 2008;43(12):983–98.
136. Jose PE, Kljakovic M, Scheib E, Notter O. The joint development of traditional bullying and victimization with cyber bullying and victimization in adolescence. J Res Adolesc. 2012;22(2):301–9.
137. Association AP, Girls TF on the S of. Report of the APA Task Force on the sexualization of girls. 2008 [cited 2025 May 7]. Available from: http://www.apa.org/pi/women/programs/girls/report-full.pdf.
138. Bor W, Dean AJ, Najman J, Hayatbakhsh R. Are child and adolescent mental health problems increasing in the 21st century? A systematic review. Aust N Z J Psychiatry. 2014;48(7):606–16.
139. Teasdale JD. Cognitive vulnerability to persistent depression. Cogn Emot. 1988;2(3):247–74.
140. Nolen-Hoeksema S. The role of rumination in depressive disorders and mixed anxiety/depressive symptoms. J Abnorm Psychol. 2000;109(3):504–11.
141. Abramson LY, Metalsky GI, Alloy LB. Hopelessness depression: a theory-based subtype of depression. Psychol Rev. 1989;96(2):358–72.
142. Mac Giollabhui N, Hamilton JL, Nielsen J, Connolly SL, Stange JP, Varga S, et al. Negative cognitive style interacts with negative life events to predict first onset of a major depressive episode in adolescence via hopelessness. J Abnorm Psychol. 2018;127(1):1–11.
143. Alloy LB, Abramson LY, Hogan ME, Whitehouse WG, Rose DT, Robinson MS, et al. The Temple-Wisconsin Cognitive Vulnerability to Depression Project: lifetime history of axis I psychopathology in individuals at high and low cognitive risk for depression. J Abnorm Psychol. 2000;109(3):403–18.
144. Huang C. Relation between attributional style and subsequent depressive symptoms: a systematic review and meta-analysis of longitudinal studies. Cogn Ther Res. 2015;39(6):721–35.
145. Silverstein B, Edwards T, Gamma A, Ajdacic-Gross V, Rossler W, Angst J. The role played by depression associated with somatic symptomatology in accounting for the gender difference in the prevalence of depression. Soc Psychiatry Psychiatr Epidemiol. 2013;48(2):257–63.
146. Kühner C. Mental disorders in pregnancy and postpartum: prevalence, course, and clinical diagnostics. Nervenarzt. 2016;87(9):926–36.

147. Mezulis AH, Hyde JS, Abramson LY. The developmental origins of cognitive vulnerability to depression: temperament, parenting, and negative life events in childhood as contributors to negative cognitive style. Dev Psychol. 2006;42(6):1012–25.
148. Calogero RM. Objectification theory, self-objectification, and body image. In: Encyclopedia of body image and human appearance [Internet]. Elsevier; 2012 [cited 2025 May 7]. p. 574–80. Available from: https://linkinghub.elsevier.com/retrieve/pii/B9780123849250000912.
149. McKinley NM, Hyde JS. The objectified body consciousness scale: development and validation. Psychol Women Q. 1996;20(2):181–215.
150. Grabe S, Hyde JS, Lindberg SM. Body objectification and depression in adolescents: the role of gender, shame, and rumination. Psychol Women Q. 2007;31(2):164–75.
151. Petersen JL, Hyde JS. Peer sexual harassment and disordered eating in early adolescence. Dev Psychol. 2013;49(1):184–95.
152. Lindberg SM, Hyde JS, McKinley NM. A measure of objectified body consciousness for preadolescent and adolescent youth. Psychol Women Q. 2006;30(1):65–76.
153. Jones BA, Griffiths KM. Self-objectification and depression: an integrative systematic review. J Affect Disord. 2015;171:22–32.
154. Lyubomirsky S, Layous K, Chancellor J, Nelson SK. Thinking about rumination: the scholarly contributions and intellectual legacy of Susan Nolen-Hoeksema. Annu Rev Clin Psychol. 2015;11:1–22.
155. Olatunji BO, Naragon-Gainey K, Wolitzky-Taylor KB. Specificity of rumination in anxiety and depression: a multimodal meta-analysis. Clin Psychol Sci Pract. 2013;20(3):225–57.
156. Rood L, Roelofs J, Bögels SM, Nolen-Hoeksema S, Schouten E. The influence of emotion-focused rumination and distraction on depressive symptoms in non-clinical youth: a meta-analytic review. Clin Psychol Rev. 2009;29(7):607–16.
157. Johnson DP, Whisman MA. Gender differences in rumination: a meta-analysis. Personal Individ Differ. 2013;55(4):367–74.
158. Michl LC, McLaughlin KA, Shepherd K, Nolen-Hoeksema S. Rumination as a mechanism linking stressful life events to symptoms of depression and anxiety: longitudinal evidence in early adolescents and adults. J Abnorm Psychol. 2013;122(2):339–52.
159. Rose AJ, Rudolph KD. A review of sex differences in peer relationship processes: potential trade-offs for the emotional and behavioral development of girls and boys. Psychol Bull. 2006;132(1):98–131.
160. Kendler KS, Karkowski LM, Prescott CA. Causal relationship between stressful life events and the onset of major depression. Am J Psychiatry. 1999;156(6):837–41.
161. Shore L, Toumbourou JW, Lewis AJ, Kremer P. Review: longitudinal trajectories of child and adolescent depressive symptoms and their predictors – a systematic review and meta-analysis. Child Adolesc Ment Health. 2018;23(2):107–20.
162. Dahlqvist HZ, Landstedt E, Young R, Gådin KG. Dimensions of peer sexual harassment victimization and depressive symptoms in adolescence: a longitudinal cross-lagged study in a Swedish sample. J Youth Adolesc. 2016;45(5):858–73.
163. Organization WH. Responding to intimate partner violence and sexual violence against women: WHO clinical and policy guidelines. World Health Organization; 2013. 66 p.
164. Nemeroff CB. Paradise lost: the neurobiological and clinical consequences of child abuse and neglect. Neuron. 2016;89(5):892–909.
165. Stoltenborgh M, Bakermans-Kranenburg MJ, Alink LRA, van IJzendoorn MH. The prevalence of child maltreatment across the globe: review of a series of meta-analyses. Child Abuse Rev. 2015;24(1):37–50.
166. Howard LM, Oram S, Galley H, Trevillion K, Feder G. Domestic violence and perinatal mental disorders: a systematic review and meta-analysis. PLoS Med. 2013;10(5):e1001452.
167. Tiggemann M, Slater A. The role of self-objectification in the mental health of early adolescent girls: predictors and consequences. J Pediatr Psychol. 2015;40(7):704–11.
168. Marazziti D, Baroni S, Picchetti M, Piccinni A, Carlini M, Vatteroni E, et al. Pharmacokinetics and pharmacodynamics of psychotropic drugs: effect of sex. CNS Spectr. 2013;18(3):118–27.

169. Damoiseaux VA, Proost JH, Jiawan VCR, Melgert BN. Sex differences in the pharmacokinetics of antidepressants: influence of female sex hormones and oral contraceptives. Clin Pharmacokinet. 2014;53(6):509–19.
170. Romanescu M, Buda V, Lombrea A, Andor M, Ledeti I, Suciu M, et al. Sex-related differences in pharmacological response to CNS drugs: a narrative review. J Pers Med. 2022;12(6):907.
171. Williams AV, Trainor BC. The impact of sex as a biological variable in the search for novel antidepressants. Front Neuroendocrinol. 2018;50:107–17.
172. Beery AK, Zucker I. Sex bias in neuroscience and biomedical research. Neurosci Biobehav Rev. 2011;35(3):565–72.
173. Kokras N, Dalla C, Papadopoulou-Daifoti Z. Sex differences in pharmacokinetics of antidepressants. Expert Opin Drug Metab Toxicol. 2011;7(2):213–26.
174. Fadiran EO, Zhang L. Effects of sex differences in the pharmacokinetics of drugs and their impact on the safety of medicines in women. In: Harrison-Woolrych M, editor. Medicines for women [Internet]. Cham: Springer International Publishing; 2015 [cited 2025 May 1]. p. 41–68. Available from: https://doi.org/10.1007/978-3-319-12406-3_2.
175. Sramek JJ, Murphy MF, Cutler NR. Sex differences in the psychopharmacological treatment of depression. Dialogues Clin Neurosci. 2016;18(4):447–57.
176. Nicolas JM, Espie P, Molimard M. Gender and interindividual variability in pharmacokinetics. Drug Metab Rev. 2009;41(3):408–21.
177. Kristensen CB. Imipramine serum protein binding in healthy subjects. Clin Pharmacol Ther. 1983;34(5):689–94.
178. Bebawy M, Chetty M. Gender differences in P-glycoprotein expression and function: effects on drug disposition and outcome. Curr Drug Metab. 2009;10(4):322–8.
179. Nicolson TJ, Mellor HR, Roberts RRA. Gender differences in drug toxicity. Trends Pharmacol Sci. 2010;31(3):108–14.
180. Meibohm B, Beierle I, Derendorf H. How important are gender differences in pharmacokinetics? Clin Pharmacokinet. 2002;41(5):329–42.
181. Sarginson JE, Lazzeroni LC, Ryan HS, Ershoff BD, Schatzberg AF, Murphy GM. ABCB1 (MDR1) polymorphisms and antidepressant response in geriatric depression. Pharmacogenet Genomics. 2010;20(8):467–75.
182. Cheung C, Yu AM, Ward JM, Krausz KW, Akiyama TE, Feigenbaum L, et al. The cyp2e1-humanized transgenic mouse: role of cyp2e1 in acetaminophen hepatotoxicity. Drug Metab Dispos. 2005;33(3):449–57.
183. Relling MV, Lin JS, Ayers GD, Evans WE. Racial and gender differences in N-acetyltransferase, xanthine oxidase, and CYP1A2 activities. Clin Pharmacol Ther. 1992;52(6):643–58.
184. Jin Y, Pollock BG, Frank E, Cassano GB, Rucci P, Müller DJ, et al. Effect of age, weight, and CYP2C19 genotype on escitalopram exposure. J Clin Pharmacol. 2010;50(1):62–72.
185. Ilic K, Hawke RL, Thirumaran RK, Schuetz EG, Hull JH, Kashuba ADM, et al. The influence of sex, ethnicity, and CYP2B6 genotype on bupropion metabolism as an index of hepatic CYP2B6 activity in humans. Drug Metab Dispos. 2013;41(3):575–81.
186. Kuo HW, Liu SC, Tsou HH, Liu SW, Lin KM, Lu SC, et al. CYP1A2 genetic polymorphisms are associated with early antidepressant escitalopram metabolism and adverse reactions. Pharmacogenomics. 2013;14(10):1191–201.
187. Kim JM, Kim SW, Stewart R, Kim SY, Yoon JS, Jung SW, et al. Predictors of 12-week remission in a nationwide cohort of people with depressive disorders: the CRESCEND study. Hum Psychopharmacol. 2011;26(1):41–50.
188. Huezo-Diaz P, Uher R, Smith R, Rietschel M, Henigsberg N, Marusic A, et al. Moderation of antidepressant response by the serotonin transporter gene. Br J Psychiatry. 2009;195(1):30–8.
189. Naito S, Sato K, Yoshida K, Higuchi H, Takahashi H, Kamata M, et al. Gender differences in the clinical effects of fluvoxamine and milnacipran in Japanese major depressive patients. Psychiatry Clin Neurosci. 2007;61(4):421–7.
190. Morgan ML, Cook IA, Rapkin AJ, Leuchter AF. Estrogen augmentation of antidepressants in perimenopausal depression: a pilot study. J Clin Psychiatry. 2005;66(6):774–80.

191. Nagata H, Nozaki M, Nakano H. Short-term combinational therapy of low-dose estrogen with selective serotonin re-uptake inhibitor (fluvoxamine) for oophorectomized women with hot flashes and depressive tendencies. J Obstet Gynaecol Res. 2005;31(2):107–14.
192. Bigos KL, Pollock BG, Stankevich BA, Bies RR. Sex differences in the pharmacokinetics and pharmacodynamics of antidepressants: an updated review. Gend Med. 2009;6(4):522–43.
193. Kornstein SG, McEnany G. Enhancing pharmacologic effects in the treatment of depression in women. J Clin Psychiatry. 2000;61(Suppl 11):18–27.
194. Katz D, Toner B. A systematic review of gender differences in the effectiveness of mindfulness-based treatments for substance use Disorders. Mindfulness. 2013;4(4):318–31.
195. Hanlon CA, McCalley DM. Sex/gender as a factor that influences transcranial magnetic stimulation treatment outcome: three potential biological explanations. Front Psychiatry [Internet]. 2022 [cited 2025 May 7];13. Available from: https://www.frontiersin.org. https://www.frontiersin.org/journals/psychiatry/articles/10.3389/fpsyt.2022.869070/full.

Bipolar Disorders

18

Ana González-Pinto and Guillermo Cano Escalera

18.1 Introduction

Bipolar disorder is a lifelong serious mental disorder that causes extreme dysregulation in mood, energy, and functioning. Lifetime prevalence is estimated to be 0.6% for bipolar disorder type I (BPI), 0.4% for bipolar disorder type II (BPII), and 2.4% for bipolar spectrum disorders [1]. Both genders are equally at risk of developing the illness. The onset of bipolar disorder usually occurs in adolescence or early adulthood, but it can appear during other periods in a lifetime, such as childhood. It affects familial relationships, social aspects, and employment, causing a general worsening in the quality of life.

The clinical course of bipolar disorder is characterized by the occurrence of one or more manic episodes, and often individuals also have recurrent episodes of major depression. Manic episodes are periods of abnormally and persistently elevated, irritable, or expansive mood and abnormal and persistent activity or energy increasing. During this period the patient may experience the following symptoms: inflated self-esteem or grandiosity feelings; decreased need for sleep; being more talkative than usual or feeling pressure to keep talking; flight of ideas or subjective experience of racing thoughts; distractibility; psychomotor agitation; or excessive involvement in pleasurable activities that can likely have painful consequences [2]. The diagnostic symptoms for major depressive episodes are the presence of a depressed

A. González-Pinto (✉)
Department of Psychiatry, Santiago Hospital, Vitoria, Spain
e-mail: ANAMARIA.GONZALEZ-PINTOARRILLAGA@osakidetza.eus

G. C. Escalera
Department of Psychiatry, Alava University Hospital, Vitoria, Spain

UPV/EHU, CIBERSAM, Spain
e-mail: Guillermo.canoescalera@osakidetza.eus

M. López-Atanes, M. Sáenz-Herrero (eds.), *Applying the Gender Perspective in Psychiatry and Psychotherapy*, https://doi.org/10.1007/978-3-032-17883-1_18

mood and loss of interest/pleasure, significant weight loss or appetite changes; insomnia or hypersomnia; fatigue or loss of energy; markedly diminished interest or pleasure in (almost) all activities; psychomotor agitation or retardation; feelings of worthlessness or excessive or inappropriate guilt; diminished ability to think, concentrate, or make decision; and recurrent thoughts of death or suicide [2]. Usually, a person with bipolar disorder only has some of these symptoms; it is very uncommon that they all manifest at the same time.

Bipolar I disorder is characterized by recurrent episodes of mania and depression, whereas bipolar II disorder is defined as recurrent episodes of depression and hypomania [2].

Many aspects of bipolar disorder have been investigated in several studies, including diagnosis, course of illness, psychiatric and physical comorbidity, suicide attempts, rapid cycling, and mixed states [3, 4]. However, the role gender could play in all those aspects remains unclear. In this chapter, we review all the information currently available on the matter.

18.2 Gender Differences in Bipolar Disorder

Although the lifetime prevalence of bipolar disorder appears to be roughly equal in both genders, some studies have shown that women are more likely to be diagnosed with bipolar II disorder, while men are more likely to be diagnosed with Bipolar I disorder [1, 5–7]. Recently it has been suggested that bipolar disorder is increasing in women [8].

18.3 Course and Clinical Characteristics of Illness

The biggest gender differences are seen for bipolar I disorder, especially when we refer to clinical features, course of illness, and comorbidity (Table 18.1) [9]. In women with BPI, the disease is characterized by a predominance of depression [2,

Table 18.1 Gender differences in bipolar disorder

Characteristics	Women	Men
More common episode	Depressive	Manic
Onset episode	Depressive	Manic
Subsyndromal depressive symptoms	More frequent	Less frequent
Age of onset	Older	Younger
Mixed episodes	More frequent	Less frequent
Seasonal episodes	More frequent	Less frequent
Rapid cycling	More frequent	Less frequent
Physical comorbidity	More frequent (thyroid diseases)	Less frequent
Psychiatric comorbidity	Eating disorder, anxiety disorders	Drug abuse

Adapted from López-Zurbano et al. [4]

10, 11]; both at the onset [12] and during lifetime course. Studies show that women spend more time in the depressed phase, with longer hospitalization for this reason [9, 13]. They also have more depressive symptoms in manic phases; thus, they are more likely to experience mixed episodes [2, 10]. This way, women also experience more suicidal ideation and more suicide attempts (whereas men make fewer attempts, but they are more violent and lethal) [9, 10, 14]. Women also have a higher probability of experiencing mood instability [10], seasonal episodes, and rapid cycling [2, 13]. On the other hand, men tend to have a predominance of manic components: their temperament is hyperthymic more frequently than in women, and the rates of mania at onset of the illness are higher [9, 10, 12, 13]. The disorder begins at a younger age in men, with an earlier first hospitalization [9]. This may explain why men are more often single [10].

Women are more often hospitalized than men and take more antidepressive and sedative/hypnotic treatments [10, 13, 14]. Women seek more treatment, probably because of their depressive polarity, as bipolar patients ask for help during depressive phases. In addition, women are more frequently married and their relatives bring women to healthcare facilities more easily [15]. Men have a higher rate of substance abuse comorbidity; therefore, they can be misdiagnosed. Finally, as women experience more suicide attempts and have more mixed episodes, they are more usually hospitalized to prevent the risk of suicide [10]. At the level of neurocognitive functioning, recent findings suggest that female patients with bipolar disorder show better performance in learning and memory, both verbal and visual, compared to men with TB. However, in psychosocial functioning, no significant gender differences were found [16]. Men performed better in working memory [17].

18.3.1 Bipolar Depression in Women and Misdiagnosis

The higher risk of depressive episodes in women than men with bipolar disorder is responsible for the frequent misdiagnosis of bipolar disorder with unipolar major disorder in women [8–10]. They have a greater number of depressive and cyclothymic temperaments and have more depressive subsyndromal symptoms [10].

The clinical characteristics of bipolar depression in women are different from those in men with regard to both bipolar I and bipolar II disorders. Women more commonly suffer from psychotic depression [9] and atypical symptoms (such as hypersomnia, increased appetite, or incongruent psychotic symptoms) [10, 12, 18]. This can explain why they are later diagnosed [9, 19] and why they take more antidepressants and benzodiazepines than men [14].

Precise establishment of a proper diagnosis by the first manifestations of bipolar depression is one of the biggest challenges in psychiatry these days. The depressive episode of bipolar disorder is many times indistinguishable from that of unipolar depression, especially if familial and personal history is not taken into account. Now there are also attempts to investigate biomarkers to help differentiate the two diagnoses [20, 21] or from healthy subjects [22]. The misdiagnosis often leads to the prescription of only antidepressants and in high doses, as what often happens in bipolar women [19], and this causes the destabilization of the course of the disorder. This incorrect prescription can provoke switches to mania/hypomania and increase the number of episodes with occurrence of rapid cycles or the development of mixed states [23]. It is estimated that it takes about 9.6 years from the onset of symptoms to the formal diagnosis of bipolar disorder [19]. Moreover, it has been observed that this delay is longer in patients with a younger age at onset, especially when they do not show psychotic symptoms or social dysfunction during the first episode [24].

According to Hirschfeld [25], more than a third of bipolar patients seek professional help during the first year after the onset of symptoms. Unfortunately, 69% are misdiagnosed and often receive the diagnosis of unipolar depression. Those who are misdiagnosed usually consult four therapists before receiving the correct diagnosis, and over a third of those have to wait for 10 years. This delay in the diagnosis and in the prescription of the correct treatment often brings significant psychosocial problems, such as conflicts with family and friends, professional or academic problems, and alcohol and substance abuse, with the corresponding worsening of patients' quality of life.

18.3.2 Suicide Risk

One of the most serious consequences associated with the misdiagnosis in bipolar patients is the increased suicide risk. The risk is higher during the first 5 years after the affective symptoms emerge [26]. In fact, about 40% of bipolar patients attempt suicide at 8.6 ± 6.6 years after the onset of affective symptoms. The suicide rate in the bipolar population ranges from 10% to 20% [27]. There is evidence that bipolar depressed patients attempt suicide earlier than unipolar patients during a specific episode. However, the patients with the highest risk of suicide are those experiencing mixed symptoms. This is because they combine the hopelessness of depression and the anxiety and impulsivity of mania. Some authors report that patients with bipolar II disorder make more suicide attempts than bipolar I and unipolar patients, although there is some controversy about this [27, 28]. The clinical variables most associated with an increased risk of suicide are the presence of severe depressive episodes, drug use, family background of affective disorders, younger age at onset, and the presence of mixed symptoms. We should pay special attention if there are behavior disorders or a history of suicidal behavior comorbidity [29]. Studies show that women tend to attempt suicide more frequently than men, but men's attempts are more violent (Table 18.2) [9, 10].

18.3.3 Rapid Cycling in Women

Rapid cycling is one of the specifiers included in the *Diagnostic and Statistical Manual of Mental Disorders*, DSM 5 [2], for bipolar disorder and related disorders. The main characteristic of rapid cycling is the occurrence of four or more mood episodes during the previous 12 months. Episodes can occur in any combination and

Table 18.2 Factors associated with suicidal risks

Risk factors	Suicidal acts	Suicidal ideation
More mixed episodes	√	√
Female sex	√	
Predominantly depressed	√	√
Latency to bipolar diagnosis	√	
Melancholic at any time		√
Hospitalization for depression	√	

Adapted from López-Zurbano et al. [4]

order. They have to meet the diagnostic criteria (symptoms and duration) for a major depressive manic or hypomanic episode, and can be delimited by a remission or by a change in polarity. The only exception in a rapid cycling bipolar disorder is that episodes occur more often than in a nonrapid cycling pattern. It appears that rapid cycling is a temporary evolution form in bipolar disorder.

Typically, rapid cycling and mood fluctuation has been considered to be associated with the female gender, but there has always been controversy about this [30–34].

18.3.4 Mania and Mixed Symptoms in Women

As women's polarity is often depressive, they usually experience more depressive symptoms: mood lability, depressed mood, greater guilt, and higher suicide and anxiety scores, even in mania episodes. This leads to the fact that women experience more manias with mixed symptoms [10, 12, 15, 35–37]. Some theories explain that they can be mediated by the predominance of anxiety symptoms in the female sex. Men, on the other hand, experience higher motor activity, grandiosity, and contact [15]. They are more likely to report "behavioral problems" and "being unable to hold a conversation" [12].

Mixed symptoms are characterized by the presence of different combinations of opposite directions in mood, motor activation, and thinking. Mood is more frequently irritable, but sometimes it is depressed. Infrequently euphoria is present, and in these cases motor activity and thinking are inhibited. The most frequent presentations of mixed symptoms in women are characterized by irritability and anxiety. Negative self-evaluation, suicide, dysphoria, psychic and somatic anxiety, social withdrawal, indecisiveness, worry, self-reproach, phobia, fatigue, discouragement, dullness of thought, loss of interest, depersonalization, panic, feelings of inadequacy, and ruminations are also frequent symptoms associated with irritable mood.

An important issue to recognize mixed symptoms is to consider not only the actual clinical presentation but to observe the changes present during 24 h or during few days. Mood changes sometimes from one pole to the opposite, and lability is present in combination with anxiety. Women with mixed symptoms are tearful, and it is important to consider this symptom as a part of the disease [38].

In relation with activity, it is more usual to see motor hyperactivity, although when there is euphoria, the patient can be inhibited. It is possible to see mixed symptoms with depression and inhibition but with accelerated thinking and flight of ideas.

The most frequent presentation of thinking in mixed symptoms in women is with rapid thinking and flight of ideas. These symptoms are accompanied by distractibility and the absence of goal. As the clinical presentations are broad, following Kraepelin's descriptions and modern ones, there are some patients with slow thinking, generally accompanied by psychomotor inhibition and euphoria or irritability. The presence of delusions is common, especially at younger ages. Mood congruent and mood incongruent symptoms are possible in the clinical presentations of mixed mania. It is important to ask patients about delusions, as some of them do not talk about their ideas. Patients with mixed states are usually more conscious about having a mental illness than other bipolar patients. Nevertheless, they do not capture exactly what is wrong, with a bad insight in the first stages of the disease [39]. Some studies find that 67% [40] of women who present a first bipolar episode presented concomitant mixed symptoms according to ICD-10 criteria for a mixed episode, obtaining similar rates (62%) when the diagnosis is established using DSM-IV criteria, as data registered in González-Pinto's study [41]. In 2010 Diflorio and Jones [42] performed a systematic review between January 1980 and 2010 on gender differences in bipolar disorder, manic depression, and mania. In this review, we found a number of studies focused on mixed episodes, appreciating that most of these episodes were more frequent in women with bipolar disorder [43, 44]. More recent research have shown a higher prevalence of mixed episodes in hospitalized women with BD, compared to men [41]. Clinical studies on manic dimension report the association of female gender to depressive dimension [9], hovering around 66% in the study by Cassidy [45] and 60% in the work of Sato et al. [46]. Significant associations have been found between suicide risk and women with mixed episodes versus men in young adult populations, as well as higher rates of suicide risk in mixed episodes versus depression or mania/hypomania [47].

According to the latest changes in DSM-5 classification regarding mixed states, we have focused in reviewing the most recent evidence to determine gender differences.

18.4 Major Depression with Mixed Features

(Appearing commonly in previous literature as "mixed depression")

According to Miller study in 2016 [36], women were more likely than men to experience subthreshold hypomanic symptoms during depressive episodes (40.7% compared to 34.4%) and pure hypomanic symptoms (17.2% compared to 14.7%). They could observe that in general terms, women were more likely than men to present mixed features. This has been a controversial subject in the past years as in some previous studies these differences were demonstrated, while in others no gender differences were found [48].

18.5 Comorbid Conditions

In psychiatric comorbidity, women tend to have more comorbid eating [2, 11, 49], anxiety, especially phobias [10, 13], and personality disorders [9]. Bipolar women suffer more frequently than men from panic disorder, obsessive–compulsive disorder, and specific phobia [14].

It is also known that even social phobias are equally prevalent among female and male populations; women suffering bipolar disorder and social phobia are four times more prone to have comorbid alcohol abuse [14]. Comorbid drug abuse is more common in men with bipolar disorder (alcohol, cocaine, cannabis) [10, 12, 14, 49], However, bipolar women have greater probability of suffering from alcohol use disorder than general population women [2].

Patients with bipolar disorder have a greater comorbidity of physical pathological conditions, as the disease and its treatment increase the risk of cardiovascular, metabolic, and endocrine diseases [50]. Women suffer higher comorbidity of thyroid disease, obesity, or being overweight [10]. Lifetime prevalence of thyroid disease (excluding thyroid cancer) is four to ten times higher in women, which links with the fact that bipolar disorder treatment (lithium salts) increases the risk of thyroid diseases itself. Women with thyroid diseases and bipolar disorder are more likely to have eating disorders, which may explain the more frequent obesity among women. Bipolar men are more prone to suffer from neurological cancer disorders, which may be due to the higher comorbidity with substance abuse [10]. However, there are no gender differences in the risk of experiencing cardiovascular diseases [10].

18.6 Adherence to Treatment

Nonadherence to medication in bipolar disorder is estimated to range from 12% to 64%, and studies with longer follow-up intervals have higher rates of nonadherence [51]. Lithium, the gold standard treatment in bipolar disorder, has a high rate of discontinuation as shown in a 6-year follow-up study, where the median adherence time to treatment was only 76 days [52]. Polypharmacy can be excessively complex and costly in bipolar disorder creating excess adverse effects and poor adherence [53].

Although men have been described to be less adherent than women [7], there are few specific studies on bipolar disorder patients showing gender differences in adherence to treatment. Substance abuse is associated with nonadherence, as patients use it as self-medication. Some studies find that all kinds of drug abuse are linked to nonadherence [54, 55]. Already in 1976, Himmelhoch [56] considered "abuse of alcohol and other substances, including organic factors may be necessary for the development of mixed mania in men."

Another factor related to treatment of nonadherence in bipolar disorder is the subjective experience of illness [57]. Some researchers have demonstrated that a good illness experience can be a primary and effective motivator for patients to keep to their treatment plan, whereas a poor subjective experience of illness often leads to lowered treatment adherence.

18.7 Discussion

Bipolar disorder (BD) presents notable gender differences in clinical manifestation, comorbidities, and treatment response. Women with BD tend to exhibit a predominance of depressive polarity, both at onset and throughout their lifetime, spending more time in depressive phases and experiencing more depressive symptoms even during manic episodes. This contributes to a higher likelihood of experiencing mixed mania, mood instability, rapid cycling, and seasonal mood episodes. In contrast, men show a lower frequency of depressive episodes but engage in more violent suicide attempts, whereas women report a higher prevalence of suicidal ideation and non-lethal suicide attempts.

Depressive symptoms in women are often accompanied by psychotic and atypical features, such as hypersomnia, increased appetite, and incongruent psychotic symptoms. Women are also more frequently misdiagnosed with unipolar depression and are prescribed antidepressants and benzodiazepines more often than men. The use of antidepressants in bipolar women increases the risk of mood destabilization, leading to a shift towards manic or hypomanic states, particularly in cases with an underlying depressive temperament.

Women tend to present higher comorbidity with anxiety disorders (such as panic disorder, obsessive-compulsive disorder, and specific phobias), eating disorders, and personality disorders. Notably, bipolar women with social phobia are four times more prone to alcohol abuse compared to men. Additionally, medical comorbidities such as thyroid disease, obesity, and being overweight are more prevalent among women with BD.

Substance use disorder is significantly more frequent among men with BD, particularly during acute manic episodes. This suggests that manic symptoms in some men may be exacerbated or triggered by substance use. Given the established cognitive differences between genders that women have better performance in verbal fluency clinical assessments may be inherently biased, leading to an underestimation of male depressive symptoms. Since language is a primary means of communication in clinical evaluations, the stronger verbal abilities in women may contribute to more accurate recognition and reporting of depressive symptoms in female patients.

From an evolutionary and social perspective, traditional gender roles may have influenced temperament and clinical presentations in BD. Historically, men have been perceived as predisposed to aggression and women to caregiving, potentially shaping gender-related differences in emotional regulation and behavioral responses. However, social changes, including women's empowerment and evolving child-rearing practices, indicate that temperament and behavioral patterns may be modifiable rather than biologically fixed. Future research should explore the impact of these sociocultural changes on BD presentation, aiming to provide more individualized and gender-sensitive approaches to treatment.

Women generally show better adherence to treatment but are more concerned about medication side effects, particularly weight gain, and require stronger social support networks. Pregnancy and the postpartum period are significant risk factors for mood disorder relapse, with depressive relapses being particularly frequent. Treatment discontinuation during pregnancy is contraindicated, necessitating a careful balance between medication risks and the dangers of affective relapse. Further research is needed to optimize treatment strategies for women with BD during pregnancy and lactation to improve outcomes for both mother and child.

In conclusion, gender differences in BD are evident in clinical presentation, comorbidities, and treatment response. The need for further studies remains crucial to deepening our understanding of these gender differences and to develop tailored interventions that ensure optimal and equitable treatment outcomes for both men and women in modern society.

References

1. Merikangas KR, Jin R, He J-P, Kessler RC, Lee S, Sampson NA, et al. Prevalence and correlates of bipolar spectrum disorder in the world mental health survey initiative. Arch Gen Psychiatry. 2011;68(3):241–51.
2. American Psychiatric Association. Diagnostic and statistical manual of mental disorders (DSM-5®). Arlington: American Psychiatric Pub; 2013.
3. Gonzalez-Pinto A, Gutierrez M, Mosquera F, Ballesteros J, Lopez P, Ezcurra J, et al. First episode in bipolar disorder: misdiagnosis and psychotic symptoms. J Affect Disord. 1998;50(1):41–4.
4. López-Zurbano S, González-Pinto A, López P. Gender differences in bipolar disorder. In: Psychopathology in women. Cham: Springer; 2015. p. 641–59.
5. Karanti A, Bobeck C, Osterman M, Kardell M, Tidemalm D, Runeson B, et al. Gender differences in the treatment of patients with bipolar disorder: a study of 7354 patients. J Affect Disord. 2015;174:303–9.
6. Popovic D, Torrent C, Goikolea JM, Cruz N, Sánchez-Moreno J, González-Pinto A, et al. Clinical implications of predominant polarity and the polarity index in bipolar disorder: a naturalistic study. Acta Psychiatr Scand. 2014;129(5):366–74.
7. Vega P, Hernández M, Martinez-Cengotitabengoa M, Gonzalez I. Why do bipolar men not comply with treatment? Int Clin Psychopharmacol. 2011;26(39):63–9.
8. Dell'Osso B, Cafaro R, Ketter TA. Has Bipolar Disorder become a predominantly female gender related condition? Analysis of recently published large sample studies. Int J Bipolar Disord. 2021;9(1):3. https://doi.org/10.1186/s40345-020-00207-z. PMID: 33392912; PMCID: PMC7779377.
9. Nivoli AMA, Pacchiarotti I, Rosa AR, Popovic D, Murru A, Valenti M, et al. Gender differences in a cohort study of 604 bipolar patients: the role of predominant polarity. J Affect Disord. 2011;133(3):443–9.

10. Azorin J-M, Belzeaux R, Kaladjian A, Adida M, Hantouche E, Lancrenon S, et al. Risks associated with gender differences in bipolar I disorder. J Affect Disord. 2013;151(3):1033–40.
11. Rasgon N, Bauer M, Glenn T, Elman S, Whybrow PC. Menstrual cycle related mood changes in women with bipolar disorder. Bipolar Disord. 2003;5(1):48–52.
12. Kawa I, Carter JD, Joyce PR, Doughty CJ, Frampton CM, Wells JE, et al. Gender differences in bipolar disorder: age of onset, course, comorbidity, and symptom presentation. Bipolar Disord. 2005;7(2):119–25.
13. Altshuler LL, Kupka RW, Hellemann G, Frye MA, Sugar CA, McElroy SL, et al. Gender and depressive symptoms in 711 patients with bipolar disorder evaluated prospectively in the Stanley Foundation bipolar treatment outcome network. Am J Psychiatry. 2010;167(6):708–15.
14. Saunders EFH, Fitzgerald KD, Zhang P, McInnis MG. Clinical features of bipolar disorder comorbid with anxiety disorders differ between men and women. Depress Anxiety. 2012;29(8):739–46.
15. Bhattacharya A, Khess CRJ, Munda SK, Bakhla AK, Praharaj SK, Kumar M. Sex difference in symptomatology of manic episode. Compr Psychiatry. 2011;52(3):288–92.
16. Serra-Navarro M, Clougher D, Oliva V, Valenzuela-Pascual C, De Prisco M, Forte MF, Garriga M, Solé B, Sánchez-Moreno J, Verdolini N, Menculini G, Tortorella A, Bernardo M, Ramos-Quiroga JA, Martinez-Aran A, Vieta E, Amoretti S, Torrent C. Sex differences in psychosocial functioning and neurocognition in bipolar disorder: a systematic review and meta-analysis. Eur Psychiatry. 2025;68(1):e45.
17. Solé B, Varo C, Torrent C, Montejo L, Jiménez E, Bonnin CDM, Clougher D, Verdolini N, Amoretti S, Piazza F, Borràs R, Pomarol-Clotet E, Sáiz PA, García-Portilla MP, Vieta E, Martínez-Arán A. Sex differences in neurocognitive and psychosocial functioning in bipolar disorder. J Affect Disord. 2022;296:208–15.
18. Benazzi F. Gender differences in bipolar II and unipolar depressed outpatients: a 557-case study. Ann Clin Psychiatry. 1999;11(2):55–9.
19. Drancourt N, Etain B, Lajnef M, Henry C, Raust A, Cochet B, et al. Duration of untreated bipolar disorder: missed opportunities on the long road to optimal treatment. Acta Psychiatr Scand. 2013;127(2):136–44.
20. Lyu N, Wang H, Zhao Q, Fu B, Li J, Yue Z, Huang J, Yang F, Liu H, Zhang L, Li R. Peripheral biomarkers to differentiate bipolar depression from major depressive disorder: a real-world retrospective study. BMC Psychiatry. 2024;24(1):543.
21. Miranda-Mendizabal A, Vetter D, Zambrano J, Zarp J, Chavarría V, Giménez-Palomo A, Gonzalez-Campos M, Valenti M, Walczer Baldinazzo L, Siddi S, Ferrari M, Weissmann D, Henry C, Haro JM, Vedel Kessing L, Vieta E. RNA editing-based biomarker blood test for the diagnosis of bipolar disorder: protocol of the EDIT-B study. Ann Gen Psychiatry. 2025;24(1):7. https://doi.org/10.1186/s12991-024-00544-8. PMID: 39915772; PMCID: PMC11803998.
22. Chart-Pascual JP, Cano-Escalera G, Graña M, Zorrilla I, Lopez-Peña P, Requena CM, Ceballos AF, Landaluce IP, Urcola H, Alvarez-Mon MA, Blumberg HP, Radua J, Gonzalez-Pinto A. Retinal thickness: a window into cognitive impairment in bipolar disorder. Span J Psychiatry Ment Health. 2025:S2950-2853(25)00004-3. https://doi.org/10.1016/j.sjpmh.2025.01.001. Epub ahead of print. PMID: 40081818.
23. Hirschfeld RMA, Vornik LA. Recognition and diagnosis of bipolar disorder. J Clin Psychiatry. 2004;65(Suppl 15):5–9.
24. Goldberg JF, Ernst CL. Features associated with the delayed initiation of mood stabilizers at illness onset in bipolar disorder. J Clin Psychiatry. 2002;63(11):985–91.
25. Hirschfeld RMA, Lewis L, Vornik LA. Perceptions and impact of bipolar disorder: how far have we really come? Results of the national depressive and manic-depressive association 2000 survey of individuals with bipolar disorder. J Clin Psychiatry. 2003;64(2):161–74.
26. González-Pinto A, Aldama A, González C, Mosquera F, Arrasate M, Vieta E. Predictors of suicide in first-episode affective and nonaffective psychotic inpatients: five-year follow-up of patients from a catchment area in Vitoria, Spain. J Clin Psychiatry. 2007;68(2):242–7.
27. Undurraga J, Baldessarini RJ, Valenti M, Pacchiarotti I, Vieta E. Suicidal risk factors in bipolar I and II disorder patients. J Clin Psychiatry. 2012;73(6):778–82.

28. Dev DA, Le GH, Kwan ATH, Wong S, Arulmozhi A, Ceban F, Teopiz KM, Meshkat S, Rosenblat JD, Guillen-Burgos HF, Rhee TG, Ho RC, Cao B, d'Andrea G, Sundberg I, McIntyre RS. Comparing suicide completion rates in bipolar I versus bipolar II disorder: a systematic review and meta-analysis. J Affect Disord. 2024;361:480–8.
29. López P, Mosquera F, de León J, Gutiérrez M, Ezcurra J, Ramírez F, et al. Suicide attempts in bipolar patients. J Clin Psychiatry. 2001;62(12):963–6.
30. Perris C. A study of bipolar (manic-depressive) and unipolar recurrent depressive psychoses. Introduction. Acta Psychiatr Scand Suppl. 1966;194:9–14.
31. Coryell W, Endicott J, Keller M. Rapidly cycling affective disorder. Demographics, diagnosis, family history, and course. Arch Gen Psychiatry. 1992;49(2):126–31.
32. Rasgon N, Bauer M, Grof P, Gyulai L, Elman S, Glenn T, et al. Sex-specific self-reported mood changes by patients with bipolar disorder. J Psychiatr Res. 2005;39(1):77–83.
33. Burt VK, Rasgon N. Special considerations in treating bipolar disorder in women. Bipolar Disord. 2004;6(1):2–13.
34. Miola A, Fountoulakis KN, Baldessarini RJ, Veldic M, Solmi M, Rasgon N, Ozerdem A, Perugi G, Frye MA, Preti A. Prevalence and outcomes of rapid cycling bipolar disorder: mixed method systematic meta-review. J Psychiatr Res. 2023;164:404–15.
35. Bräunig P, Sarkar R, Effenberger S, Schoofs N, Krüger S. Gender differences in psychotic bipolar mania. Gend Med. 2009;6(2):356–61.
36. Miller S, Suppes T, Mintz J, Helleman G, Frye MA. Mixed depression in bipolar disorder: prevalence rate and clinical correlates during naturalistic follow-up in the Stanley bipolar network. Am J Psychiatry. 2016;173(10):1015–23.
37. Suppes T, Mintz J, McElroy SL, et al. Mixed hypomania in 908 patients with bipolar disorder evaluated prospectively in the Stanley Foundation bipolar treatment network: a sex-specific phenomenon. Arch Gen Psychiatry. 2005;62:1089–96.
38. Gonzalez-Pinto A, Aldama A, Pinto AG, Mosquera F, Perez de Heredia JL, Ballesteros J, et al. Dimensions of mania: differences between mixed and pure episodes. Eur Psychiatry. 2004;19(5):307–10.
39. Gonzalez-Pinto A, Aldama A, Mosquera F, Gonzalez GC. Epidemiology, diagnosis and management of mixed mania. CNS Drugs. 2007;21(8):611–26.
40. Dell'Osso L, Placidi GF, Nassi R, Freer P, Cassano GB, Akiskal HS. The manic-depressive mixed state: familial, temperamental and psychopathologic characteristics in 108 female inpatients. Eur Arch Psychiatry Clin Neurosci. 1991;240(4–5):234–9.
41. Gonzalez-Pinto A, Barbeito S, Alonso M, Alberich S, Haidar MK, Vieta E, et al. Poor long-term prognosis in mixed bipolar patients: 10-year outcomes in the Vitoria prospective naturalistic study in Spain. J Clin Psychiatry. 2011;72(5):671–6.
42. Diflorio A, Jones I. Is sex important? Gender differences in bipolar disorder. Int Rev Psychiatry. 2010;22(5):437–52.
43. Hawton K, Sutton L, Haw C, Sinclair J, Harriss L. Suicide and attempted suicide in bipolar disorder: a systematic review of risk factors. J Clin Psychiatry. 2005;66(6):693–704.
44. Lopez P, Mosquera F, de Leon J, Gutierrez M, Ezcurra J, Ramirez F, et al. Suicide attempts in bipolar patients. J Clin Psychiatry. 2001;62(12):963–6.
45. Cassidy F, Yatham LN, Berk M, Grof P. Pure and mixed manic subtypes: a review of diagnostic classification and validation. Bipolar Disord. 2008;10(1 Pt 2):131–43.
46. Sato T, Bottlender R, Kleindienst N, Moller HJ. Syndromes and phenomenological subtypes underlying acute mania: a factor analytic study of 576 manic patients. Am J Psychiatry. 2002;159(6):968–74.
47. Sverdlichenko I, Jansen K, Souza LDM, da Silva RA, Kapczinski F, Cardoso TA. Mixed episodes and suicide risk: a community sample of young adults. J Affect Disord. 2020;266:252–7.
48. Reinares M, Bonnín Cdel M, Hidalgo-Mazzei D, Undurraga J, Mur M, Nieto E, Sáez C, Vieta E. Making sense of DSM-5 mania with depressive features. Aust N Z J Psychiatry. 2015;49(6):540–9.

49. Loftus J, Scott J, Vorspan F, Icick R, Henry C, Gard S, Kahn JP, Leboyer M, Bellivier F, Etain B. Psychiatric comorbidities in bipolar disorders: an examination of the prevalence and chronology of onset according to sex and bipolar subtype. J Affect Disord. 2020;267:258–63.
50. Gonzalez-Pinto A, Mosquera F, Alonso M, López P, Ramírez F, Vieta E, et al. Suicidal risk in bipolar I disorder patients and adherence to long-term lithium treatment. Bipolar Disord. 2006;8(5 Pt 2):618–24.
51. Colom F, Vieta E, Martínez-Arán A, Reinares M, Benabarre A, Gastó C. Clinical factors associated with treatment noncompliance in euthymic bipolar patients. J Clin Psychiatry. 2000;61(8):549–55.
52. Johnson RE, McFarland BH. Lithium use and discontinuation in a health maintenance organization. Am J Psychiatry. 1996;153(8):993–1000.
53. Kim AM, Salstein L, Goldberg JF. A systematic review of complex polypharmacy in bipolar disorder: prevalence, clinical features, adherence, and preliminary recommendations for practitioners. J Clin Psychiatry. 2021;82(3):20r13263.
54. Lang K, Korn J, Muser E, Choi JC, Abouzaid S, Menzin J. Predictors of medication nonadherence and hospitalization in Medicaid patients with bipolar I disorder given long-acting or oral antipsychotics. J Med Econ. 2011;14(2):217–26.
55. Oladunjoye AF, Kaleem SZ, Suresh A, Sahni V, Thoonkuzhy MJ, Anugwom G, Oladunjoye O, Otuada D, Ikekwere J, Espiridion ED. Cannabis use and medication nonadherence in bipolar disorder: a nationwide inpatient sample database analysis. J Affect Disord. 2022;299:174–9.
56. Hasin D, Carpenter KM, McCloud S, Smith M, Grant BF. The alcohol use disorder and associated disabilities interview schedule [AUDADIS]: reliability of alcohol and drug modules in a clinical sample. Drug Alcohol Depend. 1997;44(2–3):133–41.
57. Kriegshauser K, Sajatovic M, Jenkins JH, Cassidy KA, Muzina D, Fattal O, et al. Gender differences in subjective experience and treatment of bipolar disorder. J Nerv Ment Dis. 2010;198(5):370–2.

Anxiety Disorders 19

Margarita Saenz-Herrero, Mayte López-Atanes, Ana Espiga Izuzquiza, and Luis Urgoiti González

19.1 Introduction

It is increasingly argued that being a man or woman influences not only the prevalence of mental disorders but also the manifestation and expression of symptoms, the willingness to seek medical and psychological assistance, the course of the disease, and even the response to treatment [1, 2]. The WHO argues that not enough attention was being paid to the specific determinants of each sex in the mechanisms that promote and protect mental health and enhance resistance to stress and adversity [3].

Sex is defined as the biological features distinguishing male and female animals and humans, whereas gender refers to the socio-cultural aspects of identity in relation to sex. Certain attributes have historically been given to women and men; these inexorably represent the roles of each, circumscribed on the basis of these attributes. While male sex is related to public space, the abstract, the word, and the active female sex is related to the private, passive, and submission. In this way the social, economic, political roles, among others, to which each gender is assigned are different and lie below a dichotomy construct between opposites [4].

From an anthropological perspective Marilyn Strathern and Carol Cormack [5, 6] have stated a discourse about nature and culture that usually portrays nature as feminine; it must be subordinated to a culture that is constantly presented as active and abstract. Mind and reason are related to masculinity, whereas the body and nature are associated with femininity, awaiting significance provided by an opposing subject.

M. Saenz-Herrero · M. López-Atanes (✉) · A. E. Izuzquiza · L. U. González
Cruces University Hospital, Bilbao, Spain

Basque Country University, Santsoena, Spain
e-mail: M.lopezatanes@centra.hamburg

M. López-Atanes, M. Sáenz-Herrero (eds.), *Applying the Gender Perspective in Psychiatry and Psychotherapy*, https://doi.org/10.1007/978-3-032-17883-1_19

Thus, so-called symbolic domination emerges, often taking the form of bodily emotions—shame, humiliation, shyness, anxiety, and guilt—or passions and feelings—love, admiration, respect—and sometimes more painful emotions that manifest visibly as flushing, verbal confusion, clumsiness, shaking, anger, or impotent rage. These emotions represent ways of being subjected, often unconsciously, to the underlying complicity of societal norms and willpower, which sustain social structures with inherent censure.

Therefore, these constructs influence the way men and women experience and express anxiety. Different roles may influence the psychopathological expression of mental disorders, highlighting the importance of conducting a global analysis from a gender perspective to explain the differential prevalence of different pathologies and their symptomatology, as well as to develop more effective therapeutic approaches.

19.2 Epidemiological Data

Anxiety disorders are more prevalent in women than in men [7, 8], potentially due to genetic, hormonal, and psychosocial factors. Women report poorer psychological well-being and a higher risk of anxiety-related disability, with symptoms being more disabling [9–12]. In general, there are predisposing factors (genetics, somatic diseases, psychological trauma during development, lack of coping mechanisms, distorted thinking, beliefs, and cognitive processing) and precipitating factors (somatic or toxic problems, external and intense long-term stress, stress affecting vulnerability, and other factors [13, 14]).

From a methodological perspective, differences in prevalence may be an artefact related to men's reluctance to report symptoms, stemming from societal standards of masculinity. The type of self-report measure used may influence the degree to which sex differences emerge. Furthermore, the relationship between psychopathology and femininity is itself a matter of discussion, because one may assume that masculine behaviour is often, but erroneously, taken as the standard for mental health [15].

19.3 Psychological Models of Anxiety Disorders

Bekker and Van Mens-Verhulst [15] explain the psychological theories of anxiety disorders. They begin with the learning perspective, which is the theory that is most extensively studied in the field of anxiety disorders, then sex-role theories, and finally attachment and schema theory.

From a learning perspective, it has been argued that women, due to their greater exposure to trauma (such as sexual violence and poverty), are more vulnerable to developing fear and phobic avoidance responses.

Gender role theory posits that Western culture encourages dependency and a lack of assertiveness in women, prescribing a stress response characterised by dependency and helplessness [16, 17]. This perspective has been studied since the 1970s, mainly with agoraphobia. It was hypothesised that agoraphobia in women would decrease in prevalence as Western culture placed greater demands on women to work outside the home and to be self-reliant and assertive. This was confirmed by two epidemiological studies.

Finally, attachment and schema theory. While the original attachment theory is gender-neutral, with feminist neo-psychoanalytic theory, a gender-specific version of attachment theory has become available [18]. The authors consider the fact that the primary attachment figure is often a woman—their mother—which provides sex differences in the development of autonomy [19–21]. Considered from this perspective, the early same-sex mother-daughter relationship would imply that the symbiotic phase with the mother is more enduring and intense for girls than for boys. Consequently, girls would have more problems with individuation and separation, while boys may face challenges with attachment and expressing their need for dependency.

These models highlight the interaction between biological and socio-cultural factors in the manifestation of anxiety, and it is suggested that research should further investigate the role of gender in the development and treatment of these disorders.

19.4 Biological Factors

Anxiety disorders are associated with a common genetic vulnerability to panic disorder, generalised anxiety, and affective disorders [22]. This vulnerability involves a neurobiological response of hyperactivity to stress, characterised by a chronic increase in the function of neurochemical systems responsible for the stress response, such as corticotropin-releasing factor and adrenaline [23]. These systems act on different regions of the brain, such as the hippocampus and prefrontal cortex, areas involved in emotional regulation. Gender differences also play an important role in emotional response, with studies showing increased activity in the right amygdala in men and the left amygdala in women when exposed to emotionally disturbing images [24, 25]. In addition, serotonin has been observed to be a key factor in the predisposition of women to develop anxiety and mood disorders, making it a promising area of research [26, 27].

In addition, epigenetics is beginning to illuminate how environmental factors may influence the development of anxiety disorders [28]. For example, DNA methylation studies have shown that individuals with social anxiety disorder or panic disorder have epigenetic changes that may contribute to the development of these disorders [29–31].

Another important issue is the influence of sex hormones on the stress response [32]. For example, oestrogens can affect the noradrenaline-mediated stress response and facilitate the serotonergic response [33]. Women of reproductive age are two to three times more likely than men to develop anxiety disorders [34, 35], which may be partly due to the influence of sex hormones on brain structure and function.

Hormones such as progesterone also play a key role, as allopregnanolone (a metabolite of progesterone) has been shown to have anxiolytic effects that may help to moderate the amygdala response to stressful stimuli [36, 37].

Finally, hormonal changes during the menstrual cycle, pregnancy, and menopause are known to affect anxiety symptomatology. For example, anxiety tends to decrease during pregnancy [38], whereas many women experience a worsening of anxiety symptoms during the premenstrual phase [39]. Premenstrual tension syndrome is also associated with anxiety disorders, suggesting a complex interaction between reproductive hormones and anxiety [40], and highlighting the need to consider these factors when treating anxiety disorders in women.

19.5 Subtypes of Anxiety Disorders

The diagnostic categorical criteria usually used are subject to continual modifications in the different versions of international classifications such as the DSM5. The DSM-5 [41] comprises disorders that share features of excessive fear and anxiety and related behavioural disturbances. Fear is the emotional response to real or perceived imminent threat, whereas anxiety is anticipation of future threat.

Anxiety disorders in DSM-5 are arranged developmentally, with disorders sequenced according to the typical age at onset. DSM-5 contains specific phobia, social anxiety disorder (social phobia), panic disorder, agoraphobia without a history of panic disorder, generalised anxiety disorder, anxiety disorder due to a medical disease, anxiety disorder induced by substances, and unspecified anxiety disorder [41]. This edition also includes separation anxiety disorder and selective mutism. Obsessive compulsive disorder (OCD) and related disorders are in another section of DSM-5 classification.

We try hereby to explain the different subtypes, emphasising the anxiety disorders that from a gender perspective deserve particular attention.

Separation anxiety disorder is characterised by an intense fear of separation from attachment figures, with symptoms that may persist from childhood into adulthood [41]. According to a study by Silove et al., the lifetime prevalence of separation anxiety disorder is 4.8%, with 43.1% of cases occurring after the age of 18 years. They also identify female gender (1.3:1), childhood adversity, and traumatic events as predictors [42].

Selective mutism is characterised by the inability to speak in social situations, even when speaking in other situations. It mainly affects early childhood and has a prevalence of about 0.71% [43]. It is more common in girls (1.5:1) and its aetiology is multifactorial, involving genetic, environmental, and developmental factors [44, 45].

The DSM-5 distinguishes social phobia, specific phobia, and agoraphobia as the primary entities constituting *phobic disorders* in general. According to Lepine and Chignon [46], the diagnosis of this entity requires the presence of the feared object and situation, anxious manifestations that are of particular relevance.

Although there is a predominance of phobic disorders in the female sex, there seem to be differences according to the type of phobia. These differences can be explained by the various mechanisms that may influence them, such as ideological factors, the social facilitation of aggressive behaviour in men, and the greater tendency of men not to admit fear because it damages self-esteem and social consideration.

On the one hand, *social phobia* manifests itself as a persistent fear of social situations in which the individual feels exposed to people who are not part of their familiar environment or to possible evaluation by others [14].

According to the DSM-5 [41], hypersensitivity to criticism of the evaluation of others, difficulty in asserting oneself, low self-esteem, and feelings of inferiority are some of the characteristics of this type of phobia. Several authors seem to agree that both environmental and genetic factors influence social phobia [14, 47, 48].

It has a high comorbidity, 70–80%, with other psychiatric disorders, especially anxiety, depression, personality disorders, and substance abuse [49]. Yonkers et al. observed a greater tendency towards substance abuse in men, whereas women were more likely to present with agoraphobia [50]. They also described that women with a history of suicide attempts and poorer premorbid adjustment had a worse prognosis. According to Asher and Aderka, women are more likely to have the disorder across the lifespan and have a more variable and severe course of sever anxiety disorders (SAD) [51].

Specific phobia, on the other hand, is characterised by an intense, persistent, and irrational fear of the presence or anticipation of a specific object or situation, resulting in active avoidance and significant distress [14]. It is the third most common psychiatric disorder in the general population, with a prevalence of 12.5%, and the age of onset is one of the earliest, with an average age of onset of around 7 years [52].

Women are more likely to experience animal phobia, while men are more prone to height phobia (acrophobia) [53]. Comorbidity in specific phobia is relatively common, with the most commonly reported disorders being social phobia, substance abuse, and depression [54]. In women, comorbidity was reported in 28.3% of anxiety disorders, 13.7% of affective disorders, 3.2% of somatoform disorders, 2.2% of substance-related disorders, and 4% of eating disorders [53]. In terms of etiopathogenesis, genetic load may be more influential in men, whereas socio-familial factors are more relevant in women. However, there is insufficient evidence on the heritability of phobias and specific anxieties and more research is needed [55].

Agoraphobia is characterised by an intense fear of situations from which it may be difficult to escape, with an irrational fear of public places. In contrast to the previous conceptualisation in DSM-IV, where it was defined in terms of its relationship to panic disorder, DSM-5 establishes agoraphobia as a separate diagnosis [56]. The prevalence of this disorder is higher in women, with rates ranging from 7 to 9%, compared to 3 to 4% in men, with worse quality of life also observed in women [57, 58].

There is high comorbidity with panic disorder, generalised anxiety disorder, major depression, and substance abuse [59]. While alcohol abuse is more common in men, women are more likely to abuse tranquillisers [58–60]. Socio-cultural factors play an important role in agoraphobia, especially in women.

Panic disorder is defined by the presence of recurrent panic attacks, characterised by a sudden onset of symptoms of intense autonomic activation, accompanied by a fear of imminent death or loss of control [14]. The lifetime prevalence of panic disorder is 4.7% and it is twice as common in women as in men [34, 61–63]. The age of onset is estimated to be between 25 and 34 years in women, and later in men, between 35 and 44 years [64]. Clinically, women are more likely to report psychological symptoms of panic disorder [65]. Anticipatory anxiety is more common in women [64], whereas men are more concerned about somatic symptoms [66]. According to several studies, women have a worse course of the illness, and a poor prognostic factor for women has been identified [67]. Women have higher relapse rates [68, 69] and the disease is more disabling [59, 62].

Generalised anxiety disorder is defined as excessive worry about different events or activities on most days for at least 6 months, sometimes accompanied by somatic symptoms such as muscle tension, restlessness, fatigue, and insomnia [70]. Its lifetime prevalence is 5.7%, with a 2:1 female to male sex ratio and onset in the second decade of life [61, 71].

In women, GAD is associated with specific psychosocial factors, such as the dual burden of work and domestic responsibilities, the glass ceiling in the workplace, and exposure to gender-based violence. This leads to psychological distress and may in itself explain the "excessive worry" in which they are involved in some way, from our point of view. What is normal or healthy is very close to what is unhealthy or abnormal. In a sense, illness does not exist until we have allowed it to exist, until we name it, perceive it, and act on it from our point of view.

Substance/medication-induced anxiety disorder is anxiety due to substance intoxication or withdrawal or drug treatment. In anxiety disorder due to another medical condition, the anxiety symptoms are the physiological consequences of the other medical condition [41].

DSM-5 includes another category, "*other specified anxiety disorders*," in which symptoms characteristic of an anxiety disorder cause significant distress [41].

In DSM-5, *obsessive-compulsive disorder* has been reclassified from the spectrum of anxiety disorders; previously it was included in the spectrum of panic disorders. Regarding gender differences, Lochner et al. [72] find no difference in prevalence, whereas the CSN-R 2007 indicates a higher likelihood in women. However, they do agree on the early onset in men, with a high percentage starting before the age of 25 [73].

Differences in disease course and response to treatment have also been reported [74]. However, more similarities than differences have been described in the clinical status of the disease [75]. In terms of symptoms, women show more intrusive obsessions with cleanliness, whereas men show more nervous tics, greater overall symptom severity, and a poorer prognosis [72]. The course of the illness tends to be chronic [76].

Specific symptom changes have been observed in women with OCD, both in the premenstrual/menstrual phase and after pregnancy and menopause, confirming the relationship between cyclical menstrual/reproductive changes and relapses and fluctuations in OCD symptoms [72]. Women with OCD report worsening symptoms during the menopausal and premenstrual periods [77–79]. During the perinatal period, more than half of the women reported symptoms related to the baby, with obsessions about harming the baby being more intense after childbirth [77].

In terms of comorbidity with the disorder, eating disorders, depression or panic attacks are more common in women [33], while phobias and nervous tics are more common in men [73].

19.6 Treatment

Throughout the chapter we have discussed gender differences in anxiety disorders. Although there is enough evidence about the existence of these differences, publications often continue to neglect sex-based considerations and analyses in the studies. In 2014 was published an article announcing that all National Institutes of Health funded research will be required to consider sex influences [80]. According to Cahill, behind this event "is the rapidly burgeoning weight of evidence proving that sex matters in different ways, from the level of the intact human down to the level of ion-channel function, and everywhere in between" [81]. Also in the treatment.

Women often receive higher doses of psychotropic medications [82] and are prescribed anxiolytics at twice the rate of men, even when not formally diagnosed with an anxiety disorder. In fact, the diagnosis may go unnoticed for an extended period if symptoms are overt [83, 84].

Decreased hepatic metabolism of certain benzodiazepines and fluctuations in plasma levels of some antidepressants during the menstrual cycle have been observed [85]. Of particular note is the combined use of these drugs with oral contraceptives, where an increase in their plasma levels has been observed [86, 87]. selective serotonin reuptake inhibitors (SSRI) such as fluvoxamine and sertraline have higher concentrations in women, which may explain the difference in adverse effects.

The overall assessment that both pharmacological therapy and cognitive behavioural therapy (CBT) contribute to improvement of anxiety disorders seems to be effective for women and men. However, there is a remarkable lack of information regarding the sex-specific effects, not to mention the gender-specific effects, of treatments.

Unfortunately, existing sex-specific studies on psychosocial treatment are deficient in at least two key areas. From a gender point of view, they lack a thorough reflection on possible gender bias in sampling procedures, measurement, and analysis, and they disregard the gender-specific context. From a treatment research point of view, they do not meet one of the criteria for inclusion in a meta-analysis: that of being a randomised controlled trial. Moreover, most of the available meta-analyses appear to fail to systematically consider the sex distribution of the studies included, much less the calculation of possible sex differences in effect sizes [15].

Butler et al. [88] highlighted this deficiency in their review of meta-analysis. Butler also mentioned inattention to possible moderator variables (gender differences) as a frequent limitation of the meta-analysis procedure.

19.7 Conclusions

Gender and social, cultural, and economic factors affect health. Women have a substantially higher risk of developing lifetime anxiety disorders compared with men. In addition, research evidence has generally observed an increased symptom severity, chronic course, and functional impairment in women with anxiety disorders in comparison to men. However, the reasons for the increased risk in developing an anxiety disorder in women are still unknown and have yet to be adequately investigated including a gender perspective. Not only genetic factors and female reproductive hormones may play important roles in the expression of these gender differences but sex and gender affect who we are, what we do, and how we are treated. Evidence of gender differences in treatment response across anxiety disorders varies and remains largely inconclusive. Future research incorporating a gender perspective is essential for advancing scientific understanding.

References

1. Phillips KA, First MB. Introduction. In: Narrow WE, First MB, Sirovatka PJ, Regier DA, editors. Diary research for DSM-V. Considerations on the age and gender in psychiatric diagnosis. Barcelona: Elsevier Masson; 2009. p. 3–6.
2. Wisner KL, Dolan-Sewell R. Why is gender important? In: Regier DA, editor. Considerations on the age and gender in psychiatric diagnosis. Diary research for DSM-V. Barcelona: Elsevier Masson; 2009. p. 7–17.
3. WHO. Women's mental health: an evidence based review. Report on the world health; 2000.
4. Bourdieu P. Masculine domination. Barcelona: Anagrama; 2000.
5. MacCormack C, Strathern M. Nature, culture and gender. New York: Routledge; 1990.
6. Marylin Strathern M. An anthropological perspective. In: Harris O, Young K, editors. Feminist anthropology. Barcelona: Anagrama; 1979.
7. Wasserman GA, McReynolds LS, Ko SJ, Laura M. Gender differences in psychiatric disorders at juvenile probation intake. Am J Public Health. 2005;95:131–7.
8. Robins LN, Helzer JE, Weissman NM, Orvaschel H, et al. Lifetime prevalence of specific disorders in three sites. Arch Gen Psychiatry. 1984;41:949–58.
9. Linzer M, Spitzer R, Kroenke K, et al. Gender, quality of life, and mental disorders in primary care: results from the PRIME-MD 1000 study. Am J Med. 1996;101:526–33.
10. Gamma A, Angst J. Concurrent psychiatric comorbidity and multimorbidity in a community study: gender differences and quality of life. Eur Arch Psychiatry Clin Neurosci. 2001;251(Suppl 2):S1143–6.
11. Cloitre M, Yonkers KA, Pealstein T, Aletmus M, Davidson KW, Pigott A. Women and anxiety disorders: implications for diagnosis and treatment. CNS Spectr. 2004;9(Suppl 8):S1–16.
12. McLean CP, Asnaani A, Litz BT, Hofmann SG. Gender differences in anxiety disorders: prevalence, course of illness, comorbidity and burden of illness. J Psychiatr Res. 2011;45(8):1027–35.
13. Stein MB, et al. Childhood physical and sexual abuse in patients with anxiety disorders and in a community sample. Am J Psychiatry. 2004;153:275–7.
14. Ballús-Creus C, Bernardo M, Bioque Alcazar M, et al. Introduction to psychopathology and psychiatry. In: Vallejo Ruiloba J, editor. . 7th ed. Spain: Elsevier Masson; 2011.
15. Bekker M, van Mens-Verhulst J. Anxiety disorders: sex differences in prevalence, degree, and background, but gender-neutral treatment. Gend Med. 2007;4(Suppl B):S178–93.
16. Al-Ilssa I. The psychopathology of women. Englewood Cliffs: Prentice-Hall; 1980.

17. Wolfe BE. Gender ideology and phobias in women. In: Spatz Widom C, editor. Sex roles and psychopathology. New York: Plenum; 1984. p. 51–72.
18. Bekker MH. The development of an autonomy scale based on recent insights into gender identity. Eur J Personal. 1993;7:177–94.
19. Chodorw NJ. The reproduction of mothering: psychoanalysis and the sociology of gender. Berkeley: University of California Press; 1978.
20. Chodorw NJ. Feminism and psychoanalytic theory. Cambridge, MA: Pility Press; 1989.
21. Jordan JV, Kaplan AG, Miller JB, et al. Women's growth in connection: writings from the stone center. New York: Guildford; 1991.
22. Hettema JM, Prescott CA, Myers JM, Neale MC, Kendler KS. The structure of genetic and environmental risk factors for anxiety disorders in men and women. Arch Gen Psychiatry. 2005;62:182–9.
23. Barlow DH. Behavioral and cognitive models of post-traumatic stress disorder. Sante Ment Que. 1996;21(1):129–44. [Review] [57 refs] [French]
24. Cahill L, Haier RJ, White NS, Fallon J, Kilpatrick L, et al. Sex-related difference in amygdale activity during emotionally influenced memory storage. Neurobiol Learn Mem. 2001;75:1–9.
25. Cahill L. Sex-and hemisphere-related influences on the neurobiology of emotionally influenced memory. Prog Neuro-Psychopharmacol Biol Psychiatry. 2003;27:1235–41.
26. Cahill L. Why sex matter for neuroscience. Nat Rev Neurosci. 2006;7:477–84.
27. Cahill L. Brain sexual dimorphism. Sexual instinct. Tems 56: sexual instinct. Sexual Instinct Res Sci. 2009;56:62–70.
28. Nieto SJ, Patriquin MA, Nielsen DA, Kosten TA. Don't worry; be informed about the epigenetics of anxiety. Pharmacol Biochem Behav. 2016;146–147:60–72.
29. Murphy TM, O'Donovan A, Mullins N, O'Farrelly C, McCann A, Malone K. Anxiety associated with higher levels of global DNA methylation and altered expression of epigenetic and interleukin-6 genes. Psychiatr Genet. 2015;25(2):71–8.
30. Ziegler C, Dannlowski U, Bräuer D, Stevens S, Laeger I, Wittmann H, et al. Oxytocin receptor gene methylation: converging multilevel evidence for a role in social anxiety. Neuropsychopharmacology. 2015;40(6):1528–38.
31. Domschke K, Tidow N, Schrempf M, Schwarte K, Klauke B, Reif A, et al. Epigenetic signature of panic disorder: a role of glutamate decarboxylase 1 (GAD1) DNA hypomethylation? Prog Neuro-Psychopharmacol Biol Psychiatry. 2013;46:189–96.
32. Mitev YA, Darwish M, Wolf SS, Holsboer F, Almeida OF, Patchev VK. Gender differences in the regulation of 3 alpha-hydroxysteroid dehydrogenase in rat brain and sensitivity to neurosteroid-mediated stress protection. Neuroscience. 2003;20:541–9.
33. Piggot TA. Gender differences in the epidemiology and treatment of anxiety disorders. J Clin Psychiatry. 1999;60(Suppl 18):S4–15.
34. Alonso J, Angermeyer MC, Bernert S, Bruffaerts R, Brugha TS, Bryson H, et al. Prevalence of mental disorders in Europe: results from the European Study of the Epidemiology of Mental Disorders (ESEMED) project. Acta Psychiatr Scand Suppl. 2004;109(420):S21–7.
35. Carrasco-Galán I, Espinar-Fellmann I. Anxiety disorders and gender. Mind Brain. 2008;31:12–21.
36. Biggio G, Pisu MG, Biggio F, Serra M. Allopregnanolone modulation of HPA axis function in the adult rat. Psychopharmacology. 2014;231(17):3437–44.
37. Sripada RK, Welsh RC, Marx CE, Liberzon I. The neurosteroids allopregnanolone and dehydroepiandrosterone modulate resting-state amygdala connectivity. Hum Brain Mapp. 2014;35(7):3249–61.
38. Heron J, et al. The course of anxiety and depression through pregnancy and the postpartum in a community sample. J Affect Disord. 2004;80:65–73.
39. McLeod D, Hoehn-Saric R, Foster G, Hipsley P. The influence of premenstrual syndrome on rating of anxiety in woman with generalized anxiety disorder. Acta Psychiatr Scand. 1993;88:248–51.
40. Freeman EW. Premenstrual syndrome and premenstrual dysphoric disorder: definitions and diagnosis. Psychoneuroendocrinology. 2003;28(Suppl 3):S25–37.

41. Diagnostic and statistical manual of mental disorders. 5th ed. Arlington: American Psychiatric Association; 2013.
42. Silove D, Alonso J, Bromet E, Gruber M, Sampson N, Scott K, et al. Pediatric-onset and adult-onset separation anxiety disorder across countries in the world mental health survey. Am J Psychiatry. 2015;172(7):647–56. Epub 2015 Jun 5
43. Bergman RL, Piacentini J, McCracken JT. Prevalence and description of selective mutism in a school-based sample. J Am Acad Child Adolesc Psychiatry. 2002;41(8):938–46.
44. Kristensen H. Selective mutism and comorbidity with developmental disorder/delay, anxiety disorder, and elimination disorder. J Am Acad Child Adolesc Psychiatry. 2000;39(2):249–56.
45. Hua A, Major N. Selective mutism. Curr Opin Pediatr. 2016;28(1):114–20.
46. Sanchez PMG, Eguiluz UI. Thought content. In: Eguiluz UI, Segarra RE, editors. Introduction of the psychopathology, an integrative view. 3rd ed. Madrid: Panamericana; 2012. p. 98.
47. Chavina D, Stein M. Phenomenology of social phobia. In: Estein A, Hollander E, editors. Anxiety disorders treaty. Barcelona: Ars Medica; 2004.
48. Marcin M, Nemeroff C. The neurobiology of social anxiety disorder: the relevance of fear and anxiety. Acta Psychiatr Scand Suppl. 2003;108(417):S51–64.
49. Liebowitz M. Easing the burden of social anxiety disorder. J Clin Psychiatry. 2008;69(9):1485–96.
50. Yonkers KA, et al. An eight-year longitudinal comparison of clinical course and characteristics of social phobia among men and women. Psychiatr Serv. 2001;52:637–43.
51. Asher S, Aderka IM. Gender differences in social anxiety disorder: a review of the literature. J Anxiety Disord. 2017;49:23–31. https://doi.org/10.1016/j.janxdis.2017.03.004.
52. Kessler RC, et al. Prevalence, severity, and comorbidity of 12-month DSM-IV disorder in the National Comorbidity Survey Replication. Arch Gen Psychiatry. 2005;62:617–27.
53. Becker ES, et al. Epidemiology of specific phobia subtypes: findings from the Dresden Mental Health Study. Eur Psychiatry. 2007;22:69–74.
54. Wythilingun B, Stein D. Specific phobia. In: Stein D, editor. Clinical manual of anxiety disorders. Washington, DC: American Psychiatric Public; 2004.
55. Van Houtem CM, Laine ML, Boomsma DI, Ligthart L, van Wijk AJ, De Jongh A. A review and meta-analysis of the heritability of specific phobia subtypes and corresponding fears. J Anxiety Disord. 2013;27(4):379–88.
56. Seo D, Ahluwalia A, Potenza MN, Sinha R. Gender differences in neuralcorrelates of stress-induced anxiety. J Neurosci Res. 2017;95(1–2):115–25.
57. Altemus M, Epstein L. Sex differences in anxiety disorders. In: Becker JB, Berkley KJ, Geary N, Hampson E, Herman JP, Young EA, editors. Sex differences in the brain. New York: Oxford University Press; 2008. p. 397–404.
58. Kessler RC, McGonagle KA, Zhao S, et al. Lifetime and 12 month prevalence of DSM-III-R psychiatric disorders in the United States: results from the national comorbidity survey. Arch Gen Psychiatry. 1994;51(1):8–19.
59. Starcevic V, Djordjevic A, Latas M, Bogojevic G. Characteristics of agoraphobia in woman and men with panic disorder with agoraphobia. Depress Anxiety. 1998;8:8–13.
60. Cox BJ, Swinson RP, Shulman ID, et al. Gender effects and alcohol use in panic disorder with agoraphobia. Behav Res Ther. 1993;31(4):413–6.
61. NCS-R. Lifetime prevalence of GSM-IV/WMH-CIDI disorders by de sex and cohort. NCS-Update. Jun 17 2007.
62. Weissman M, Bland R, Canino G, Faravelli C, et al. The cross-national epidemiology of panic disorder. Arch Gen Psychiatry. 1997;54(4):305–9.
63. Eaton W, Kramer M, Anthony JC. The incidence of specific DIS/DSM-III mental disorders: data from the NIMH Epidemiologic Catchment Area Program. Acta Psychiatr Scand. 1989;79(2):163–78.
64. Scheibe G, Albus M. Age at onset, precipitating events, sex distribution, and co-occurrence of anxiety disorders. Psychopathology. 1992;25:11–8.
65. Sheikh JI, et al. Gender differences in panic disorder: findings from the National Comorbidity Survey. Am J Psychiatry. 2002;159:55–8.

66. Turgeon L, Marchand A, Dupuis G. Clinical features in panic disorder with agoraphobia: a comparison of men and women. J Anxiety Disord. 1998;12(6):539–42.
67. Kendler K, Walters E, Neale M, Kessler R, et al. The structure of genetic and environmental risk factors for six major psychiatric disorders in women. Phobia, generalized anxiety disorder, panic disorder, bulimia, major depression, and alcoholism. Arch Gen Psychiatry. 1995;52(5):374–83.
68. Yonkers KA, et al. Chronicity, relapse, and illness-course of panic disorder, social phobia, and generalized anxiety disorder: findings in men and women from 8 years of follow-up. Depress Anxiety. 2003;17:173–9.
69. Yonkers KA, Zlotnick C, Allsworth J, et al. Is the course of panic disorder the same in men and women? Am J Psychiatry. 1998;155:596–602.
70. Sadock BJ, Sadock VA. Kaplan and Sadock's synopsis of psychiatry. 10th ed. New York: Wolters Kluwer; 2012.
71. Kessler RC, et al. The epidemiology of generalized anxiety disorder. Psychiatr Clin North Am. 2001;24:19–39.
72. Lochner C, Hemmings SM, Kinnear CJ, Moolman-Smook JC, Corfield VA, Knowles JA, et al. Gender in obsessive-compulsive disorder: clinical and genetic findings. Eur Neuropsychopharmacol. 2004;14:105–13.
73. Bogetto F, Venturello S, Albert U, Maina G, Gand L, Ravizza A. Gender-related clinical differences in obsessive-compulsive disorder. Eur Psychiatry. 1999;14:434–41.
74. Torresan RC, Ramos-Cerqueira AT, De Mathis MA, Diniz J-B, Ferra˜o YA, Miguel EC, Torres AR. Sex differences in the phenotypic expression of obsessive-compulsive disorder: an exploratory study from Brazil. Compr Psychiatry. 2009;50:63–9.
75. Tukel R, Polat A, Genc A, Bozkurt O, Atli H. Gender-related differences among Turkish patients with obsessive-compulsive disorder. Compr Psychiatry. 2004;45:362–6.
76. Alonso P, et al. Long-term follow up and predictors of clinical outcome in obsessive- compulsive patients treated with serotonin reuptake inhibitors and behavioral therapy. J Clin Psychiatry. 2001;62:535–40.
77. Labad J, et al. Female reproductive cycle and obsessive-compulsive disorder. J Clin Psychiatry. 2005;66:428–35.
78. Williams KE, Koran LM. Obsessive-compulsive disorder in pregnancy, the puerperium, and the premenstruum. J Clin Psychiatry. 1997;58:330–4.
79. Vulink NC, et al. Female hormones affect symptom severity in obsessive-compulsive disorder. Int Clin Psychopharmacol. 2006;21:171–5.
80. Clayton JA, Collins FS. Policy: NIH to balance sex in cell and animal studies. Nature. 2014;509(7500):282–3.
81. Cahill L, Aswad D. Sex influences on the Brain: an issue whose time has come. Neuron. 2015;88(6):1084–5.
82. Hamilton J, Yonkers K. Sex differences in pharmacokinetics of psychotropic medications. In: Jensvold M, Halbreich U, Hamilton J, editors. Psychopharmacology and woman. Washington, DC: American Psychiatric Press; 1996.
83. Van der Waals FW, et al. Sex differences among recipients of benzodiazepines in Dutch general practice. Br Med J. 1993;307:363–6.
84. Wang PS, et al. Failure and delay in initial treatment contact after first onset of mental disorders in the National Comorbidity Survey Replication. Arch Gen Psychiatry. 2005;62:603–13.
85. Kimmel S, Gonsalves L. Fluctuating level of antidepressants premenstrually. J Psychosom Obstet Gynaecol. 1992;13:277–80.
86. Ellinwood EH, Easler ME, Linnoila M. Effects of oral contraceptives on diazepam induced psychomotor impairment. Clin Pharmacol Ther. 1994;35:360–6.
87. Abernethy DR, Greenblatt DJ, Shader RI. Imipramine and desipramine disposition in the elderly. J Pharmacol Exp Ther. 1985;232:183–8.
88. Butler AC, Chapman JE, Forman EM, Beck AT. The empirical status of cognitive-behavioral therapy: a review of meta-analyses. Clin Psychol Rev. 2006;26:17–31.

The Gender Perspective in Trauma Spectrum Disorders

20

Mayte López-Atanes, Ingo Schäfer, Maria Jolin Rodrigo, and Leire Erkoreka

20.1 Introduction

Over the past several decades, the adverse effects of psychological trauma have received increasing attention. Post-traumatic stress disorder (PTSD) was first officially defined in 1980 in the third edition of the APA classification system, DSM-3. However, the actual criteria for what constitutes psychological trauma have varied over time. Currently, the DSM-5 mentions a major traumatic event such as exposure to actual or threatened death, serious injury, or sexual violence, while the recently approved International Classification of Diseases (ICD)-11 diagnostic

M. López-Atanes (✉)
Department of Psychiatry, University Hospital Galdakao-Usansolo, Galdakao, Spain

University of the Basque Country, Bilbao, Spain

Center of Interdisciplinary Addiction Research, University of Hamburg, Hamburg, Germany
e-mail: M.lopezatanes@centra.hamburg

I. Schäfer
Center of Interdisciplinary Addiction Research, University of Hamburg, Hamburg, Germany

Department of Psychiatry and Psychotherapy, University Medical Center Hamburg-Eppendorf, Hamburg, Germany
e-mail: i.schaefer@uke.de

M. J. Rodrigo
University Hospital Galdakao-Usansolo, Galdakao, Spain
e-mail: maria.jolinrodrigo@osakidetza.eus

L. Erkoreka
University Hospital Galdakao-Usansolo, Galdakao, Spain

University of the Basque Country, Bilbao, Spain
e-mail: leire.erkorekagonzalez@osakidetza.eus

M. López-Atanes, M. Sáenz-Herrero (eds.), *Applying the Gender Perspective in Psychiatry and Psychotherapy*, https://doi.org/10.1007/978-3-032-17883-1_20

guidelines for PTSD mention an "extremely distressing or life-threatening event or series of events, such as sexual abuse or a serious accident" [1, 2].

There are three sets of symptoms that are common to both ICD-11 and DSM-5 criteria and are usually considered to be the core symptoms of PTSD. These are intrusions or re-experiencing of the event (such as intrusive memories, repetitive acting out of the event or aspects of it, nightmares, flashbacks, distress triggered by reminders of the event(s)); avoidance (such as avoiding thoughts, feelings, or reminders of the event(s), or avoiding people, places, conversations, or situations associated with the event(s)); and arousal and reactivity or feelings of current threat (such as irritability, hypervigilance, easily startled, difficulty concentrating, difficulty sleeping) [2, 3].

Exposure to a traumatic event, defined according to the diagnostic guidelines, is required for the diagnosis of post-traumatic stress disorder (PTSD), making PTSD a psychiatric disorder that, by definition, is related to and occurs because of a stressful or traumatic event. However, the consequences of psychological trauma are not limited to PTSD. In addition to PTSD, patients with other disorders have high rates of traumatic experiences, including patients with depression, drug and alcohol abuse, anxiety disorders, borderline personality disorder (BPD), and somatic disorders [4, 5]. Although the diagnosis of these latter disorders does not necessarily require exposure to a traumatic event, epidemiological studies have provided strong evidence that stressful life experiences and trauma are major risk factors for their development [5–7].

Additionally, in the last ICD-11 guidelines the diagnosis of complex PTSD has been recognized, as some people's reactions to traumatic events go beyond previous definitions of PTSD [1, 8]. To receive this diagnosis, one must have the core symptoms of PTSD and experience disturbances in self-identity (e.g., negative self-concept), emotional dysregulation (e.g., emotional reactivity, violent outbursts), and persistent difficulties in relationships [1, 2]. In recent years, complex post-traumatic stress disorder has been the subject of numerous investigations which have confirmed its close relationship with child sexual abuse, although it can also arise after other traumas such as torture [9]. Furthermore, it has been determined that it is a different entity to borderline personality disorder, despite the large number of overlapping symptoms and frequent comorbidity [10–12].

20.2 Epidemiology of Traumatic Experiences and Trauma-Related Disorders

Studies show that a large percentage of the population has been exposed to traumatic events [13]. The National Comorbidity Survey (NCS) by Kessler and co-workers [14] examined trauma exposure in a nationwide probability sample of 5877 adult residents of the United States and found that 61% of men and 51% of women had experienced at least one traumatic event during their lifetime. However, only a fraction of individuals goes on to develop post-traumatic stress disorder, and most recover to pre-trauma levels of psychological functioning [15]. The exact prevalence of this disorder is not known as the literature provides very different results, ranging from 2.5 to 74%, but it is probably around 10%, depending on the population studied [16]. Additionally, not all potential events have the same risk of developing subsequent psychopathology: natural disasters are linked to a much lower risk of developing PTSD (5–10%) compared to interpersonal trauma, such as a sexual assault (40%) [17, 18]. Long-term, repeated interpersonal trauma, which includes intimate partner violence, carries the highest risk of developing severe forms of PTSD, especially complex PTSD [17, 19].

Sex/gender differences in PTSD are well established, with women having twice the prevalence of men and a higher risk of developing PTSD after experiencing a traumatic event [20, 21]. Men are more likely than women to report an overall history of potentially traumatic events [14], but certain types of traumata, such as childhood sexual abuse, sexual assault, and intimate partner violence occur more often in women and have also been linked to a higher odd of PTSD development [17, 19, 22]. However, studies have shown that a higher proportion of sexual and interpersonal trauma not clearly explains the different risk respecting gender [21, 23]. Other factors, such as a higher prevalence of depression in this group, the type of cognitive appraisal, the sum of social difficulties, and differences in the hormonal stress response, are also hypothesized to play a role [22–24]. Among LGTBQ populations, transgender people are 2.52 times more likely to have PTSD than their cis counterparts, followed by bisexual people in terms of increased risk (OR: 2.44) [25].

Because the type of trauma experienced determines the clinical presentation and therapeutic approach, gender differences in the types of traumata experienced deserve special attention. In high-income countries, women are more likely to report childhood sexual abuse (7–34% vs. 3–29% of men) [26], in contrast to other types of childhood maltreatment that show no gender difference. In low-income countries, girls are at greater risk of infanticide, sexual abuse, and neglect, while boys appear to be at greater risk of harsh corporal punishment [27]. Throughout adulthood, women continue to experience more episodes of interpersonal trauma, particularly intimate partner violence and sexual abuse. To get a clear picture of the scope of violence against women, Eurostat conducted a comprehensive survey on gender-based violence involving 114,023 women (aged 18 to 74) from across the EU. The results show that in the EU-27, 17.7% of women have experienced physical violence or threats and/or sexual violence by an intimate partner during their lifetime. The prevalence rate of lifetime intimate partner violence is higher (31.8%) when psychological violence is included. In the 12 months prior to the survey, 5.3% of women in the EU had experienced physical violence or threats, sexual violence, and/or psychological violence by an intimate partner [28]. In addition, 30.8% of women have experienced sexual harassment at work and 12.9% have experienced sexual violence since the age of 15. In other contexts, the situation is even more dramatic: for example, almost 90% of women in Afghanistan have experienced at least one form of domestic violence, 17% have experienced sexual violence, and 52% have experienced physical violence [29]. The data show that violence against women is systematic and universal.

20.3 Violence Against Women as Collective Traumatization

In recent years, there has been growing attention to gender-based violence (GBV), which is "the violence directed against a person because of that person's gender or violence that disproportionately affects people of a particular gender" [28]. Due to the magnitude of the problem and the emergence of feminist activism, several public institutions and governments have increased their efforts to study and prevent gender-based violence. Feminist activism recognizes the collective experience of GBV and therefore promotes women's empowerment. The American Psychological Association (APA) also cites gender-based violence as an example of collective trauma [30], which contrasts with the few studies that academically examine the collective experience of gender-based trauma [31, 32], and the standard approach as an individual trauma in clinical practice.

Collective trauma refers to the psychological reactions to violence perpetrated against a particular group, making it a shared experience of violence with ongoing repercussions on a group's identity and social memory. Collective memory of trauma differs from individual memory because collective memory persists beyond the lives of the direct survivors of the events and is remembered by group members who may be far removed in time and space from the traumatic events. These subsequent generations of trauma survivors, who never experienced the actual events, may remember the events differently than the direct survivors, and then the construction of these past events may take different forms and shapes from generation to generation [33]. It also differs from the definition of individual trauma in that collective trauma reflects the long-term social and political implications of a traumatic history that are transmitted across time and space and does not refer to individual psychopathological reactions to trauma. Victims of collective trauma experience losses of group power, status, and control, which can contribute to feelings of anxiety, fear, sadness, mistrust, perceived loss of control, avoidance, social isolation, and loneliness that persist across generations [34, 35].

Rachel Pain tries to frame GBV as collective trauma providing arguments supporting this conceptualization [31]. First, she points to the universal nature of violence against women, due to a united sense of suffering, the fact that GBV is an endemic condition of many cultures and its collective dimensions (such as societal judgments of how survivors behave, tell their stories, and seek help, whether they are believed and how culpable they are held). She also mentions the collective control that GBV exerts, because only some violent acts are needed to raise wider awareness of danger. From childhood, women are warned of the dangers of men, even before they experience violence themselves. These warnings are meant to protect girls and women from acts of violence that previous generations have already experienced. As a result, many women feel hypervigilant when potentially exposed to such situations, even if they haven't experienced violent acts themselves [36, 37]. Sexual violence and the fear of sexual violence have a clear, empirically documented impact on women's lives. Research shows that women often position themselves in relation to feelings of vulnerability, spatially protecting themselves from unknown men in public spaces [38, 39]. The classic example is walking alone at night and feeling anxious and hyperalert to any potential threat. If a man comes along, women may already feel in danger and react as if they are already in danger of being raped, even if the man has no intention of doing so. Men, however, do not experience this when walking alone at night, unless they have experienced a traumatic event. Fear associated with nighttime, or poorly lit, commuting has been shown to negatively impact female students' physical, emotional, and social health [40], and feelings of safety also affect sleep patterns and academic performance [41].

Feminist sociologists have already argued that rape works to disempower women. As Campbell A. discussed, rape-prevention strategies usually focus on women's safety, suggesting safety strategies primarily for women in public. Thus, the focus is on the victim instead of the perpetrator [38]. Due to this, after a disclosure of rape, it is still common that the focus is not on the perpetrator but on how the victim failed to protect herself, receiving negative reactions, even from family members and being socially stigmatized [42–44]. Safe-keeping strategies become acts of self-surveillance, as women position themselves as anxious and at risk, seeming to authenticate their vulnerable nature [38]. However, it can also be argued that women's fear of crime is a rational response to a real threat in terms of the amount and variety of violence that women experience at different points in their lives. Women tend to avoid doing certain things or going to certain places as part of their risk-avoidance behavior. These concerns are compounded by women's past exposure to various forms of threat and violence and the collective experiences of other women, which can reinforce a sense of threat [45].

Another important aspect is that most acts of sexual violence against women are perpetrated by men in the victim's social network, such as a family member, romantic partner, or work colleague. In college women, up to 85–90% of assaults are committed by someone known, and only a minority by strangers [46]. However, women are most concerned about possible assault by men they do not know. They are less concerned about assault by a range of other people they know, including current and former partners [45]. In many cases, women do not even recognize these acts as violence because they do not fit into their scheme of things. Research shows that when the assault is perpetrated by an acquaintance, it may occur in situations that are considered normal socializing, such as dating or parties. Optimistic bias, or the thought that "it won't happen to me," can also lead women to underestimate the risk of acquaintance assault [47]. Additionally, nonconsensual sex may be perceived as rape by the victim if the perpetrator is unknown but not if the perpetrator is a romantic partner. In fact, rape within marriage is still permitted in many countries. As a result, victims of intimate partner sexual violence are more likely to suffer from feelings of guilt, victimization, and shame, as well as difficulty communicating the experience [48].

20.4 Reactions of the Practitioner in the Treatment of Traumatized Patients

Therapists working with people who have experienced trauma often experience emotions or reactions of their own during the therapy process. These reactions may be temporary, such as a counter-traumatic reaction, or they may cause a transformation in the therapist's experience or perception of the world, which is called vicarious trauma. Traumatic countertransference is a term coined by Judith Herman, who in 1992 published *Trauma and Recovery*, which outlined new concepts for understanding, defining, and treating post-traumatic stress disorder (PTSD) [49]. Herman's theory was based on years of work with people who had suffered trauma, including survivors of sexual assault, domestic violence, natural disasters, and military combat. Despite the limited conceptual clarity surrounding counter-traumatic reactions in trauma therapy, research suggests that therapists may experience complex emotional responses when working with trauma survivors, including identification with clients' helplessness and heightened awareness of their own vulnerability. These reactions may produce a sense of disconnection from the environment, sadness, hopelessness, or anger [50].

In contrast to traumatic countertransference, which is temporarily linked to a particular session, event or problem that reacts with the internal or external life of the therapist, vicarious traumatization is the result of the cumulative effect of ongoing exposure to traumatic experiences by mental health professionals. Its effects are persistent and are felt beyond a particular therapy, both in other therapeutic relationships and in the therapist's personal and professional life [51, 52]. Symptoms of vicarious traumatization are multiple. Emotional symptoms of vicarious trauma can consist of prolonged grief, sadness, or irritability or anger. Therapist can feel easily distracted or experience mood swings. Behavioral symptoms consist of sense of isolation, substance abuse, or risk-taking behaviors. Cognitive symptoms may be cynicism and negativity, difficulty with concentration or focus, or memory problems [53]. Although some individuals experience positive psychological changes as a result of working with trauma survivors, therapists need to be aware that vicarious traumatization can have a negative impact on therapy, leading to disruption of the therapeutic alliance, boundary overstepping, conflict within professional teams, and the urge to rescue or control clients [54].

20.5 Gender in PTSD Treatment Interventions

There are a number of possible treatments for PTSD, including trauma-focused interventions, non-trauma-focused interventions, and pharmacological approaches. Treatment guidelines typically recommend various types of trauma-focused psychotherapeutic treatments as first-line treatments for PTSD, as several studies have shown them to be effective in reducing PTSD symptoms [55–57]. However, evidence on whether there are gender differences in response to psychological and other interventions for PTSD is scarce. In one meta-analysis, [58] evaluated gender differences in the outcomes of trauma-focused therapy for PTSD. They found that although trauma-focused therapy was effective in both men and women, women showed greater reductions in both clinician-rated and self-rated PTSD symptoms compared to men [58]. However, they pointed that more than 30% of studies could not be included in the analysis due to lack of sex/gender disaggregated data, which could have affected these results. Also, there was heterogeneity in the type of traumatic experiences and method of exposure therapy included. Blain et al. [59] also found that only a small minority of RCTs that included participants of both genders examined gender differences in treatment outcomes, but those that did showed equivalent outcomes for primary PTSD symptoms.

Regarding the LGBT+ population, there are no established guidelines for the treatment of PTSD due to the lack of studies that specifically focus on this population, even though they are disproportionally affected by trauma. However, quality patient-centered communication is recommended, as LGBT+ individuals are more likely than the general population to experience discrimination both in daily life and when seeking mental and physical health care [60]. This makes these patients more likely to show distrust on the medical system. Clinicians and their practices can take steps to create an environment of safety and inclusion by establishing clear nondiscrimination policies, providing training on LGBT+ health, and establishing a formal process for LGBT+ clients to raise concerns or complaints. In addition, clinicians should strive to be gender inclusive. For example, asking for preferred pronouns and talking about relationships in an inclusive way (i.e., not assuming a heterosexual or cisgender identity) [61]. The effectiveness of specific trauma exposure therapies has been largely unexplored. Narrative exposure therapy has some evidence of effectiveness in this population, with results showing statistically significant reductions in post-traumatic stress symptoms and increases in resilience and positive well-being at discharge from treatment [62, 63].

20.6 Conclusions

Post-traumatic stress disorder and stress-related disorders are highly prevalent in the general population. However, women have a higher prevalence of these disorders and a higher risk of developing PTSD following a traumatic event. Although the reasons for this are likely to be both social and biological, the fact that they are exposed to a greater number of interpersonal traumas from childhood influences the development of the disorder. The same is true for non-binary populations, who suffer from hate crimes and discrimination in addition to other types of potential traumatic events. When treating PTSD, it is necessary to consider the influence of gender: gender-based violence must be recognized as a systemic phenomenon that not only affects at an individual level. Gender influences social interactions, how others respond, and how women experience violence. Given the universal and systemic nature of violence against women, many women presenting for treatment have experienced this violence at some point in their lives. While treatment for traumatic exposure is necessary and has been shown to be effective, there is also a need to promote the empowerment and dignity of discriminated groups, such as women and non-binary individuals, who may be particularly distrustful of the health care system due to previous experiences of discrimination. In addition, many of these patients will also require psychosocial support, so a multidisciplinary approach is needed to introduce the gender perspective in trauma care.

References

1. Maercker A, Eberle DJ. Disorders specifically associated with stress in ICD-11. Vol. 4, Clin Psychol Eur PsychOpen; 2022.
2. Bryant RA. Post-traumatic stress disorder: a state-of-the-art review of evidence and challenges. World Psychiatry. 2019;18(3):259–69.
3. Heim C, Douglas Bremner J, Nemeroff CB. Trauma spectrum disorders. In: Runge MS, Patterson C, editors. Principles of molecular medicine [Internet]. Totowa: Humana Press; 2006. p. 1203–10. Available from: https://doi.org/10.1007/978-1-59259-963-9_127.
4. Copeland WE, Shanahan L, Hinesley J, Chan RF, Aberg KA, Fairbank JA, et al. Association of Childhood Trauma Exposure with adult psychiatric disorders and functional outcomes. JAMA Network Open [Internet]. 2018;1(7):e184493. Available from: https://doi.org/10.1001/jamanetworkopen.2018.4493
5. Bailey M, Fairchild G, Hammerton G, Bauer A, Carpena MX, Murray J, et al. Associations between childhood trauma and adolescent psychiatric disorders in Brazil: a longitudinal, population-based birth cohort study. Lancet Glob Health [Internet]. 2025;13(2):e309–18. Available from: https://doi.org/10.1016/S2214-109X(24)00452-2
6. Lewis SJ, Arseneault L, Caspi A, Fisher HL, Matthews T, Moffitt TE, et al. The epidemiology of trauma and post-traumatic stress disorder in a representative cohort of young people in England and Wales. Lancet Psychiatry [Internet]. 2019;6(3):247–56. Available from: https://doi.org/10.1016/S2215-0366(19)30031-8
7. Webb RT, Antonsen S, Carr MJ, Appleby L, Pedersen CB, Mok PLH. Self-harm and violent criminality among young people who experienced trauma-related hospital admission during childhood: a Danish national cohort study. Lancet Public Health [Internet]. 2017;2(7):e314–22. Available from: https://doi.org/10.1016/S2468-2667(17)30094-4
8. Reed GM, First MB, Kogan CS, Hyman SE, Gureje O, Gaebel W, et al. Innovations and changes in the ICD-11 classification of mental, behavioural and neurodevelopmental disorders. World Psychiatry. 2019;18(1):3–19.
9. Nickerson A, Cloitre M, Bryant RA, Schnyder U, Morina N, Schick M. The factor structure of complex posttraumatic stress disorder in traumatized refugees. Eur J Psychotraumatol. 2016;7(1)
10. Cloitre M, Garvert DW, Weiss B, Carlson EB, Bryant RA. Distinguishing PTSD, complex PTSD, and borderline personality disorder: a latent class analysis. Eur J Psychotraumatol. 2014;5
11. Cloitre M, Garvert DW, Brewin CR, Bryant RA, Maercker A. Evidence for proposed ICD-11 PTSD and complex PTSD: a latent profile analysis. Eur J Psychotraumatol. 2013;4(SUPPL)
12. Knefel M, Donn WG, Marylene C, Lueger-Schuster B. Update to an evaluation of ICD-11 PTSD and complex PTSD criteria in a sample of adult survivors of childhood institutional abuse by Knefel & Lueger-Schuster (2013): a latent profile analysis. Eur J Psychotraumatol [Internet]. 2015;6(1):25290. Available from: https://doi.org/10.3402/ejpt.v6.25290
13. Knipscheer J, Sleijpen M, Frank L, de Graaf R, Kleber R, Ten Have M, et al. Prevalence of potentially traumatic events, other life events and subsequent reactions indicative for posttraumatic stress disorder in The Netherlands: a general population study based on the trauma screening questionnaire. Int J Environ Res Public Health. 2020;17(5)

14. Kessler RC, Sonnega A, Bromet E, Hughes M, Nelson CB. Posttraumatic stress disorder in the National Comorbidity Survey. Arch Gen Psychiatry [Internet]. 1995;52(12):1048–60. Available from: https://doi.org/10.1001/archpsyc.1995.03950240066012
15. Littleton H, Danny A, Grills-Taquechel AE. Longitudinal evaluation of the relationship between maladaptive trauma coping and distress: examination following the mass shooting at Virginia Tech. Anxiety Stress Coping [Internet]. 2011;24(3):273–90. Available from: https://doi.org/10.1080/10615806.2010.500722
16. Schincariol A, Orrù G, Otgaar H, Sartori G, Scarpazza C. Posttraumatic stress disorder (PTSD) prevalence: an umbrella review. Psychol Med. Cambridge University Press. 2024;54:1.
17. Liu H, Petukhova MV, Sampson NA, Aguilar-Gaxiola S, Alonso J, Andrade LH, et al. Association of DSM-IV posttraumatic stress disorder with traumatic experience type and history in the World Health Organization World Mental Health Surveys. JAMA Psychiatr [Internet]. 2017;74(3):270–81. Available from: https://doi.org/10.1001/jamapsychiatry.2016.3783
18. Creamer M, Burgess P, McFarlane AC. Post-traumatic stress disorder: findings from the Australian National Survey of Mental Health and Well-being. Psychol Med [Internet]. 2001;31(7):1237–47. Available from: https://www.cambridge.org/core/product/E3BC3B438AA652411395CC4F2CE59653
19. Fernández-Fillol C, Pitsiakou C, Perez-Garcia M, Teva I, Hidalgo-Ruzzante N. Complex PTSD in survivors of intimate partner violence: risk factors related to symptoms and diagnoses. Eur J Psychotraumatol. 2021;12(1)
20. Tolin DF, Foa EB. Sex differences in trauma and posttraumatic stress disorder: a quantitative review of 25 years of research. Psychol Bull. 2006 Nov;132(6):959–92.
21. Christiansen DM, Berke ET. Gender- and sex-based contributors to sex differences in PTSD. Curr Psychiatry Rep. Springer. 2020;22
22. Ditlevsen DN, Elklit A. Gender, trauma type, and PTSD prevalence: a re-analysis of 18 nordic convenience samples. Ann Gen Psychiatry [Internet]. 2012;11(1):26. Available from: https://doi.org/10.1186/1744-859X-11-26
23. Christiansen DM, Hansen M. Accounting for sex differences in PTSD: a multi-variable mediation model. Eur J Psychotraumatol. 2015;6:1–10.
24. Olff M, Langeland W, Draijer N, Gersons BPR. Gender differences in posttraumatic stress disorder. Psychol Bull. 2007;133:183–204.
25. Marchi M, Travascio A, Uberti D, De Micheli E, Grenzi P, Arcolin E, et al. Post-traumatic stress disorder among LGBTQ people: a systematic review and meta-analysis. Epidemiol Psychiatric Sci. Cambridge University Press. 2023;32
26. Finkelhor D. The international epidemiology of child sexual abuse. Child Abuse Negl [Internet]. 1994;18(5):409–17. Available from: https://www.sciencedirect.com/science/article/pii/0145213494900264
27. Gilbert R, Widom CS, Browne K, Fergusson D, Webb E, Janson S. Burden and consequences of child maltreatment in high-income countries. Lancet [Internet]. 2009;373(9657):68–81. Available from: https://doi.org/10.1016/S0140-6736(08)61706-7
28. European Union Agency for fundamental rights. EU gender-based violence survey -.
29. Afghanistan Multiple Indicator Cluster Survey. 2010.
30. Psychological Association A. APA Presidential Task Force Culturally Informed Trauma and Grief Recovery Toolkit Collective Trauma.
31. Pain R. Collective trauma? Isolating and commoning gender-based violence. Gend Place Cult. 2022;29(12):1788–809.
32. Salter M, Woodlock D, Dragiewicz M, Conroy E, Ussher J, Burke J, et al. "I see it running through my family": the intergenerational and collective trauma of gender-based violence. J Family Trauma Child Custody Child Develop. 2025;22:254.
33. Hirschberger G. Collective trauma and the social construction of meaning. Front Psychol. Frontiers Media S.A. 2018;9

34. Mengyao L, Bernhard L, Gilad H, Jiyoung P. From threat to challenge: understanding the impact of historical collective trauma on contemporary intergroup conflict. Perspect Psychol Sci [Internet]. 2022;18(1):190–209. Available from: https://doi.org/10.1177/17456916221094540
35. Lykes MB, Beristain CM, Pérez-Armiñan MLC. Political violence, impunity, and emotional climate in Maya communities. J Soc Issues [Internet]. 2007;63(2):369–85. Available from: https://doi.org/10.1111/j.1540-4560.2007.00514.x
36. Christine B, Linda S. Feeling safe in the dark: examining the effect of entrapment, lighting levels, and gender on feelings of safety and lighting policy acceptability. Environ Behav [Internet]. 2012;46(2):193–212. Available from: https://doi.org/10.1177/0013916512453838
37. Chaney RA, Baer A, Tovar LI. Gender-based heat map images of campus walking settings: a reflection of lived experience. Violence Gend [Internet]. 2023;11(1):35–42. Available from: https://doi.org/10.1089/vio.2023.0027
38. Campbell A. Keeping the "lady" safe: the regulation of femininity through crime prevention literature. Crit Criminol. 2005;13:119–40.
39. Curchin K. The dilemma of rape avoidance advice: acknowledging women's agency without blaming victims of sexual assault. Womens Stud Int Forum [Internet]. 2019;75:102240. Available from: https://www.sciencedirect.com/science/article/pii/S0277539518305582
40. Burdette AM, Needham BL. Neighborhood environment and body mass index trajectories from adolescence to adulthood. J Adolesc Health [Internet]. 2012;50(1):30–7. Available from: https://doi.org/10.1016/j.jadohealth.2011.03.009
41. Etopio AL, Berthelot ER. Defining and measuring fear of crime: a new validated scale created from emotion theory, qualitative interviews, and factor analyses. Criminol Criminal Justice Law Soc. 2022;23(1):46–67.
42. Ahrens CE. Being silenced: the impact of negative social reactions on the disclosure of rape. Am J Community Psychol. 2006;38(3–4):263–74.
43. Elliott SA, Goodman KL, Bardwell ES, Mullin TM. Reactions to the disclosure of intrafamilial childhood sexual abuse: findings from the National Sexual Assault Online Hotline. Child Abuse Negl [Internet]. 2022;127:105567. Available from: https://www.sciencedirect.com/science/article/pii/S0145213422000874
44. Jewkes R, Mhlongo S, Chirwa E, Seedat S, Myers B, Peer N, et al. Pathways to and factors associated with rape stigma experienced by rape survivors in South Africa: analysis of baseline data from a rape cohort. Clin Psychol Psychother. 2022;29(1):328–38.
45. Violence against women: an EU-wide survey Main results Violence against women: an EU-wide survey. Available from: http://europa.eu
46. National Institute of Justice. "Most Victims Know Their Attacker," [Internet]. [cited 2025 Apr 15]. Available from: https://nij.ojp.gov/topics/articles/most-victims-know-their-attacker#0-0
47. Nurius PS. Risk perception for acquaintance sexual aggression: a social-cognitive perspective. Aggress Violent Behav. Elsevier Ltd. 2000;5:63–78.
48. Kennedy AC. Sexual Violence within Intimate Relationships [Internet]. Available from: https://www.researchgate.net/publication/349255308
49. Herman JL. Trauma and recovery. New York NB Books, editor. 1992.
50. Phillips SBD. Group Interventions for Treatment of Psychological Trauma Module 7: Countertransference: Effects on the Group Therapist Working with Trauma.
51. Cavanagh A, Wiese Batista E. Countertransference in trauma therapy. J Trauma Stress Disord Treat. 2015;04(04)
52. Baird K, Kracen AC. Vicarious traumatization and secondary traumatic stress: a research synthesis*. Couns Psychol Q [Internet]. 2006;19(2):181–8. Available from: https://doi.org/10.1080/09515070600811899
53. Jimenez RR, Andersen S, Song H, Townsend C. Vicarious trauma in mental health care providers. J Interprof Educ Pract [Internet]. 2021;24:100451. Available from: https://www.sciencedirect.com/science/article/pii/S2405452621000380

54. McNeillie N, Rose J. Vicarious trauma in therapists: a meta-ethnographic review. Behav Cogn Psychother [Internet]. 2021;49(4):426–40. Available from: https://www.cambridge.org/core/product/CF4E8B70A0DCF3D74D84122251178E9A
55. APA. Guideline Development Panel for the Treatment of Posttraumatic Stress Disorder in Adults Adopted as APA Policy PTSD Clinical Practice Guideline for the Treatment of. 2017.
56. Post-traumatic stress disorder NICE guideline [Internet]. 2018. Available from: www.nice.org.uk/guidance/ng116
57. Hamblen JL, Norman SB, Sonis JH, Phelps AJ, Bisson JI, Nunes VD, et al. A guide to guidelines for the treatment of posttraumatic stress disorder in adults: an update. Psychotherapy.. American Psychological Association Inc. 2019;56:359–73.
58. Wade D, Varker T, Kartal D, Hetrick S, O'Donnell M, Forbes D. Gender difference in outcomes following trauma-focused interventions for posttraumatic stress disorder: systematic review and meta-analysis. Psychol Trauma. 2016;8(3):356–64.
59. Blain LM, Galovski TE, Robinson T. Gender differences in recovery from posttraumatic stress disorder: a critical review. Aggress Violent Behav. 2010;15:463–74.
60. Livingston NA, Berke D, Scholl J, Ruben M, Shipherd JC. Addressing diversity in PTSD treatment: clinical considerations and guidance for the treatment of PTSD in LGBTQ populations. Curr Treat Options Psychiatry. Springer. 2020;7:53–69.
61. PTSD: National Center for PTSD. Assessment and Treatment Considerations for Working With LGBTQ+ Clients With PTSD.
62. Julian JM, Conn BM, Chavez M, Zubareva N, Wages E. Narrative exposure therapy to reduce posttraumatic stress symptoms among transgender and gender diverse adolescents and young adults: a pilot study. Psychol Sex Orientat Gend Divers. 2024; No Pagination Specified-No Pagination Specified
63. Casas MA, Conn BM. Narrative exposure therapy for treating post-traumatic stress among transgender youth of color with selective mutism. Clin Case Stud. 2024;23(1):63–81.

Eating Disorders

21

Margarita Sáenz-Herrero, Olatz Napal Fernández, Luis Urgoiti González, and Ana Espiga Izuzquiza

21.1 Historical-Anthropological Perspective on Eating Behaviour

In various cultures, the female body has been considered a symbol of high social status, reflecting nutrition and fertility, as seen in the Venus of Willendorf. In tribal societies, obese women were perceived as more attractive and having greater reproductive capacity, while thinness, associated with famine, was linked to death [7]. For men, attractiveness depended more on skills and social power [8]. In Classical Greece, the idealization of the male body preceded that of the female, with Hippocrates and Aristophanes describing bulimic practices [9]. Hippocrates had already noted the link between obesity, infertility, and other health issues [10]. In Rome, vomiting to regulate weight was common, particularly among the upper classes [11]. During the Middle Ages, fasting was regarded as a religious practice and a path to spiritual purity [12]. Holy anorexia, as a phenomenon of food refusal, is observed in religious figures such as Saint Liberata [13]. During the Renaissance, physical appearance gained social relevance, and anorexia became secularized [6]. In the eighteenth century, more cases of bulimia and anorexia were documented, although the understanding of these disorders was still limited [14]. The nineteenth century reinforced the culture of thinness within a context of urbanization and industrialization [8]. Anorexia and bulimia were described as mental disorders, with women increasingly diagnosed with anorexia nervosa [1]. Social and familial changes were linked to these conditions, and by the end of the century, obesity began to be understood in terms of energy balance and genetics [15]. The twentieth century saw a surge in research on eating disorders (EDs). From the 1950s onwards,

M. Sáenz-Herrero (✉) · O. N. Fernández · L. U. González · A. E. Izuzquiza
Cruces University Hospital, Barakaldo, Spain

University of the Basque Country, Bilbao, Spain

M. López-Atanes, M. Sáenz-Herrero (eds.), *Applying the Gender Perspective in Psychiatry and Psychotherapy*, https://doi.org/10.1007/978-3-032-17883-1_21

obesity was associated with emotional conflicts [16], while in the 1960s, it began to be treated with diets and surgery [7]. Today, globalized food markets create a paradox of simultaneous hunger and obesity, exacerbating body dissatisfaction and EDs, particularly among women [5]. The COVID-19 lockdown worsened EDs in two-thirds of cases and contributed to weight gain in more than 50% of obese individuals [2]. Isolation and stress had a negative impact, intensifying eating disorders, especially in those with anorexia nervosa and bulimia [17].

21.2 Body Image and Associated Psychopathology

21.2.1 Body and Corporeality: Phenomenology

Corporeality and body awareness, according to Jaspers, have a descriptive foundation based on the simultaneous experience of the body as both an object and an internal experience [18]. The body we are and the body we have are connected through bodily sensations and the feelings derived from them [19]. The body schema structures all bodily experiences, providing a reference for our identity [20]. In Jaspers' psychopathology (1913), consciousness and corporeality are key concepts for the experience of the Self, which recognizes itself through unity, identity, and opposition to the external world [18].

Ortega y Gasset distinguishes between the extracorporeal body, as an anatomical and physiological entity, and the intracorporeal body, as a phenomenological experience [21]. Sartre, on the other hand, differentiates between the body as being-for-itself and as being-for-others [22]. In this sense, the body is a way of being in the world, of inhabiting it, projecting it, and sharing it, giving meaning to reality [19]. Health is reflected in the silent body, while illness turns the body into a strange object, highlighting its ambivalence. It is not only a source of mastery and power, but also of fragility and finitude. Merleau-Ponty emphasizes that illness reminds us that we do not just have a body, but that we are a lived body, which sometimes escapes our control [19]. For Janet, personality does not reside in the soul but in the body, making it essential to understand the body in the study of identity [23]. The body integrates doing, feeling, thinking, and wanting in an inseparable way [24]. From birth, we seek connection with others, which includes an emotional dimension [4]. Thus, emotions are bodily dispositions, and the body is the medium through which we experience the world and learn [25]. In psychopathology and neurology, various terms such as self-concept, body image, body schema, and body cathexis have been used to describe how a person conceptualizes themselves, each with distinct nuances [26] (Table 21.1).

21.2.2 Body and Postmodernity

Current culture is marked by the omnipresence of body aesthetics, leading to dissatisfaction and constant body modification, especially among women, who are affected by unattainable ideals [20]. Foucault notes that the body can be transformed

Table 21.1 Body and Corporeality. Phenomenology

Term	Description
Self-concept	Abstract and fully conscious awareness of oneself. It can refer both to the bodily concept (physical) and to the conscious self beyond the body
Body image	Includes cognitive, perceptual, affective, and behavioural dimensions of body awareness
Body schema	Contains a spatial element that encompasses more than just the body itself. Example: clothing and glasses are part of the body schema when imagining oneself in a context
Body cathexis	Related to strength, power, and libido. It represents the energy of the self that enables action

Created by the authors of this chapter

and perfected, and in postmodernity, the body extends beyond its physical dimensions, including clothing and adornments as an extension of identity [27]. This is particularly relevant for women, where body image influences subjectivity. Artists like Marina Abramović and Frida Kahlo use their bodies as artistic mediums, reflecting how the body is a manifestation in the world [8, 28].

21.2.3 Body and Gender

Gender is a cultural construct that determines each individual's identity, and there are different ways of experiencing the body between men and women [28]. While men are socialized with a more instrumental focus, female identity is heavily influenced by body image, relationships, and caregiving [8]. Judith Butler argues that gender is a complex construct, and femininity is not something natural, but acquired [28]. The Hegelian tradition links desire to social recognition, a process marked for women by abuse and degradation [29]. The female body is both exalted and demeaned, which, in some cases, leads to voluntary subordination, the result of social determinism [30]. Furthermore, the pathologization of the female body has been a constant in the history of psychiatry.

21.2.4 Body Schema

Schilder defines the body schema as the three-dimensional representation of our body based on our interaction with the world [20]. Slade describes it as the mental image of the body's size, shape, and structure, along with the feelings towards each part [20]. Wallon, in turn, emphasizes the childhood origins of body awareness, noting that a child initially recognizes others' organs better than their own, and the awareness of the body develops from the relationship with the mother [32]. The symbolic function of the body is not acquired until 6–7 years of age [33]. For Merleau-Ponty, the body has three dimensions: in itself, for itself, and for others, being essential for human communication and language [19]. Phenomenology has overcome the body/mind dualism, showing that the bodily experience is linked to time, space, the Self, and the world [19]. The body and the world are inseparable, and bodily experience is directed towards the world. The brain integrates sensory and motor information through mirror neurons, allowing adaptation and social interaction [34]. Body image is learned and shaped throughout life, especially during childhood and adolescence, when corresponding neural networks are fixed. Each person develops a unique perception of their body, influenced by past experiences. According to Damasio, somatic markers are emotional processes associated with the bodily state that modulate the organism's response, anticipating rational processes [26].

21.2.5 Body Schema and Corporeality Disorders (Table 21.2)

Table 21.2 Body Schema and Corporeality Disorders

Psychological disorders	Description
Cotard syndrome	Experience of the disappearance of body parts or the entire body (body denial). Objective in conditions like melancholia
Hypochondriacal delusion	Denial of organs or bodily functions, common in schizophrenia
Heautoscopy phenomenon	Perception of the body as a second self, outside oneself (can occur in febrile states, dreamlike states, brain lesions, or schizophrenia).
Cenesthetic hallucinations and Ekbom syndrome	Hallucinations where the body perceives internal parasites, such as worms. May be accompanied by visual hallucinations
Depersonalization	Sensation of displacement or disconnection from the body, common in anxiety disorders
Dysmorphophobia	Excessive concern over a perceived deformity, common in eating disorders

Created by the authors of this chapter

21.3 Psychopathology of Eating Behaviour

Eating disorders (ED) are severe mental illnesses with high mortality rates and significant psychiatric comorbidities. According to the DSM5, anorexia nervosa (AN) is characterized by low body weight and body image disturbance; bulimia nervosa (BN) by episodes of binge eating followed by compensatory behaviours; and binge-eating disorder (BED) by excessive food intake without compensatory behaviours, leading to distress [17]. Additionally, evidence suggests that many individuals exhibit significant psychopathology related to ED without fully meeting diagnostic criteria, and that symptoms such as body dissatisfaction or binge eating are present in the general population, even in the absence of a formal diagnosis [7].

21.3.1 Body Image in Eating Disorders

Body image (BI) encompasses cognitive, perceptual, affective, and behavioural dimensions, existing along a continuum of positive and negative experiences. Its development is influenced by cultural, interpersonal, and biological factors. A key concept is symbolic body capital (SBC), which explains how physical appearance is valued in different social and economic contexts [35]. Positive body image (PBI) is a protective factor that promotes self-esteem and connection with one's body. In contrast, negative body image (NBI) is associated with body dissatisfaction (BD), perceptual distortion, and increased vulnerability to eating disorders (ED) [31]. BD is highly prevalent, especially among women, and is influenced by sociocultural pressures, low self-esteem, and social comparison [35]. Three explanatory models have been proposed:

- The sociocultural model, which highlights the influence of media, peers, and family on the internalization of beauty ideals.
- The biopsychosocial model, which integrates biological and psychological factors.
- Objectification theory, which explains how evaluating one's body through an external gaze reinforces self-objectification and body dissatisfaction.

BD emerges in childhood and intensifies during adolescence, where social media amplify comparison and aesthetic pressure. Among young and adult women, it is linked to restrictive dieting, compulsive exercise, and a higher risk of ED. In men, BD can manifest as a pursuit of muscularity, with specific patterns depending on gender identity, sexual orientation, and ethnic minority status [36]. Trans men present a high prevalence of disordered eating behaviours. Research underscores the need to address BI from a gender perspective to better understand its impact on mental health and ED throughout the lifespan [8, 28].

21.3.2 Body Image Distortion (BID)

Body image distortion (BID) is defined as the inaccurate perception of body size and shape and is a key diagnostic criterion in anorexia nervosa (AN) and bulimia nervosa (BN). Although it is not included in binge-eating disorder (BED), the overvaluation of weight and shape is associated with its severity and prognosis [8, 17]. AN is a severe psychiatric disorder, with a prevalence of up to 1% in women and the highest mortality rate among mental illnesses (up to 10%). BID plays a central role in its development, treatment, and relapse, to the extent that some have proposed renaming it "body image disorder." Addressing BID is crucial for improving therapeutic outcomes. Studies suggest that patients with AN overestimate their body size more than those with BN and that this overestimation persists even when controlling for anxiety and depression [1, 31].

21.3.3 Other Psychopathological Aspect of Eating Behaviour (Table 21.3)

Table 21.3 Other Psychopathological Aspects of Eating Disorders

	Definition	Relationship with ED
Rumination	Repetitive thoughts about negative experiences and emotions, focusing on their meaning, causes, and consequences [37] Differences from other cognitive processes: Worry: future-oriented, related to threats, perceived as uncertain but controllable Obsessions: future-oriented, ego-dystonic, and unacceptable, whereas rumination can be ego-syntonic	Associated with ED, depression, and anxiety Maintenance factor in ED In AN, reinforces the sense of control and food restriction Emotional avoidance strategy No significant differences in rumination between AN and BN May contribute to the persistence of ED symptoms
Perfectionism	Striving for high standards with self-criticism when they are not met [38]. Can be divided into: Perfectionistic concerns: linked to maladaptive outcomes (stress, anxiety, depression) Perfectionistic strivings: may have adaptive or maladaptive outcomes	Key risk and maintenance factor in ED Direct relationship with depressive symptoms Core component in cognitive-behavioural and interpersonal treatment models for ED

Created by the authors of this chapter

21.3.4 Quantitative Eating Disorders Due to Excess

Quantitative eating disorders due to excess include various psychopathological manifestations that may be associated with severe psychiatric disorders, impulsive eating patterns, and dysfunctional emotional regulation strategies [5, 17].

21.3.4.1 Potomania

Potomania consists of a compulsive and sustained desire to consume large volumes of liquid, especially water. It has been described in patients with obsessive disorders, schizophrenia, and severe intellectual disabilities, where it may be part of a ritualization pattern or a self-induced behaviour without a clear medical justification.

21.3.4.2 Dipsomania

Dipsomania is characterized by intermittent and compulsive episodes of alcohol consumption without establishing a habitual drinking pattern. It typically arises in response to stressors and is associated with poor impulse control, leading to maladaptive behaviours.

21.3.4.3 Polydipsia

Polydipsia is defined as an increased frequency and quantity of liquid intake, observed in medical conditions such as diabetes mellitus but also in psychiatric disorders like psychosis and eating disorders (ED). In patients with AN, polydipsia may function as a strategy to induce satiety or artificially manipulate body weight, while in BN and obesity, it can be linked to impulsive eating patterns. Resulting water intoxication can lead to dilutional hyponatremia with severe neurobiological consequences, including confusion, lethargy, disorientation, seizures, and even coma.

21.3.4.4 Bulimia Nervosa (BN)

BN is a disorder characterized by recurrent episodes of excessive and compulsive food intake within a short period, followed by inappropriate compensatory behaviours (self-induced vomiting, laxative or diuretic abuse, fasting, or excessive exercise). There is a significant body image disturbance and a pathological fear of weight gain, reinforcing a self-evaluation focused on thinness. Binge episodes often occur in the afternoon or evening, typically preceded by increased anxiety and dysphoria, acting as a dysfunctional emotional regulation attempt. Following the loss of control over food intake, feelings of guilt, shame, and fear of weight gain emerge, reinforcing purging behaviours. These patients frequently present with anxiety and depressive symptoms, as well as high comorbidity with personality disorders (especially borderline traits), substance abuse, and other impulsive behaviours such as kleptomania. The course of BN is fluctuating, with a risk of chronicity if not addressed early. Psychological and psychiatric interventions are essential to break the pathological cycle and improve prognosis.

21.3.4.5 Binge-Eating Disorder (BED)

Formally described in 1992 by Spitzer, BED is characterized by recurrent episodes of compulsive eating without the presence of compensatory behaviours. Its diagnosis is particularly relevant in patients with obesity, in whom it is highly prevalent. Unlike BN, the core feature of BED is not the quantity of food consumed but the subjective feeling of loss of control over eating [39]. Psychopathological manifestations include an accelerated eating pace, an inability to stop eating despite satiety, and the presence of guilt and dysphoria after binge episodes. Although diagnostic criteria do not include body dissatisfaction as a central symptom, in clinical practice, it is frequently observed as an associated factor, often exacerbated by experiences of discrimination and social rejection due to weight.

21.3.4.6 Polyphagia

Polyphagia refers to a pathological increase in appetite secondary to an alteration in satiety perception. Some authors propose differentiating it from bulimia (which involves a compulsive pattern) and hyperorexia (a more nonspecific term) due to its stronger association with dysregulation of the homeostatic hunger mechanism.

21.3.4.7 Phagomania

Phagomania refers to the tendency to consume food repeatedly between meals without physiological hunger to justify it. It is associated with emotional factors such as anxiety, boredom, or feelings of loneliness and can range from a cultural habit to a pathological manifestation within EDs or other affective disorders.

21.3.5 Quantitative Eating Disorders Due to Deficit

21.3.5.1 Anorexia Nervosa (AN)

Anorexia nervosa is a disorder characterized by persistent food refusal due to an irrational fear of weight gain, leading to significant weight loss and refusal to maintain a minimally normal body weight. It is accompanied by body image distortion [1]. Anorexia as an isolated symptom is insufficient for an AN diagnosis, as it may be part of the symptomatology of various psychiatric disorders, particularly melancholic depression and delusional disorders, as well as other medical conditions [17]. In the restrictive type of AN, weight loss occurs through dieting, fasting, or excessive exercise. In the purging type, self-induced vomiting, laxative abuse, diuretics, or enemas are used to counteract potential weight gain. These subtypes may alternate throughout the course of the illness [1]. Cognitive alterations observed in EDs, as described by Garner and Bemis, include overgeneralization (*When I ate sweets, I was fat, so I must never eat them again*), magnification of negative consequences (*If I gain a kilo, I'll die*), dichotomous thinking (*If I don't control my diet completely, I won't be able to control anything*), ideas of reference (*When I eat, everyone is looking at me*), and superstitious thinking (*If I eat sweets, they will turn into fat*) [40]. Anxiety is a constant emotional factor, appearing from the onset of AN as diffuse anxiety that tends to increase as the disorder progresses. Phobic anxiety is likely the central pathogenic mechanism of AN. Anxiety-provoking stimuli range from morbid fear of gaining weight to loss of control, body image concerns, low self-esteem, and social and familial pressures [1]. Affective disorders occur in most cases during the illness, with some patients showing symptoms from the beginning. These include sadness, anhedonia, insomnia, feelings of worthlessness, hopelessness, guilt, and low self-esteem. Thoughts about body image, food, or weight are intrusive and recurrent, consuming much of the patient's time and triggering anxiety in the form of *ruminations, worries, or obsessions* [17].

21.3.5.2 Adipsia

Adipsia is a rare disorder characterized by a diminished sense of thirst and reduced fluid intake. It is generally caused by organic hypothalamic dysfunction, but in psychiatric contexts, it may be associated with oppositional behaviours, psychotic disorders with delusional or hallucinatory experiences, or secondary gain [5].

21.3.5.3 Avoidant/Restrictive Food Intake Disorder (ARFID)

Included in the DSM-5, ARFID is characterized by the avoidance of certain foods, leading to nutritional deficiencies, significant weight loss, and psychosocial impairment. Unlike AN or BN, it is not associated with body image distortions or other psychiatric conditions. ARFID is common in childhood but can also occur in adulthood [17].

21.3.6 Qualitative Eating Disorders

21.3.6.1 Sitophobia/Siteophobia

A rare disorder characterized by an irrational and obsessive fear of certain foods in specific circumstances, which may develop into phobias or delusions related to food intake [17].

21.3.6.2 Neophobia

Fear of consuming new foods, which is a normal part of child development as a defensive mechanism to avoid potentially dangerous foods. It is associated with reduced intake of certain foods [41].

21.3.6.3 Disorexias

Appetite alterations linked to significant emotional situations, such as pregnancy cravings or individuals in extreme situations (e.g., death row inmates). These behaviours reflect emotional gratification through food consumption [5].

21.3.6.4 Allotriophagy

A disorder involving abnormal eating behaviours, including *pica*, which involves the ingestion of non-food substances (e.g., dirt, hair, faeces). It is generally associated with psychotic disorders, autism, or intellectual disabilities and may be linked to nutritional deficiencies and specific syndromes [42].

21.3.6.5 Pica

A severe disorder characterized by the persistent ingestion of non-nutritive substances (e.g., dirt, hair, faeces). If it persists beyond age two, it may indicate an underlying psychopathological disorder, such as autism or psychosis. It is also associated with mineral deficiencies, particularly iron or zinc [42].

21.3.6.6 Rumination Syndrome (Merycism)

The voluntary and repetitive regurgitation of food, common in early childhood but rare in adults, except in cases of intellectual disability. It is associated with high mortality due to malnutrition or respiratory complications [5].

21.3.6.7 Orthorexia Nervosa (ON)

An obsessive concern with healthy eating, leading to the exclusion of foods perceived as unhealthy. This restrictive lifestyle negatively impacts quality of life and often coexists with obsessive-compulsive traits [43].

21.3.6.8 Muscle Dysmorphia (Bigorexia)

An obsession with muscular appearance, where individuals perceive themselves as weak despite having a muscular body. It involves excessive exercise, strict dieting, and the use of supplements or steroids. It can lead to severe health issues, including depression and cardiac problems.

21.3.6.9 Night Eating Syndrome (NES)

A condition where individuals wake up to engage in binge-eating episodes. It is not fully defined as a disorder but may be related to sleep disorders or eating disorders [44].

21.4 Key Points

1. *Hunger* is an urgent biological need, while *appetite* is influenced by cultural and social factors. The body is inseparable from doing, feeling, and thinking, serving as the medium for experience and learning.
2. *Body dissatisfaction*, common in women and girls, involves a negative self-evaluation of weight and shape, making it a strong predictor of depression and a key factor in eating disorders (EDs).
3. *Body image distortion (BID)* is a central criterion in EDs, influencing onset, treatment, and relapse, to the point that it has been suggested to rename anorexia nervosa (AN) as *body image disorder*.

References

1. Bruch H. Perceptual and conceptual disturbances in anorexia nervosa. Psychosom Med. 1962;24:187–94.
2. Sideli L, Micali N. Effects of COVID-19 lockdown on eating disorders and obesity: a systematic review and meta-analysis. Eur Eat Disord Rev. 2021;29:826–41.
3. Contreras J. Antropología de la alimentación. Madrid: Ed Eudema; 1993.
4. Bowlby J. Attachment and loss, vol. 1. New York: Basic Books; 1969.
5. Patel R. Obesos y famélicos. Barcelona: Ed Los libros del lince; 2008.
6. Brumberg JJ. Fasting girls. The emergence of anorexia nervosa as a modern disease. Cambridge: Harvard University Press; 1988.
7. Brownell KD. History of obesity. In: Brownell KD, Fairburn CG, editors. Eating disorders and obesity. Nueva York: The Guilford Press; 1995.
8. Gordon RA. Anorexia and bulimia: anatomy of a social epidemic. Oxford: Blackwell; 1990.
9. Giannini AJ. A history of bulimia. In: Giannini AJ, Slaby AE, editors. The eating disorders. New York: Springer; 1993.
10. Hippocrates. On airs, waters, and places. Cambridge: Harvard University Press; 1923.
11. Bell RM. Holy anorexia. Chicago: University of Chicago Press; 1985.
12. Bynum CW. Holy feast and holy fast. Berkeley: University of California Press; 1987.
13. Noordenbos G. Door dik en dun. In: Allagaert P, Cailleau A, editors. Vastenheiligen, wondermeisjes en hongerkunstenaars. Gante: Museum Dr Guislain; 1991.
14. Gull WW. Anorexia nervosa. Lancet. 1888;i:516–7.

15. Bray GA. Obesity: historical development of scientific and cultural ideas. Int J Obes. 1990;14:909–26.
16. Stunkard AJ. A history of binge eating. In: Fairburn CG, Wilson GT, editors. Binge eating: nature, assessment and treatment. Nueva York: Guilford Press; 1993.
17. American Psychiatric Association. DSM-5 Development. Feeding and Eating Disorders. [Internet]. Disponible en: www.dsm5.org.
18. Jaspers K. Psicopatología general. Buenos Aires: Editorial Beta; 1977.
19. Merleau-Ponty M. Fenomenología de la percepción. Barcelona: Editorial Península; 1975.
20. Schilder P. Imagen y apariencia del cuerpo humano. Buenos Aires: Editorial Paidós; 1977.
21. Ortega y Gasset J. Meditaciones del Quijote o experimentos de nueva España (1914). In: Obras completas, vol. Tomo II. 4th ed. Madrid: Revista de Occidente; 1957. p. 322.
22. Sartre JP. El ser y la nada. Buenos Aires: Ed Losada; 1977.
23. Janet P. L'évolution psychologique de la personnalité. París: Chahine; 1929.
24. Damasio AR. Descartes' error: emotion, reason and the human brain. New York: G.P. Putnam; 1994.
25. Varela FJ, Thompson E, Rosch E. The embodied mind. Cognitive science and human experience. Cambridge: MIT Press; 2004.
26. Damasio AR. The somatic marker hypothesis and the possible functions of the prefrontal cortex. Philos Trans R Soc Lond Ser B Biol Sci. 1996;351(1346):1413–20.
27. Foucault M. Discipline and punish. New York: Vintage Books; 1977.
28. Butler J. El género en disputa. Madrid: Paidós-Ibérica; 2007.
29. Hegel GWF. Fenomenología del espíritu. Madrid: Fondo de Cultura Económica; 1966.
30. Beauvoir S. El segundo sexo. Madrid: Cátedra; 2008.
31. Slade PD. Body image in anorexia nervosa. Br J Psychiatry. 1988;153:20–2.
32. Wallon H. Les origines du caractère chez l'enfant. París: Presses Universitaires de France; 1930.
33. Piaget J. The origins of intelligence in children. New York: International Universities Press; 1952.
34. Rizzolatti G, Craighero L. The mirror-neuron system. Annu Rev Neurosci. 2004;27:169–92.
35. Fallon A. Culture in the mirror: sociocultural determinants of body image. In: Cash TF, Pruzinsky T, editors. Body images: development, deviance and change. New York: Guilford Press; 1990.
36. Nagata J. Eating disorders in adolescent boys and young men: an update. Curr Opin Pediatr. 2020;32(4):476–81.
37. Smith K, Lavender J. Rumination and eating disorder psychopathology: a meta-analysis. Clin Psychol Rev. 2018;61:9–23.
38. Limburg K, Watson H, Egan S. The relationship between perfectionism and psychopathology: a meta-analysis. J Clin Psychol. 2017;73(10):1301–26.
39. Spitzer RL, Devlin M, Walsh BT, Hasin D. Binge eating disorder: a multisite field trial of the diagnostic criteria. Int J Eat Disord. 1992;11:191–203.
40. Garner DM, Olmsted MP, Polivy J. Development and validation of a multidimensional eating disorder inventory for anorexia nervosa and bulimia. Int J Eat Disord. 1983;2:15–34.
41. Russell CG, Worsley A. A population-based study of preschoolers' food neophobia and its association with food preferences. J Nutr Educ Behav. 2008;40(1):11–9.
42. Moore DF Jr, Sears DA. Pica, iron deficiency, and the medical history. Am J Med. 1994;97:390–3.
43. Yilmaz FC. Orthorexia and eating attitudes in health sciences students. Niger J Clin Pract. 2023;26:502–7.
44. Striegel-Moore R, Dohm F, Hook J, Schreiber G, Crawford P, et al. Night eating syndrome in young adult women: prevalence and correlates. Int J Eat Disord. 2005;37:200–6.

Sex and Gender Differences in Psychosis

22

Beatriz Isabel Molina Cañas, María Santaolalla Sánchez, and Oihane Mentxaka Solozabal

22.1 Introduction

Sex and gender differences in schizophrenia provide a critical framework for understanding disparities in incidence, clinical presentation, and outcomes, shaped by biological (e.g., hormonal) and psychosocial interactions [1]. While traditional views suggested similar prevalence between sexes, contemporary studies reveal nuanced differences. Restrictive diagnostic criteria (e.g., Feighner criteria: female-male ratio 0.41:1; ICD: 0.92:1) and meta-analyses highlight lower incidence rates in women, particularly when excluding late-onset cases over 45 years [1, 2]. Prevalence parity in general populations may reflect higher male treatment nonadherence, suicide rates, or methodological biases in study designs [2].

A hallmark difference is the later age of onset in women, consistent across cultures and diagnostic criteria [1]. Females also exhibit better premorbid adjustment, including higher educational attainment and social functioning, with fewer behavioral or neurocognitive deficits—differences emerging more clearly in chronic than first-episode cases [3]. Clinically, women demonstrate more affective and positive symptoms (e.g., paranoid subtype predominance) and higher rates of

B. I. M. Cañas
Department of Psychiatry, Cruces University Hospital, Barakaldo, Biscay, Spain

M. S. Sánchez
Department of Psychiatry, Reina Sofía University Hospital, Córdoba, Spain

O. M. Solozabal (✉)
Department of Psychiatry, Cruces University Hospital, Barakaldo, Biscay, Spain

Biobizkaia Health Research Institute, Cruces University Hospital, Barakaldo, Biscay, Spain

Department of Neuroscience, Faculty of Medicine and Nursing, University of the Basque Country, UPV/EHU, Leioa, Biscay, Spain
e-mail: oihane.mentxakasolozabal@osakidetza.eus

M. López-Atanes, M. Sáenz-Herrero (eds.), *Applying the Gender Perspective in Psychiatry and Psychotherapy*, https://doi.org/10.1007/978-3-032-17883-1_22

schizoaffective or brief psychotic disorders [3]. Prognosis favors women, with fewer relapses, lower substance use, and better occupational functioning, though antipsychotic use elevates metabolic risks (e.g., diabetes, obesity) [4]. Cognitive profiles diverge, with women outperforming men in memory tasks but men excelling in visuospatial functions; executive functioning shows no sex differences [5].

Biological hypotheses, such as estrogen's neuroprotective role in modulating dopamine, contrast with psychosocial theories that remain context-dependent and less replicated [1, 6]. Early-onset psychosis (EOP, onset <18 years) further illustrates sex disparities: males typically develop psychosis earlier (18–25 years) with longer untreated periods (duration of untreated psychosis, DUP) and substance use, whereas females exhibit later onset (25–35 years), depressive precursors, and better remission rates [7–9]. Longitudinal data identify female sex, older onset age, and shorter DUP as predictors of remission, underscoring sex/gender as key variables in etiopathogenic models [9].

This chapter synthesizes evidence on sex and gender differences in adolescent-onset psychosis, exploring implications for research and clinical practice.

22.2 Physiopathology

Schizophrenia exhibits notable sex and gender differences in epidemiology, clinical presentation, and neurobiological correlates. This article synthesizes recent evidence on these variations, focusing on age of onset, familial risk, substance use, and neuroimaging findings.

22.2.1 Age of Onset

Men typically develop schizophrenia earlier than women, with peak incidence between 20 and 29 years, compared to women's broader risk window spanning 20–39 years [10]. While women historically were thought to have a second incidence peak during menopause (45–54 years), a recalibration of 43 studies (133,693 cases) revised this to a smaller secondary peak at 30–39 years [11]. The earlier onset in men may be partially mediated by higher rates of cannabis use [12]. However, familial risk attenuates these sex differences: individuals with a family history of psychosis show no significant gender disparity in age of onset [13, 14].

22.2.2 Obstetric and Familial Risk

Perinatal complications are inconsistently linked to schizophrenia, with studies reporting higher rates in men [15], women [16], or no sex differences [17]. Similarly, maternal influenza exposure during pregnancy lacks conclusive evidence for sex-specific effects [18]. Familial risk patterns also vary: maternal psychosis is more frequently transmitted to sons, while paternal psychosis shows a daughter-predominant transmission [19, 20]. However, not all studies corroborate these associations [21].

22.2.3 Substance Use

Substance use disorders (SUDs), particularly cannabis, are more prevalent in men and correlate with earlier psychosis onset [12, 22]. Men with schizophrenia exhibit higher rates of cannabis, cocaine, and hallucinogen use than women [23, 24]. Cannabis use is associated with severe symptom trajectories, functional impairment, and relapse [25]. Notably, men with cannabis-induced psychosis have a 47.6% risk of transitioning to schizophrenia, compared to 29.8% in women [26]. Women, however, face greater challenges in quitting tobacco when co-using cannabis and may experience worse illness courses with SUDs [27, 28].

22.2.4 Epidemiological Trends in Early-Onset Psychosis (EOP) and First-Episode Psychosis (FEP)

EOP (onset <18 years) and FEP demonstrate a male predominance, with incidence ratios of 1.42:1 [29, 30]. The ABC Schizophrenia Study highlights this disparity, showing first-admission peaks at 18–25 years for men versus 25–35 years for women [31]. Diagnostic criteria influence these trends; excluding schizoaffective disorders reduces female representation [32].

22.2.5 Substance Abuse

Global data indicate men are three times likelier to use cannabis, a key psychosis risk factor [33]. In FEP, 52.8% of ultra-high-risk individuals report lifetime cannabis exposure, rising to 60–80% in first-episode cohorts [34, 35]. Early adolescent use (<14 years) heightens psychosis vulnerability and correlates with poorer treatment outcomes [36]. Neuroimaging studies suggest sex-specific neurodevelopmental effects, such as enlarged amygdala volumes in female users linked to anxiety and depression [37].

22.2.6 Genetic Factors

Sex-specific genetic risks are emerging. Maternal psychosis predisposes sons, while paternal psychosis elevates daughters' risk [19, 20]. Genome-wide analyses implicate X-chromosome loci and sex-dependent expression of risk genes [38].

22.2.7 Hormonal Influences

Estradiol may delay onset in women via neuroprotective effects [39]. Conversely, hypoestrogenism is common in female patients, even pre-treatment [40]. Antipsychotic-naïve EOP patients exhibit hypothalamic-pituitary-gonadal axis dysregulation, including hyperprolactinemia and low testosterone in men [41].

22.2.8 Neuroimaging

Sexual dimorphism in brain structure is altered in schizophrenia. Men show greater ventricular enlargement and corpus callosum abnormalities, while women have larger pituitary volumes, potentially reflecting HPA-axis dysregulation [42, 43]. Regional volumetric differences also predict symptom severity: frontal atrophy correlates with disorganization in men, whereas diffuse atrophy associates with positive symptoms in women [44, 45].

Schizophrenia's sex and gender differences arise from complex interactions between genetic, hormonal, and environmental factors. While men face earlier onset and higher SUD prevalence, women exhibit unique risk windows and hormonal vulnerabilities. Future research should prioritize longitudinal designs to clarify neurodevelopmental trajectories and sex-specific treatment pathways.

22.3 Trauma and Gender

Exposure to adverse childhood experiences, including abuse, neglect, and bullying, is strongly linked to an elevated risk of psychosis, as evidenced by meta-analyses and large population-based studies [46–48]. While sexual and physical abuse have historically been highlighted as risk factors, recent research underscores gender-specific patterns in trauma exposure. For instance, male patients with first-episode psychosis (FEP) report higher rates of physical or emotional neglect, whereas female patients exhibit significantly greater prevalence of emotional abuse [49]. These findings contrast with earlier studies reporting higher rates of sexual and physical abuse among women compared to same-sex controls [50]. This discrepancy may stem from methodological differences, as Pruessner et al. [49] compared male and female patients directly, while Fisher et al. [50] analyzed trauma exposure relative to gender-matched controls. Notably, the prevalence of sexual abuse in Pruessner et al.'s cohort (24.2% in women, 16.7% in men) was lower than the weighted averages reported in prior reviews [47], potentially due to stricter criteria excluding mild trauma [49]. Similarly, the total childhood trauma rate in Pruessner et al. (54.3%) was lower than rates exceeding 70% in other studies [51–54], further emphasizing the impact of assessment methodologies.

Childhood sexual abuse (CSA) is associated with more severe hallucinations and delusions in FEP, aligning with trauma-related intrusion models, and correlates with earlier psychosis onset, particularly among women [55, 56]. Women with physical abuse histories also demonstrate earlier onset than men, consistent with evidence suggesting that childhood abuse increases schizophrenia risk more prominently in women [50, 57]. Beyond abuse, bullying victimization is linked to subclinical psychotic symptoms and mental health challenges, with women in FEP samples reporting higher bullying rates than men [58–60]. This may reflect gender differences in coping mechanisms, as women are more prone to internalizing behaviors like rumination—a response style linked to psychopathology—while men tend to externalize distress [50, 61, 62]. Internalizing behaviors also mediate the relationship between bullying and psychotic symptoms, potentially heightening psychosis risk in women exposed to stressors [63].

22.4 Clinical Course and Gender Differences

The clinical course of schizophrenia exhibits significant gender-based heterogeneity, with notable differences in age of onset, symptom profiles, and long-term outcomes. Men typically experience an earlier onset (late teens to early twenties), linked to poorer cognitive and functional prognoses, while women present a delayed onset (mid-to-late twenties), associated with better social integration and outcomes [64, 65]. Longitudinal studies indicate that women have shorter hospital stays, lower relapse rates, and higher community tenure after first admission compared to men [66, 67]. Men, however, demonstrate higher institutionalization rates, prolonged recovery times, and a sevenfold increased suicide risk, partly due to comorbid substance abuse and weaker social networks [68, 69].

22.4.1 Symptomatology and Cognitive Functioning

Men predominantly exhibit negative symptoms (e.g., anhedonia, affective flattening) and cognitive deficits, whereas women show more positive symptoms (e.g., hallucinations, delusions) and affective disturbances [64, 70]. These differences influence diagnostic patterns, with women more frequently classified under paranoid subtypes and men under residual subtypes [64, 71]. Cognitive performance diverges by gender: women outperform men in verbal memory, attention, and executive functioning, while men retain better visuospatial skills, mirroring patterns in healthy populations [72, 73]. Social cognition, including mentalizing and emotion recognition, is also more preserved in women, contributing to their adaptive resilience [74].

22.4.2 Hormonal Influences and Neuroprotection

Estrogens may underpin these disparities through neuroprotective mechanisms. Lower serum estradiol levels in women with schizophrenia correlate with symptom severity, while higher levels attenuate negative symptoms and cognitive decline [75, 76]. Premenopausal women or those receiving hormone therapy exhibit fewer negative symptoms, suggesting estrogen's role in mitigating neuronal atrophy [77, 78]. Postmenopausal women experience symptom exacerbation, aligning with declining estrogen levels, whereas men maintain stable but severe symptom profiles [79].

22.4.3 Premorbid Adjustment and Social Functioning

Women demonstrate superior premorbid adjustment, marked by better educational attainment, employment history, and social relationships prior to illness onset [80, 81]. These factors, combined with later onset, enhance their baseline social functioning and marital rates [64, 82]. Men, conversely, face insidious premorbid decline, characterized by academic and social dysfunction, linked to neurodevelopmental anomalies [83, 84]. Despite similar marital rates at first episode, women are more likely to marry and parent as the illness progresses, reflecting greater social adaptability [85].

22.4.4 Duration of Untreated Psychosis (DUP) and Outcomes

While some studies report longer DUP in men, meta-analyses suggest no consistent gender effect, highlighting methodological variability across studies [86, 87]. Adolescent-onset males exhibit prolonged DUP, often compounded by cannabis use, which may accelerate psychosis onset [88]. Early intervention strategies remain critical, as delayed treatment correlates with poorer outcomes, particularly in males [89].

Gender differences in schizophrenia arise from interplay between hormonal, neurodevelopmental, and psychosocial factors. Estrogen's neuroprotective effects in women may delay onset and ameliorate symptoms, whereas men's earlier neurodevelopmental vulnerabilities predispose them to severe deficits. Addressing these differences through gender-tailored interventions could improve prognostic outcomes.

22.5 Gender and Treatment

Men and women exhibit significant differences in genetics, physiology, and lifestyle factors such as height, weight, diet, exercise, smoking, alcohol use, and illicit drug consumption [90, 91]. These differences extend to pharmacokinetics and pharmacodynamics, including metabolism, absorption, distribution, and excretion of medications. For instance, young women (aged 20–39) on maintenance treatment require lower doses of antipsychotics than men, a trend that reverses after age 40 [24, 92]. Women also tend to have higher plasma levels of antipsychotics due to factors like body size, weight, blood volume, and adipose tissue, which are generally greater in women [93, 94]. This slower release of lipophilic antipsychotics may protect women in cases of voluntary treatment cessation [95].

Smoking, which reduces plasma levels of antipsychotics, is more prevalent in men, potentially explaining their need for higher doses [96–98]. Women, on the other hand, often exhibit slower drug elimination, leading to higher plasma concentrations and increased side effects. Consequently, depot medication intervals should be longer for women [90]. Additionally, women tend to respond better to psychosocial treatments, which should be considered in their care plans [99, 100].

22.5.1 Treatment Response and Adherence

Treatment response and overall outcomes in schizophrenia are generally worse in men than in women [101–103]. Men also show poorer adherence to medical appointments and treatment [104–106]. Women's more positive attitudes toward medication and help-seeking behaviors may contribute to their better outcomes [107]. Antipsychotic response is generally better in women, while men often require higher doses for efficacy [108–112].

22.5.2 Side Effects

Side effects of antipsychotics vary significantly between genders. Women are more prone to metabolic syndrome, a risk factor for cardiovascular disease, with studies showing higher prevalence rates compared to men [113–116]. Antipsychotics also increase body mass index (BMI) more frequently in women, raising concerns about reproductive health and potential harm to newborns [117–119].

While no clear sex differences exist for acute motor side effects like dystonia or parkinsonism, older women are at higher risk for tardive dyskinesia, possibly due to declining estrogen levels after menopause [120, 121]. Women are also more susceptible to QT interval prolongation and torsade de pointes [122].

Hormonal side effects, such as elevated prolactin levels, are more common in women, even at lower antipsychotic doses [112, 123, 124]. Hyperprolactinemia is associated with sexual dysfunction, low bone mineral density, and osteoporosis, with men showing lower bone density than women in some studies [122, 125–127]. Finally, clozapine-induced agranulocytosis and eosinophilia are more frequent in women [128, 129].

22.6 Special Considerations in the Treatment of Women with Psychosis

22.6.1 Hormonal Influences and Treatment Response

Women with schizophrenia require tailored treatment approaches due to hormonal fluctuations during menstrual cycles, pregnancy, postpartum, and menopause

[130–132]. Estrogen levels significantly influence symptom severity, with positive symptoms improving during high-estrogen phases and worsening during low-estrogen periods (e.g., premenstrual or postmenopause) [133]. Premenopausal women generally respond better to antipsychotics than postmenopausal women [134].

22.6.2 Menstrual Cycle

Antipsychotics frequently cause menstrual irregularities (78%) or amenorrhea (22–50%) [135]. Despite these effects, effective contraception is critical to prevent unplanned pregnancies, which are more common in women with schizophrenia [136].

22.6.3 Pregnancy

Schizophrenia itself is associated with obstetric and neonatal risks, including preterm birth, pre-eclampsia, and congenital anomalies [137–139]. Antipsychotic use during pregnancy may further increase teratogenic or neonatal risks [137, 140]. Monotherapy at minimal effective doses is recommended. Olanzapine is most commonly prescribed, while risperidone and quetiapine are alternatives with less robust evidence [137, 140]. Clozapine, aripiprazole, and other newer agents are discouraged due to limited safety data [141, 142].

22.6.4 Postpartum and Breastfeeding

Postpartum psychosis risk rises due to abrupt estrogen decline [144, 145]. Guidelines advise avoiding antipsychotics during breastfeeding; if unavoidable, dosing should align with the infant's longest sleep period to minimize exposure [146, 147].

22.6.5 Menopause

Postmenopausal women face heightened risks of tardive dyskinesia, QTc prolongation, and metabolic side effects [148–150]. Monitoring weight, bone density, and cardiovascular markers is essential [151]. Hyperprolactinemia from antipsychotics may accelerate menopause, necessitating prolactin monitoring [152]. First-generation antipsychotics should be avoided due to adverse effect profiles [153].

Prospective studies are urgently needed to clarify gender-specific pharmacotherapy impacts, particularly during pregnancy, lactation, and menopause. Genetic and hormonal factors must be prioritized to optimize outcomes and reduce side effects [154].

22.7 Conclusion

This comprehensive analysis underscores the profound influence of sex and gender on the etiology, manifestation, and trajectory of schizophrenia. Biological factors—such as hormonal fluctuations, neurodevelopmental pathways, and genetic vulnerabilities—interact dynamically with psychosocial elements, including trauma exposure, substance use, and societal roles, to shape divergent outcomes for men and women. Women generally exhibit later onset, better premorbid adjustment, and more favorable prognoses, potentially mediated by estrogen's neuroprotective effects, yet face unique challenges such as metabolic risks from antipsychotics and hormonal vulnerabilities during reproductive transitions. Conversely, men experience earlier onset, higher rates of substance use, and poorer functional outcomes, driven in part by neurodevelopmental disruptions and social disengagement. These disparities necessitate gender-sensitive approaches in diagnosis, treatment, and long-term care, emphasizing tailored pharmacological strategies, trauma-informed interventions, and proactive monitoring of sex-specific side effects. Future research must prioritize longitudinal and mechanistic studies to unravel the interplay of biological and psychosocial factors, ensuring equitable and effective care for all individuals with schizophrenia. Addressing these differences is not merely a clinical imperative but a step toward dismantling the systemic biases that perpetuate disparities in mental health outcomes.

References

1. Riecher-Rössler A, Butler S, Kulkarni J. Sex and gender differences in schizophrenic psychoses: a critical review. Arch Womens Ment Health. 2018;21(6):627–48.
2. Ochoa S, Usall J, Cobo J, Labad X, Kulkarni J. Gender differences in schizophrenia and first-episode psychosis: a comprehensive literature review. Schizophr Res Treat. 2012;2012:916198.
3. Zhang XY, Chen DC, Xiu MH, et al. Gender differences in never-medicated first-episode schizophrenia and medicated chronic schizophrenia patients. J Clin Psychiatry. 2012;73(7):1025–33.
4. McEvoy JP, Meyer JM, Goff DC, et al. Prevalence of the metabolic syndrome in patients with schizophrenia: baseline results from the CATIE trial. Schizophr Res. 2005;80(1):19–32.
5. Chan RC, Chen EY, Cheung EF, et al. Executive functioning in chronic schizophrenia. Schizophr Res. 2006;81(2–3):173–89.
6. Cotton SM, Lambert M, Schimmelmann BG, et al. Gender differences in first-episode psychosis. Schizophr Res. 2009;114(1–3):17–24.
7. Schimmelmann BG, Conus P, Cotton S, et al. Differences between early-onset and adult-onset psychosis. Schizophr Res. 2007;95(1–3):1–8.
8. Stevens JR, Prince JB, Prager LM, et al. Psychotic disorders in children and adolescents. Prim Care Companion CNS Disord. 2014;16(2):PCC.13r01585.
9. Chang WC, Tang JY, Hui CL, et al. Prediction of remission in first-episode psychosis. Aust N Z J Psychiatry. 2012;46(2):100–8.
10. Häfner H, Maurer K, an der Heiden W. ABC Schizophrenia study: an overview of results since 1996. Soc Psychiatry Psychiatr Epidemiol. 2013;48(7):1021–31.
11. Van der Werf M, et al. Systematic review and collaborative recalculation of 133,693 incident cases of schizophrenia. Psychol Med. 2014;44(1):9–16.

12. Crocker CE, Tibbo PG. The interaction of gender and cannabis in early phase psychosis. Schizophr Res. 2018;194:18–25.
13. Esterberg ML, et al. The impact of a family history of psychosis on age-at-onset and positive and negative symptoms of schizophrenia: a meta-analysis. Schizophr Res. 2010;120(1–3):121–30.
14. Bergen SE, et al. Genetic modifiers and subtypes in schizophrenia: investigations of age at onset, severity, sex and family history. Schizophr Res. 2014;154(1–3):48–53.
15. Kirov G, et al. Do obstetric complications cause the earlier age at onset in male than female schizophrenics? Schizophr Res. 1996;20(1–2):117–24.
16. Verdoux H, Bourgeois M. A comparative study of obstetric history in schizophrenics, bipolar patients and normal subjects. Schizophr Res. 1993;9(1):67–9.
17. Forsyth JK, et al. Genetic risk for schizophrenia, obstetric complications, and adolescent school outcome: evidence for gene-environment interaction. Schizophr Bull. 2013;39(5):1067–76.
18. Preti A, et al. Risk for obstetric complications and schizophrenia. Psychiatry Res. 2000;96(2):127–39.
19. Goldstein JM, et al. Sex-specific rates of transmission of psychosis in the New England high-risk family study. Schizophr Res. 2011;128(1–3):150–5.
20. Goldstein JM, et al. Sex differences in the genetic risk for schizophrenia: history of the evidence for sex-specific and sex-dependent effects. Am J Med Genet B Neuropsychiatr Genet. 2013;162(7):698–710.
21. Maier W, et al. The impact of gender and age at onset on the familial aggregation of schizophrenia. Eur Arch Psychiatry Clin Neurosci. 1993;242(5):279–85.
22. González-Pinto A, et al. Impact of cannabis and other drugs on age at onset of psychosis. J Clin Psychiatry. 2008;69(8):1210–6.
23. Rodríguez-Jiménez R, et al. Dual diagnosis in psychiatric inpatients: prevalence and general characteristics. Investig Clin. 2008;49(2):195–205.
24. Galderisi S, et al. No gender differences in social outcome in patients suffering from schizophrenia. Eur Psychiatry. 2012;27(6):406–8.
25. Foti DJ, et al. Cannabis use and the course of schizophrenia: 10-year follow-up after first hospitalization. Am J Psychiatry. 2010;167(8):987–93.
26. Arendt M, et al. Cannabis-induced psychosis and subsequent schizophrenia-spectrum disorders: follow-up study of 535 incident cases. Br J Psychiatry. 2005;187(6):510–5.
27. González-Pinto A, et al. Psychosis and smoking cessation: difficulties in quitting associated with sex and substance abuse. Psychiatry Res. 2012;195(1–2):45–50.
28. Lange EH, et al. One-year follow-up of alcohol and illicit substance use in first-episode psychosis: does gender matter? Compr Psychiatry. 2014;55(2):274–82.
29. Aleman A, et al. Sex differences in the risk of schizophrenia: evidence from meta-analysis. Arch Gen Psychiatry. 2003;60(6):565–71.
30. Cocchi A, et al. Sex differences in first-episode psychosis and in people at ultra-high risk. Psychiatry Res. 2014;215(2):314–22.
31. Häfner H, et al. The epidemiology of early schizophrenia. Influence of age and gender on onset and early course. Br J Psychiatry Suppl. 1994;23:29–38.
32. Lewine RRJ. Effect of diagnostic criteria on the ratio of male to female schizophrenic patients. Am J Psychiatry. 1984;141(1):84–7.
33. United Nations Office on Drugs and Crime. World drug report 2016. 2016.
34. Carney R, et al. Cannabis use and symptom severity in individuals at ultra-high risk for psychosis: a meta-analysis. Acta Psychiatr Scand. 2017;136(1):5–15.
35. Myles H, et al. Cannabis use in first episode psychosis: meta-analysis of prevalence, and the time course of initiation and continued use. Aust N Z J Psychiatry. 2016;50(3):208–19.
36. Stefanis NC, et al. Age at initiation of cannabis use predicts age at onset of psychosis: the 7- to 8-year trend. Schizophr Bull. 2013;39(2):251–4.
37. McQueeny T, et al. Gender effects on amygdala morphometry in adolescent marijuana users. Behav Brain Res. 2011;224(1):128–34.

38. Riecher-Rössler A, et al. Oestrogens, prolactin, hypothalamic-pituitary-gonadal axis, and schizophrenic psychoses. Lancet Psychiatry. 2017;4(1):63–72.
39. Kulkarni J, et al. The role of estrogen in the treatment of men with schizophrenia. Int J Endocrinol Metab. 2013;11(3):129–36.
40. Haijma SV, et al. Brain volumes in schizophrenia: a meta-analysis in over 18,000 subjects. Schizophr Bull. 2013;39(5):1129–38.
41. Gruner P, et al. Pituitary volume in first episode schizophrenia. Psychiatry Res Neuroimaging. 2012;203:100–2.
42. Romo-Nava F, et al. Pituitary volume in schizophrenia spectrum disorders. Schizophr Res. 2013;146:301–7.
43. Cowell PE, et al. Sex differences in neuroanatomical and clinical correlations in schizophrenia. Am J Psychiatry. 1996;153(6):799.
44. Malla AK, et al. Computed tomographic findings in schizophrenia: relation with symptom dimensions and sex differences. J Psychiatry Neurosci. 1999;24(2):131–8.
45. Falkenburg J, Tracy DK. Sex and schizophrenia: a review of gender differences. Psychosis. 2014;6(1):61–9.
46. Varese F, Smeets F, Drukker M, et al. Childhood adversities increase the risk of psychosis: a meta-analysis of patient-control, prospective- and cross-sectional cohort studies. Schizophr Bull. 2012;38(4):661–71.
47. Morgan C, Fisher H. Environment and schizophrenia: environmental factors in schizophrenia: childhood trauma—a critical review. Schizophr Bull. 2007;33(1):3–10.
48. Read J, van Os J, Morrison AP, Ross CA. Childhood trauma, psychosis and schizophrenia: a literature review with theoretical and clinical implications. Acta Psychiatr Scand. 2005;112(5):330–50.
49. Pruessner M, King S, Vracotas N, et al. Gender differences in childhood trauma in first episode psychosis: association with symptom severity over two years. Schizophr Res. 2018;199:327–33.
50. Fisher H, Morgan C, Dazzan P, et al. Gender differences in the association between childhood abuse and psychosis. Br J Psychiatry. 2009;194(4):319–25.
51. Stumbo SP, Yarborough BJH, Paulson RI, Green CA. The impact of adverse child and adult experiences on recovery from serious mental illness. Psychiatr Rehabil J. 2015;38(4):320–7.
52. Duhig M, Patterson S, Connell M, et al. The prevalence and correlates of childhood trauma in patients with early psychosis. Aust N Z J Psychiatry. 2015;49(7):651–9.
53. Schalinski I, Fischer Y, Rockstroh B. Impact of childhood adversities on the short-term course of illness in psychotic spectrum disorders. Psychiatry Res. 2015;228(3):633–40.
54. Trotta A, Murray RM, David AS, et al. Impact of different childhood adversities on 1-year outcomes of psychotic disorder in the genetics and psychosis study. Schizophr Bull. 2016;42(2):464–75.
55. Bendall S, Hulbert CA, Alvarez-Jimenez M, et al. Testing a model of the relationship between childhood sexual abuse and psychosis in a first-episode psychosis group. J Nerv Ment Dis. 2013;201(11):941–7.
56. Kocsis-Bogár K, Mészáros V, Perczel-Forintos D. Gender differences in the relationship of childhood trauma and the course of illness in schizophrenia. Compr Psychiatry. 2018;82:84–8.
57. Gayer-Anderson C, Fisher HL, Fearon P, et al. Gender differences in the association between childhood physical and sexual abuse, social support and psychosis. Soc Psychiatry Psychiatr Epidemiol. 2015;50(10):1489–500.
58. Arseneault L, Bowes L, Shakoor S. Bullying victimization in youths and mental health problems: "much ado about nothing"? Psychol Med. 2010;40(5):717–29.
59. Kelleher I, Keeley H, Corcoran P, et al. Childhood trauma and psychosis in a prospective cohort study: cause, effect, and directionality. Am J Psychiatry. 2013;170(7):734–41.
60. Mackie CJ, O'Leary-Barrett M, Al-Khudhairy N, et al. Adolescent bullying, cannabis use and emerging psychotic experiences: a longitudinal general population study. Psychol Med. 2013;43(5):1033–44.

61. Broderick PC. Early adolescent gender differences in the use of ruminative and distracting coping strategies. J Early Adolesc. 1998;18(2):173–91.
62. Nolen-Hoeksema S, Larson J, Grayson C. Explaining the gender difference in depressive symptoms. J Pers Soc Psychol. 1999;77(5):1061–72.
63. Fisher HL, Schreier A, Zammit S, et al. Pathways between childhood victimization and psychosis-like symptoms in the ALSPAC birth cohort. Schizophr Bull. 2013;39(5):1045–55.
64. Krysta K, Murawiec S, Klasik A, et al. Sex-specific differences in cognitive functioning among schizophrenic patients. Psychiatr Danub. 2013;25:244–6.
65. McGregor C, et al. Estrogens and the cognitive symptoms of schizophrenia: possible neuroprotective mechanisms. Front Neuroendocrinol. 2017;47:19–33.
66. Uggerby P, Nielsen RE, Correll CU, et al. Characteristics and predictors of long-term institutionalization in patients with schizophrenia. Schizophr Res. 2011;131(1–3):120–6.
67. Cotton SM, Lambert M, Schimmelmann BG, et al. Gender differences in premorbid and treatment characteristics in first-episode psychosis. Schizophr Res. 2009;114(1–3):17–24.
68. Kulkarni J, Gavrilidis E, Worsley R, et al. The role of estrogen in treating men with schizophrenia. Int J Endocrinol Metab. 2013;11(3):129–36.
69. Ruiz-Veguilla M, Moreno-Granados J, Salcedo-Marin MD, et al. Sex-specific cognitive abnormalities in early-onset psychosis. Rev Bras Psiquiatr. 2017;39(1):28–35.
70. Thara R, Kamath S. Women and schizophrenia. Indian J Psychiatry. 2015;57(Suppl 2):S246–51.
71. Han M, Huang X, Xiu M, et al. Gender differences in cognitive function of chronic schizophrenia. Prog Neuro-Psychopharmacol Biol Psychiatry. 2012;39:358–63.
72. Ayesa-Arriola R, Setién-Suero E, Neergaard KD, et al. Premorbid IQ subgroups in first-episode psychosis: long-term sex differences in function and neurocognition. Schizophr Res. 2018;197:370–7.
73. Marsh R, Gerber AJ, Peterson BS. Neuroimaging studies of normal brain development. J Am Acad Child Adolesc Psychiatry. 2008;47(11):1233–51.
74. Abu-Akel A, Bo S. Superior mentalizing abilities of female patients with schizophrenia. Psychiatry Res. 2013;201(3):794–9.
75. Riecher-Rössler A. Oestrogens, prolactin, and schizophrenic psychoses. Lancet Psychiatry. 2017;4(1):63–72.
76. Kulkarni J, Riedel A, de Castella AR, et al. Estrogen in schizophrenia treatment. Schizophr Res. 2001;41(1):137–44.
77. Lindamer LA, Buse DC, Lohr JB, et al. Hormone replacement therapy in postmenopausal women with schizophrenia. Biol Psychiatry. 2001;49(1):47–51.
78. Riecher-Rössler A, Häfner H, Stumbaum M, et al. Can estradiol modulate schizophrenic symptomatology? Schizophr Bull. 1994;20(1):203–14.
79. Goldstein JM, Seidman LJ, Goodman JM, et al. Sex differences in neuropsychological functions in schizophrenia. Am J Psychiatry. 1998;155:1358–64.
80. Allen DN, Strauss GP, Barchard KA, et al. Gender differences in premorbid adjustment in schizophrenia. Schizophr Res. 2013;146(1–3):132–7.
81. Tang YL, Gillespie CF, Epstein MP, et al. Gender differences in Chinese inpatients with schizophrenia. Schizophr Res. 2007;97(1–3):88–96.
82. Häfner H. Gender differences in schizophrenia. Psychoneuroendocrinology. 2003;28(Suppl 2):17–54.
83. Larsen TK, McGlashan TH, Johannessen JO, et al. Premorbid patterns in first-episode schizophrenia by gender. Schizophr Bull. 1996;22(2):257–69.
84. Hassan GAM, Taha GRA. Long-term functioning in early-onset psychosis. Behav Brain Funct. 2011;7:28.
85. Ochoa S, Usall J, Villalta-Gil V, et al. Gender differences in social functioning in schizophrenia. Schizophr Res. 2012;141(2–3):175–81.
86. Shah J, Mizrahi R, McKenzie K. Social aetiology of psychosis. Br J Psychiatry. 2011;199(1):11–4.

87. Chang WC, Tang JYM, Hui CLM, et al. Premorbid adjustment and negative symptoms in first-episode schizophrenia. Psychiatry Res. 2013;209(3):353–60.
88. Mackie CJ, O'Leary-Barrett M, Al-Khudhairy N, et al. Adolescent bullying, cannabis use, and psychosis. Psychol Med. 2013;43(5):1033–44.
89. Riecher-Rössler A, McGorry PD. Early detection and intervention in psychosis. Key Issues Ment Health. 2016;179:179–89.
90. Seeman MV. Gender differences in the prescribing of antipsychotic drugs. Am J Psychiatry. 2004;161:1324–33.
91. Yonkers KA, et al. Gender differences in pharmacokinetics and pharmacodynamics of psychotropic medication. Am J Psychiatry. 1992;149:587–95.
92. Seeman MV. Interaction of sex, age, and neuroleptic dose. Compr Psychiatry. 1983;24(2):125–8.
93. Schwartz JB. The influence of sex on pharmacokinetics. Clin Pharmacokinet. 2003;42:107–21.
94. Sica DA, et al. Gender and its effect in cardiovascular pharmacotherapeutics. Congest Heart Fail. 2005;11(3):163–6.
95. Seeman MV. Neuroleptic expressed prescription for men and women. Soc Pharmacol. 1989;3:219–36.
96. Haring C, et al. Dose-related plasma levels of clozapine: influence of smoking behavior, sex, and age. Psychopharmacology. 1989;99(1):38–40.
97. Goff DC, et al. Cigarette smoking in schizophrenia: relationship to psychopathology and medication side effects. Am J Psychiatry. 1992;149(9):1189–94.
98. Crawford MB, et al. Issues related to sex differences in antipsychotic treatment. Curr Opin Psychiatry. 2016;29(3):211–7.
99. Haas GL, et al. Gender and schizophrenia outcome: a clinical trial of an inpatient family intervention. Schizophr Bull. 1990;16(2):277–92.
100. Davis JA, et al. Gender differences in family attitudes about schizophrenia. Psychol Med. 1996;26(4):689–96.
101. Abel KM, et al. Sex differences in schizophrenia. Int Rev Psychiatry. 2010;22:417–28.
102. Angermeyer MC, et al. Gender and the course of schizophrenia: differences in treated outcomes. Schizophr Bull. 1990;16(2):293–307.
103. da Silva TL, et al. Contribution of sex hormones to gender differences in schizophrenia: a review. Asian J Psychiatr. 2015;18:2–14.
104. Sellwood W, et al. Demographic factors associated with extreme non-compliance in schizophrenia. Soc Psychiatry Psychiatr Epidemiol. 1994;29(4):172–7.
105. Nose M, et al. How often do patients with psychosis fail to adhere to treatment programmes? A systematic review. Psychol Med. 2003;33(7):1149–60.
106. Law MR, et al. A longitudinal study of medication nonadherence and hospitalization risk in schizophrenia. J Clin Psychiatry. 2008;69:47–53.
107. Galdas PM, et al. Men and health help-seeking behaviour: literature review. J Adv Nurs. 2005;49:616–23.
108. Kulkarni J, et al. Estradiol for treatment-resistant schizophrenia: a large-scale randomized-controlled trial in women. Mol Psychiatry. 2015;20(6):695–702.
109. Begemann MJH, et al. Estrogen augmentation in schizophrenia: a quantitative review of current evidence. Schizophr Res. 2012;141(2–3):179–84.
110. Ghafari E, et al. Combination of estrogen and antipsychotics in the treatment of women with chronic schizophrenia. Clin Schizophr Relat Psychoses. 2013;6(4):172–6.
111. Melkersson KI, et al. Dose requirement and prolactin elevation of antipsychotics in male and female patients with schizophrenia. Br J Clin Pharmacol. 2001;51(4):317–24.
112. Szymanski S, et al. Gender differences in onset of illness, treatment response, course, and biologic indexes in first-episode schizophrenic patients. Am J Psychiatry. 1995;152(5):698–703.
113. Carliner H, et al. Prevalence of cardiovascular risk factors among racial and ethnic minorities with schizophrenia spectrum and bipolar disorders: a critical literature review. Compr Psychiatry. 2014;55(2):233–47.
114. Bener A, et al. A two-fold risk of metabolic syndrome in a sample of patients with schizophrenia. Diabetes Metab Syndr. 2014;8(1):24–9.

115. Huang MC, et al. Prevalence of metabolic syndrome among patients with schizophrenia in Taiwan. Acta Psychiatr Scand. 2009;120:274–80.
116. Boke O, et al. Prevalence of metabolic syndrome among inpatients with schizophrenia. Int J Psychiatry Med. 2008;38(1):103–12.
117. Xiang YT, et al. Sex differences in patients with schizophrenia: a prospective, multi-center study. Psychiatry Res. 2010;177:294–8.
118. Limosin F, et al. Body mass index and prevalence of obesity in a French cohort of patients with schizophrenia. Acta Psychiatr Scand. 2008;118(1):19–25.
119. Vieweg WV, et al. Proarrhythmic risk with antipsychotic and antidepressant drugs: implications in the elderly. Drugs Aging. 2009;26(12):997–1012.
120. Yasui N, et al. Prolactin response to bromperidol treatment in schizophrenic patients. Pharmacol Toxicol. 1998;82:153–6.
121. O'Keane V. Antipsychotic-induced hyperprolactinaemia, hypogonadism and osteoporosis in the treatment of schizophrenia. J Psychopharmacol. 2008;22(2 Suppl):70–5.
122. Stubbs B, et al. A meta-analysis of prevalence estimates and moderators of low bone mass in people with schizophrenia. Acta Psychiatr Scand. 2014;130(6):470–86.
123. Halbreich U, et al. Decreased bone mineral density in medicated psychiatric patients. Psychosom Med. 1995;57(5):485–91.
124. Alvir JM, et al. A reevaluation of the clinical characteristics of clozapine-induced agranulocytosis. J Clin Psychopharmacol. 1994;14:87–9.
125. Banov MD, et al. High risk of eosinophilia in women treated with clozapine. J Clin Psychiatry. 1993;54:466–9.
126. Auquier P, Lançon C, Rouillon F, et al. Mortality in schizophrenia. Pharmacoepidemiol Drug Saf. 2006;15(12):873–9.
127. Targum SD, Caputo KP, Ball SK. Menstrual cycle phase and psychiatric admissions. J Affect Disord. 1991;22(1):49–53.
128. Lande RG, Karamchandani V. Chronic mental illness and the menstrual cycle. J Am Osteopath Assoc. 2002;102(12):655–9.
129. Thompson KN, Kulkarni J, Sergejew AA. Extrapyramidal symptoms and oestrogen. Acta Psychiatr Scand. 2000;101(2):130–4.
130. Seeman MV. Antipsychotic-induced amenorrhea. J Ment Health. 2011;20(5):484–91.
131. Miller LJ. Sexuality, reproduction, and family planning in women with schizophrenia. Schizophr Bull. 1997;23(4):623–35.
132. Galbally M, Snellen M, Power J. Antipsychotic drugs in pregnancy: a review of maternal and fetal effects. Ther Adv Drug Saf. 2014;5(2):100–9.
133. McCauley-Elsom K, Kulkarni J. Managing psychosis in pregnancy. Aust N Z J Psychiatry. 2007;41(3):289–92.
134. Hasan A, et al. WFSBP guidelines for biological treatment of schizophrenia, part 3: special circumstances. World J Biol Psychiatry. 2015;16:142–70.
135. Mehta TM, Van Lieshout RJ. Safety of clozapine in pregnancy and lactation. Arch Womens Ment Health. 2016;20(1):1–9.
136. Kendell RE, Chalmers JC, Plats C. Epidemiology of puerperal psychosis. Br J Psychiatry. 1987;150(5):662–73.
137. Ahokas A, Aito M, Turiainen S. Association between oestradiol and puerperal psychosis. Acta Psychiatr Scand. 2000;101(2):167–9.
138. Lehman AF, et al. Practice guideline for schizophrenia treatment. Am J Psychiatry. 2004;161(2):1–56.
139. DGPPN. S3 guidelines for schizophrenia treatment. Steinkopff-Verlag; 2006.
140. Yang FD, et al. Sex differences in QTc prolongation in schizophrenia. Psychopharmacology. 2011;216(1):9–16.
141. Al-Khatib SM, et al. QT interval and clinical practice. JAMA. 2003;289(16):2120–7.
142. Lange B, et al. Gender effects in psychosis pharmacotherapy. Expert Opin Pharmacother. 2017;18(4):351–62.

Personality Disorders: Borderline Personality Spectrum

23

Olatz Napal Fernández, Laín Díaz López,
Carmen Garrido Fernández, and María Pérez Martín

23.1 Personality Disorder and Gender

Understanding personality disorders cannot be separated from a gender perspective. Gender stereotypes shape both the expression and perception of dysfunctional traits, leading to differences in presentation and diagnosis. In Cluster A, paranoid, schizoid, and schizotypal disorders are more common in men, possibly due to greater social tolerance of emotional detachment and distrust. In women, these traits are often viewed through a depressive or anxious lens [1–3]. In Cluster C, avoidant and dependent personality disorders are more frequent in women, reflecting the reinforced submissiveness and fear of rejection, whereas obsessive-compulsive personality disorder is more common in men, aligning with traits such as masculinity, control, and perfectionism [1–3]. In Cluster B, gender stereotypes are especially pronounced, particularly regarding emotional expression. It is no coincidence that these types of disorders are diagnosed more frequently in women and in people who do not conform to male heteronormative parameters. Diagnoses in this group reflect opposing gender norms: borderline and histrionic personality disorders are more frequent in women, reinforcing the link between emotionality and femininity, while antisocial and narcissistic disorders are more common in men, associated with aggression and grandiosity [1, 3–6]. These patterns highlight the socially and historically constructed nature of personality disorders, even leading to debates about the legitimacy of some, such as histrionic personality disorder [7].

From childhood, gender socialization shapes personality by promoting some traits while inhibiting others. Girls are encouraged toward emotional

O. N. Fernández (✉) · L. D. López · C. G. Fernández · M. P. Martín
Cruces University Hospital, Barakaldo, Spain

University of the Basque Country, Bilbao, Spain
e-mail: olatz.napalfernandez@osakidetza.eus

M. López-Atanes, M. Sáenz-Herrero (eds.), *Applying the Gender Perspective in Psychiatry and Psychotherapy*, https://doi.org/10.1007/978-3-032-17883-1_23

sensitivity, compliance, and dependence, whereas boys are pushed toward autonomy, aggression, and competitiveness. These patterns influence both personality expression and the processing of adverse experiences. Women, more often exposed to gender-based violence and childhood abuse, may develop coping strategies that are clinically interpreted as symptoms of personality disorders, such as hypersensitivity to rejection or emotional instability [8–10]. In contrast, men may exhibit externalizing responses like impulsivity and aggression, leading to different diagnoses [8, 11]. Thus, early experiences shape not only personality but also the clinical perception of psychopathology.

Gender stereotypes also contribute to biases in clinical practice. Traits linked to a specific gender influence how clinicians classify behaviors as "normal" or "pathological" and assign them to diagnostic categories. Studies show that simply varying a patient's gender in clinical vignettes can alter diagnostic evaluations [3–6, 12, 13]. These biases impact diagnostic accuracy and treatment access, highlighting the need for greater gender awareness in personality disorder assessment and clinical care.

23.2 Borderline Personality Disorder

The term "borderline" was first used in 1938 by the analyst Adolph Stern to describe patients who appeared to be more profoundly disturbed than those suffering from neurotic symptoms, but could not be classified as psychotic [14].

For Kernberg, the major difference between the neurotic and the borderline patient is the borderline's lack of a clear sense of identity. While neurotic patients can verbally describe themselves, borderline patients provide contradictory, incomplete self-portraits and exhibit inconsistent behavior. A core symptom is "splitting," where one holds two contradictory perceptions of the self or others as entirely good or bad, unable to integrate them into a coherent image. This pathological ego structure is rooted in early childhood, with object relations theory assigning the mother a pivotal role in shaping the infant's personality [15, 16]. In 2013, the new edition of the DSM-5 characterized borderline identity disturbance by an impoverished, unstable self-image, excessive self-criticism, chronic emptiness, and dissociative states under stress [1].

BPD has been a controversial diagnosis [17], criticized for its weighted construction, its inconsistent and unclear meaning, and its uneven, stigmatizing, and punitive application [18]. Studies cite BPD rates of approximately 0.4–1.8% among community samples [19, 20] and 10–25% among clinical samples [21, 22]. Gender differences in rates of borderline personality disorder (BPD), with approximately three females diagnosed for every male diagnosed, have been cited in the most recent edition of the DSM-5 [1, 23, 24]. These diagnostic rates and their gender differences have been noted for several other personality disorders as well; for example, both dependent and histrionic personality disorders are also said to be more prevalent among females than males [25]. BPD diagnosis has been "feminized" and has become a new "female malady" for the late twentieth century [25].

Linehan's biopsychosocial model of BPD etiology suggests that the escalated rate of BPD among women is a consequence of several factors, such as escalated rates of sexual abuse among women, invalidating cultural ideals for women, and sexism directed at girls who fail to be appropriately "feminine" or whose talents are considered "masculine" in areas like mechanics. Thus, women are more likely to encounter these forms of invalidation, and because invalidation is a critical factor leading to the development of BPD within Linehan's model, women are more likely to develop BPD in adulthood [26].

Butler critiques pre-social conceptions of identity and subjecthood, arguing that gender and selfhood are inseparable. To speak of "selves" inevitably involves gender. Butler questions the neutrality and universality of the self, showing how its concept reflects masculine subjectivity and marginalizes women's experiences [27–29]. Within patriarchal gender binaries, feminine identity is unstable, marked by paradox and contradiction—caught between essentialist femininity and psychological norms of a "healthy" self, creating a double bind of ambiguity and confusion [30].

Men constitute a minority of BPD diagnoses, with 25–30% diagnosed as male [25]. One explanation is that males exhibiting borderline traits are often diagnosed with antisocial personality disorder (ASPD) instead [31]. The frequently cited 1:3 male-to-female BPD ratio contrasts with the reverse 3:1 ratio for ASPD.

Studies indicate that women with BPD are more likely to experience chronic emptiness, suicidal behavior, self-mutilation, and affective instability, while men are more likely to exhibit impulsivity [32, 33]. Others argue that sex differences in BPD are minimal, mainly limited to a greater likelihood that women will engage in sexually abusive relationships [34]. A high proportion of those diagnosed with BPD are LGBTQ+. The question remains whether they genuinely experience identity "disturbances" characteristic of BPD or whether clinicians perceive and label them differently. Some men may escape the borderline label because their behaviors align with masculine norms, while those diagnosed as borderline often deviate from these stereotypes [30].

23.3 Gender and Madness: A Historical View

Tracing the history of madness back to the pre-modern discourse of witchcraft, some authors describe how this discourse positioned the deviant woman as a "witch/outsider" threatening social norms [25, 35]. Such women could be punished, controlling and neutralizing their perceived threat. As the religious worldview shifted to a scientific paradigm, Foucault described the emergence of a scientifically controlled concept of insanity [36]. This marked the transition from "witchcraft" as the dominant discourse on female deviancy to "hysteria" in the nineteenth century. Hysteria became the ultimate signifier of women as pathological and irrational. Showalter demonstrated the symbolic association of madness with femininity in

Western history, arguing that hysteria was not an individual pathology but a response to powerlessness arising from contradictory expectations of femininity [37]. Women labeled "hysterical" were, on the one hand, unable to meet social norms and, on the other, unable to release themselves from the force of these norms, since the norms had been internalized. Hysteria undermined the norm of female refinement in two ways: directly, through the "fits" or unseemly emotional outbursts to which hysterical individuals were prone, and indirectly, through debilitating physical symptoms that rendered the individual helpless, in a caricature of feminine delicacy [38]. Hysteria became an epidemic, with women accepting their "illness" and at the same time "finding a way to rebel against an intolerable social role" [25].

There has been an increasing recognition that the label "borderline" may function in the same way that "hysteria" did in the late nineteenth and early twentieth centuries: as a label for women. According to Jimenez MA, "the similarities between BPD and hysteria are striking. Both diagnoses delimit appropriate behavior for women and many of the criteria are stereotypically feminine" [39]. BPD is a more aggressive version of hysteria, with the distinction being the inclusion of anger and other "aggressive" characteristics in borderline personality disorder, such as shoplifting, reckless driving, and substance abuse [39]. From a social constructionist perspective, BPD (like witchcraft and hysteria) represents a deviation from rationality and individuality [40]. The diagnosis depends on a psychiatrist's judgment of emotional appropriateness, referencing the norm of "rationality." Both anger and fear of abandonment can be deemed inappropriate, rather than understandable responses to trauma [40]. The diagnosis is often applied to women who fail to conform to gender norms by expressing anger and aggression. Jimenez argues that "this successor to hysteria, in depicting the borderline patient as a 'demanding, aggressive, and angry woman' and highlighting 'promiscuity' as a feature, reflects contemporary moral judgments on female behavior" [39]. At the same time, the diagnosis is also applied to women who conform too easily, internalizing anger and expressing it through self-injury [40]. Wirth-Cauchon discusses how "women diagnosed with BPD are representing society's contradictions about femininity, with the double-bind of being denigrated for both emotionality and rationality, for active sexuality and for passive servicing of men" [30].

23.4 Social Causation of Distress and Trauma

Traumatic experiences are often reported among individuals with BPD and frequently include multiple forms of traumatization, such as physical or sexual; these stressful events can contribute to different burdensome symptoms (such as reexperiencing, avoidant behavior, and increased arousal) characteristic of posttraumatic stress disorder (PTSD) [41].

The document "Women's mental health: Into the mainstream strategic development of mental health care for women" [42] acknowledges that many women with a diagnosis of BPD have a history of trauma. At least 70% have been sexually abused as children [43]. Some studies report that 88% of people diagnosed with

BPD had experienced abuse: for 80%, this was childhood abuse; for 70%, this was early sexual abuse [44]. This can lead us to think that childhood sexual abuse is a powerful example of the social causation of distress with relation to BPD. However, the history of societal responses to childhood sexual abuse is a history of denial and distortion, and we can also find this in psychiatry's denial of etiological relevance of abuse, trauma and oppression for psychological distress [40]. Some authors consider the diagnosis of BPD a powerful new manifestation of this tendency to deny the extent and impact of childhood sexual abuse, neglect, or emotional abuse [40]. Some papers describe how the "symptoms" that define BPD can be better understood as adaptive reactions to early relational traumas. They suggest that it is much more helpful to understand people's behavior as an attempt to ensure "some measure of mastery, control and alliance with others, in the face of trauma, helplessness and inner vulnerability" than as the result of "a disorder of the personality, that is, solely as an internal deficit" [45–47].

The comorbidity of BPD and PTSD is frequent, yet not well understood. The prevalence of PTSD has been reported to be as high as 54% among individuals with BPD [41]. Lifetime comorbidity of BPD and PTSD is associated with more dysfunction than either individual disorder, with childhood sexual abuse playing an important role in the development of this comorbidity [48]. Trauma exposure and comorbid PTSD are frequently missed in this population, and the clinical presentation of these two disorders can easily be confused [41]. This may be due to similarities in domains of affect regulation, impulse control, interpersonal relationships, reality testing, and self-integration [48]. Absence of comorbid PTSD among BPD is related to faster time to remission, while a history of sexual victimization is related to a less favorable course of PTSD with a lower likelihood of remission and a higher risk of recurrence of PTSD [41]. Also, cumulative trauma has been suggested to predict current PTSD [49]. Sexual trauma, as compared to other types of trauma, has been proposed to be related to more severe PTSD [50]. In women with BPD, poly-traumatization was not significantly related to PTSD diagnosis as compared to single traumatization, whereas sexual victimization was significantly more prevalent in women with PTSD diagnosis and BPD, as compared to other types of traumatic events [51].

Herman considers that the BPD's behaviors are a form of adaptation to trauma. BPD is the most prominent psychiatric diagnosis (with somatization disorder and multiple personality disorder) given to people suffering from childhood trauma. Herman argues that even the category of PTSD is too narrowly defined, focusing on singular events such as combat, disaster, and rape, thus missing the more complex picture of prolonged abuse. She proposes a new category to encompass the spectrum of conditions related to trauma: "complex posttraumatic stress disorder" [51, 52]. The borderline's relations to other people can often be understood as strategies of adaptation held over from past relations with abusive caretakers. The patient's instability becomes understood as a response to an external event, rather than being rooted in a character or personality disorder. With the label "BPD" there is a risk of losing narrative comprehensibility, placing the patient's symptoms within a scientific-medical frame of character pathology. And yet while sexual and physical abuse is a major factor, it does not fully account for the predominance of women diagnosed as borderline, since not all individuals have histories of childhood abuse, and it happens in 20–40% of women diagnosed as borderline [25].

23.5 The Description of BPD

BPD, "*it not only causes instability, but also symbolizes it*" [31], involves instability in mood, self-image, relationships, and feelings of emptiness or rage. One diagnostic criterion for BPD pertains to a disturbance in "identity." Some authors argued that identity disturbance and unstable relationships are at the core of "borderline pathology" [53].

23.5.1 Fragmented Selves (Wirth-Caucho's Classification/ Description)

23.5.1.1 Mask Self

Borderline narratives express feelings of artificiality or falsity often accompanied by sensations of emptiness and numbness. "As a superficial, surface mask or person that is a kind of empty adaptation to the surroundings" [30]. Sometimes they try to have a closer relationship with others, relying not on others to give them a "setting and pulse," but on fragmentary feeling sensations to "anchor" their identities. Helene Deutsch described the *"as if personality"* in which persons appear to be "normal," yet, on closer observation, lack warmth or depth. There is only imitation of others, identification with the environment that facilitates "good adaptation" to the world without depth or inner life. Deutsch says that "if it is a woman, she seems to be the quintessence of feminine devotion, imparted by her passivity and readiness for identification" [54].

23.5.1.2 Lost Self

We can see the mutable meaning of the borderline label, simultaneously close to, and different from, psychosis. It also seems that the patient has a marginal presence that refuses to be integrated within the group, being inaccessible and placing herself out of the bounds of normality, without being declared psychotic [30].

23.5.1.3 Repressed Self

Women in our culture tend to repress distinctive aspects of the self that are bound up with autonomy and aggression. Whirth-Cauchon says that the construction of the self as feminine creates a double bind; on one hand, they must suppress their "non-feminine" aspects: autonomy and aggression. On the other hand, they must disavow their feminine embodiment: "The world of thought and action is the world of men; to enter it, women must leave their distinctively female bodies and sexuality 'outside'" [30].

23.5.1.4 Double Self

The alternate personality who, continuing with the 'sexual self', for example, can sometimes perform the self described before (more passive, reclusive, etc.), and at other times emerges like an alternate personality, seductive, dark, hypersensual, reproducing the cultural split between passive femininity and "forbidden" sexual autonomy, "the bitch".

23.5.1.5 Interrupted Self

The patients give descriptions of depersonalization, numbness, and emptiness. They describe a profound alienation from their body and fight against a sense that they do not exist as a flesh–blood person. Some women describe their emptiness like a response to their lack of fit with the narrow roles society offered white, middle-class, privileged girls. The feelings of inadequacy (unfitness) mixed with their resistance to these roles [55].

23.6 At the Border: Dependency and Fear of Abandonment, Anger, and Regulation of Emotion

Dependency and the Fear of Abandonment The term *dependent* has been used in a variety of ways: "to describe a need state (longing, oral needs), an affective state (feelings of helplessness, neediness), and even a personality trait (passive dependent) [56]. Stiver [56] differs dependency from the boundary confusions and fear of loss of self-experienced by those who wish to merge with another, which results from a lack of cohesive self. The trend toward merger occurs not because of a failure to separate but because of an inability to remain connected with others while asserting a distinct sense of self [57]. Karen Horney [58] said that a dependent woman literally lives "in the eyes of others." If she exists only in the eyes of others, she finds it difficult to be alone; she only has a self if she is interacting with others. For her, "being alone means both the loss of identity and the proof of being despicable." Their vulnerability to criticism, disinterest from the others, or disagreement makes any of these feel like an extreme attack. Because she is dependent on those who might mean her harm, her ability to discern harmful or abusive conditions is compromised, and she deals with such conditions by alternating between accusing the other and accusing herself [58].

Anger Dysregulated anger and its behavioral manifestations, such as physical fights, are among the defining BPD criteria [59]. Adolescent girls soon discover that expressing anger may expose them to criticism and isolation. The experience of anger itself can bring with it a sense of separateness, difference, and aloneness [60]. Anger can take forms that range along a continuum, one pole of which is self-destructive behavior [61]. The suppression of anger results in both frustration and inaction, weakness and a lack of self-esteem—further contributing to a sense of unworthiness and inferiority that, in turn, generates more anger. Women often report feeling filled with unwarranted, irrational anger, and although this description does not relay an accurate picture of their psychological situation, it is one "that the external world—so-called 'reality'—is only too ready to confirm, because any anger is 'too much anger in women'. Indeed, the risk of expressing can appear grave and disorganizing. All this can end in a kind of self-fulfilling prophecy" [62].

Men with BPD are more likely to have comorbid narcissistic, antisocial, paranoid, and schizotypal personality disorders, alcohol and substance use disorders but less likely to have dependent and obsessive–compulsive personality disorders compared to women with BPD [63]. Many women (and some men also) tend to express anxiety as a secondary elaboration of suppressed anger. When they are confronting situations that are genuinely angering, they experience acute anxiety because they are not able to permit themselves to express the anger directly or because the suppression of anger has become so automatic that they cannot feel the anger at all [25].

Regulation of Emotion In Linehan's view, BPD is a disorder of emotional dysregulation, and most borderline behaviors stem either from attempts to regulate intense emotion or are the results of affect dysregulation [26]. Linehan's theory of the etiology of BPD symptoms rests upon biological as well as social learning foundations; however, some authors defend that social learning, in itself, can help to create emotional vulnerability.

23.7 The Body Talks

The concept of "Idiom of distress" is referred to as "socially and culturally resonant means of experiencing and expressing distress in local worlds" [64]. In her analysis of "female maladies" such as hysteria, agoraphobia, BPD, and anorexia, Bordo suggests that the symptoms of these female maladies are politically symbolic: loss of mobility and voice, inability to leave the home, feeding others while starving self, taking up space and whittling down the space one's body takes up, all have symbolic and political meaning within the varying rules governing the historical construction of gender. These women can be viewed as unconsciously protesting the constraints of gender roles through their bodies, rather than through verbal articulation [65]. The author focuses in particular on dissociation, a common symptom in BPD that signifies not simply individual women's suppressed memories, but the suppression and denial of historical memories of a circulating social violence [66].

23.7.1 Self-Distructiveness

Self-Injury Many people diagnosed as having BPD drink too much, shop too much, have eating problems, and/or engage in sexually promiscuous behavior, these behaviors are more likely to be viewed as variants of "normal" behaviors, whereas cutting, burning one's skin, or trying to kill oneself are not [25]. Self-injurious behavior (SIB) may take the form of self-mutilation through cutting, burning, or other means; risk-taking behavior that could lead to self-harm; impulsivity in the form of substance or food abuse; or suicide attempts, etc. Of the different forms of self-injury, chronic self-mutilation is unarguably the behavior most readily recognized as "borderline," even though it is by no means restricted to the borderline patient [67]. SIB can become a central means by which borderline clients give expression to separation/abandonment conflicts [68] and relieve the cumulative tensions arising from the struggle for expression of anger and other emotional needs [67, 69]. "For women at the border—and also some men (and all gay people), transexuals, intersexuals, etc.—the sense that no one can comprehend the extent and intensity of her suffering is an understandable consequence of the sense of never having *been known*. The patients are saying 'it is through my pain you shall know me'" [25].

Suicide Suicide attempts occur in up to 75% of patients with BPD, and up to 10% commit suicide, a rate almost 50 times greater than in the general population [70]. In DSM-5, BPD is the only personality disorder with suicidal or self-injurious behavior explicitly included in the diagnostic criteria [1]. BPD has been shown to have greater associations with suicidal behavior than major depressive disorder, another psychiatric disorder with a suicide-related criterion [70]. Some authors found that there is a trend toward higher maximum lethality of suicide attempts in men suicide attempters compared with women suicide attempters but no difference between men and women with regard to the proportion of suicide attempters or the number of suicide attempts [52]. For Linehan, parasuicidal behaviors constitute an attempt, albeit a maladaptive one, to gain control over unbearably painful, overwhelming negative affect.

23.8 LGTBIQ+ Community and BDP

The prevalence of borderline personality disorder (BPD) is higher in the LGTBIQ+ community than in the general population. Several studies explore this issue, offering different explanations. One major factor is diagnostic bias, where gender expressions and sexual orientations that deviate from heteronormative norms are pathologized [71]. For example, gay men displaying stereotypically feminine traits are more likely to be diagnosed with BPD, given its historical association with femininity, while more stereotypically masculine behavior in lesbian women may be viewed as disruptive. A similar issue arises with transgender individuals, where clinicians may conflate gender dysphoria with identity diffusion seen in BPD, leading to frequent misdiagnoses [72].

However, aside from these diagnostic biases, there is a higher association of certain BPD traits with the LGTBIQ+ community, as observed in various studies, showing that areas related to affectivity and interpersonal relationships are altered. The association of these alterations is theorized to be linked to discriminatory events and stigma experienced by these individuals due to their sexuality and gender identity, with these experiences of rejection and violence increasing vulnerability for the development of disorders like BPD. This is particularly true considering that, many times, these experiences of rejection come from close individuals such as family members and friends, which can amplify the impact of these experiences on the individual [73].

References

1. American Psychiatric Association. Diagnostic and statistical manual of mental disorders. 5th ed. Arlington: American Psychiatric Association; 2013.
2. He H, Xu M, Fei Z, Xie Y, Gu X, Zhu H, Wang J. Sex differences in personality disorders in a Chinese clinical population. Front Psychol. 2022;13:1006740. https://doi.org/10.3389/fpsyt.2022.1006740. PMID: 36213898; PMCID: PMC9537623
3. Rienzi BM, Scrams DJ. Gender stereotypes for paranoid, antisocial, compulsive, dependent, and histrionic personality disorders. Psychol Rep. 1991;69(3 Pt 1):976–8. https://doi.org/10.2466/pr0.1991.69.3.976. PMID: 1784694
4. Bruce M, Weinraub D. Implicit gender bias in the clinical judgment of psychopathy and personality disorders among licensed psychologists in the USA. J Pers Assess. 2023;105(6):763–9. https://doi.org/10.1080/00223891.2023.2178928. Epub 2023 Mar 1. PMID: 36857100
5. Green A, MacLean R, Charles K. Clinician perception of pathological narcissism in females: a vignette-based study. Front Psychol. 2023;14:1090746. https://doi.org/10.3389/fpsyg.2023.1090746. PMID: 37151338; PMCID: PMC10157482
6. Green A, Day NJS, Hart CM, Grenyer BFS, Bach B. Gender bias in assessing narcissistic personality: exploring the utility of the ICD-11 dimensional model. Br J Clin Psychol. 2024; https://doi.org/10.1111/bjc.12503. Epub ahead of print. PMID: 39262046
7. Nuckolls CW. Toward a cultural history of the personality disorders. Soc Sci Med. 1992;35(1):37–47. https://doi.org/10.1016/0277-9536(92)90117-9. PMID: 1496411
8. Jonason PK, Davis MD. A gender role view of the dark triad traits. Pers Individ Dif. 2018;125:102–5. https://doi.org/10.1016/j.paid.2018.01.004.
9. Izdebska A. Personality disorders in adult female child sexual abuse survivors: dimensions of personality pathology and characteristics of abuse. J Interpers Violence. 2021;36(23-24):NP13487–516. https://doi.org/10.1177/0886260520903136. Epub 2020 Mar 3. PMID: 32125218
10. Scheffers F, van Vugt E, Lanctôt N, Lemieux A. Experiences of (young) women after out-of-home placement: an examination of personality disorder symptoms through the lens of child maltreatment. Child Abuse Negl. 2019;92:116–25. https://doi.org/10.1016/j.chiabu.2019.03.022. Epub 2019 Apr 8. PMID: 30974255
11. Green A, MacLean R, Charles K. Female narcissism: assessment, aetiology, and behavioural manifestations. Psychol Rep. 2022;125(6):2833–64. https://doi.org/10.1177/00332941211027322. Epub 2021 Jun 22. PMID: 34154472; PMCID: PMC9578082
12. Flanagan EH, Blashfield RK. Gender bias in the diagnosis of personality disorders: the roles of base rates and social stereotypes. J Personal Disord. 2003;17(5):431–46. https://doi.org/10.1521/pedi.17.5.431.22974. PMID: 14632376
13. Jane JS, Oltmanns TF, South SC, Turkheimer E. Gender bias in diagnostic criteria for personality disorders: an item response theory analysis. J Abnorm Psychol. 2007;116(1):166–75. https://doi.org/10.1037/0021-843X.116.1.166. PMID: 17324027; PMCID: PMC4372614
14. Stern A. Psychoanalytic investigation of and therapy in the border line group of neuroses. Psychoanal Q. 1938;7:467–89.
15. Kernberg O. Mentioned in: Wirth-Cauchon J. Women and the borderline personality disorder: symptoms and stories. New Brunswick, NJ, and London: Rutgers University Press; 2003.

16. Kernberg O. Borderline conditions and pathological narcissism. 5th ed. New York: Jason Aronson, Inc.; 2012. [Originally published in 1975]
17. Roth A, Fonagy P. What works for whom? A critical review of psychotherapy research. London and New York: Guilford Press; 1996.
18. Lewis G, Appleby L. Personality disorder: the patients psychiatrists dislike. Br J Psychiatry. 1988;153:44–9.
19. Torgersen S, Kringlen E, Cramer V. The prevalence of personality disorders in a community sample. Arch Gen Psychiatry. 2001;58:590–6.
20. Johnson DM, Shea MT, Yen S, Battle CL, Zlotnick C, Sanislow CA, Grilo CM, Skodol AE, Bender DS, McGlashan TH, Gunderson JG, Zanarini MC. Gender differences in borderline personality disorder: findings from the collaborative longitudinal personality disorders study. Compr Psychiatry. 2003;44(4):284–92.
21. American Psychiatric Association. Diagnostic and statistical manual of mental disorders. 4th ed. Washington, DC: American Psychiatric Association; 1994.
22. Gunderson JG, Zanarini MC. Current overview of the borderline diagnosis. J Clin Psychiatry. 1991;42:1015–20.
23. Zanarini MC, Williams AA, Lewis RE, Reich RB, Vera SC, Marino MF. Reported pathological childhood experiences associated with the development of borderline personality disorder. Am J Psychiatry. 1997;154:1101–6.
24. Zanarini MC, Frankenburg FR, Reich DB, Marino MF, Haynes MC, Gunderson JG. Violence in the lives of adult borderline patients. J Nerv Ment Dis. 1999;187:65–71.
25. Becker D. Through the looking glass: women and borderline personality disorder. Boulder: Westview Press; 1997.
26. Linehan M. Cognitive-behavioral treatment of borderline personality disorder. New York: Guilford Press; 1993.
27. Beauvoir S. The second sex. Trans. Parshley EM. New York: Vintage; 1989.
28. Cixous H, Clément C. The newly born woman. Trans. Wing B. Minneapolis: University of Minnesota Press; 1986.
29. Bourdieu P. La domination masculine. Paris: Éditions du Seuil; 1998. 7th ed. Barcelona: Editorial Anagrama; 2012
30. Wirth-Cauchon J. Women and the borderline personality disorder: symptoms and stories. New Brunswick, NJ, and London: Rutgers University Press; 2003.
31. Cauwels J. Imbroglio: rising to the challenges of borderline personality disorder. New York: WW Norton; 1992.
32. Holthausen BS, Habel U. Sex differences in personality disorders. Curr Psychiatry Rep. 2018;20(107) https://doi.org/10.1007/s11920-018-0975-y.
33. Hoertel N, Peyre H, Wall MM, Limosin F, Blanco C. Examining sex differences in DSM-IV borderline personality disorder symptom expression using item response theory (IRT). J Psychiatr Res. 2014;59:213–9.
34. Sansone RA, Wiederman MW. Sex and age differences in symptoms in borderline personality symptomatology. Int J Psychiatry Clin Pract. 2014;18:145–9.
35. Szasz T. The myth of mental illness. London: Paladin; 1972.
36. Foucault M. Madness and civilization: a history of insanity in the age of reason. London: Tavistock; 1967.
37. Showalter E. The female malady: women, madness and English culture 1830–1980. New York: Penguin; 1985.
38. Hale NG Jr. Freud and the Americans: the beginnings of psychoanalysis in the United States, 1876–1917. New York: Oxford University Press; 1971.
39. Jimenez MA. Gender and psychiatry: psychiatric conceptions of mental disorders in women, 1960-1994. Affilia. 1997;12(2):154–75.
40. Saw C, Proctor G. Women at the margins: a critique of the diagnosis of borderline personality disorder. Fem Psychol. 2005;15(4):483–90. https://doi.org/10.1177/0959353505057620.
41. Sinai C, Hirvikoski T, Wiklander M, Nordström AL, Nordström P, Nilsonne A, Wilczek A, Asberg M, Jokinen J. Exposure to interpersonal violence and risk of posttraumatic stress dis-

order among women with borderline personality disorder. Psychiatry Res. 2018;262:311–5. https://doi.org/10.1016/j.psychres.2018.01.047.
42. Department of Health. Women's mental health: into the mainstream—strategic development of mental health care for women. London: Department of Health; 2002.
43. Meichenbaum D. Treating post-traumatic stress disorder: a handbook and practice manual for therapy. Chichester: Wiley; 1994.
44. Castillo H. You don't know what it's like. Ment Health Care 2000;4(2):42–3, 53–8.
45. Warner S, Wilkins T. Diagnosing distress and reproducing disorder: women, child sexual abuse and borderline personality disorder. In: Reavey P, Warner S, editors. New feminist stories of childhood sexual abuse. London: Routledge; 2003. p. 167–86.
46. Wilkins TM, Warner S. Understanding the therapeutic relationship—women diagnosed as borderline personality disordered. Br J Forensic Pract. 2000;2(3):30–7.
47. Wilkins TM, Warner S. Women in special hospitals: understanding the presenting behavior of women diagnosed with borderline personality disorder. J Psychiatr Ment Health Nurs. 2001;8:289–97.
48. Schneider EM, Wood PK, Trull TJ. The comorbidity of borderline personality disorder and posttraumatic stress disorder: revisiting the prevalence and associations in a general population sample. Bord Personal Disord Emot Dysregul. 2015;2:11.
49. Briere J, Agee E, Dietrich A. Cumulative trauma and current posttraumatic stress disorder status in general population and inmate samples. Psychol Trauma. 2016;8:439–46.
50. Jacob JM, Lamp K, Rauch SA, Smith ER, Buchholz KR. The impact of trauma type or number of traumatic events on PTSD diagnosis and symptom severity in treatmentseeking veterans. J Nerv Ment Dis. 2017;205:83–6.
51. Herman J. Trauma and recovery. New York: Basic Books; 1992.
52. World Health Organization. International classification of diseases for mortality and morbidity statistics (11th revision). Geneva: World Health Organization; 2018.
53. Devita Singh MA, McMain S, Zucker KJ. J Sex Med 2011;8(2):447–454. https://doi.org/10.1111/j.1743-6109.2010.02198.x.
54. Deutsch H. Some forms of emotional disturbance and their relationship to schizophrenia. In: Stone MH, editor. Essential papers on borderline disorders: one hundred years at the border. New York: New York University Press; 1942.
55. Kaysen S. Girl, interrupted. New York: Turtle Bay Books; 1993.
56. Stiver IP. The meanings of dependency in female-male relationships. In: Jordan JV, Kaplan AG, Miller JB, Stiver IP, Surrey JL, editors. Women's growth in connection. New York: Guilford; 1991. p. 143–61.
57. Gilligan C. In a different voice. Cambridge, MA: Harvard University Press; 1982.
58. Horney K. The neurotic personality of our time. New York: WW Norton; 1937.
59. Gunderson JG, Herpertz SC, Skodol AE, Torgersen S, Zanarini MC. Borderline personality disorder. Nat Rev Dis Primers. 2018;4:18029.
60. Lerner HG. Internal prohibitions against female anger. In: Lerner HG, editor. Women in therapy. Northvale: Jason Aronson; 1988. p. 59–75. (Reprinted from: Am J Psychoanal. 1980;40(2):137–48.).
61. Westkott M. The feminist legacy of Karen Horney. New Haven: Yale University Press; 1986.
62. Miller JB. The construction of anger in women and men. In: Jordan JV, Kaplan AG, Miller JB, Stiver IP, Surrey JL, editors. Women's growth in connection. New York: Guilford; 1991. p. 181–96.
63. Sher L, Rutter SB, New AS, Siever LJ, Hazlett EA. Gender differences and similarities in aggression, suicidal behavior, and psychiatric comorbidity in borderline personality disorder. Acta Psychiatr Scand. 2018:1–9. https://doi.org/10.1111/acps.12981.
64. Nichter M. Idioms of distress: alternatives in the expression of psychosocial distress: a case study from South India. Cult Med Psychiatry. 1981;5(5):379–408.
65. Bordo S. Unbearable weight: feminism, Western culture and the body. Berkeley: University of California Press; 1997.
66. Griggers C. Becoming woman. Minneapolis: University of Minnesota Press; 1997.

67. Favazza AR. Bodies under siege. Baltimore: Johns Hopkins University Press. [año de publicación necesario]
68. Perry JC, Cooper SH. A preliminary report on defenses and conflicts in borderline personality disorder. J Am Psychoanal Assoc. 1986;34:863–93.
69. Waites E. Trauma and survival: post-traumatic and dissociative disorders in women. New York: Norton; 1993.
70. Sher L, Fisher AM, Kelliher CH. Clinical features and psychiatric comorbidities of borderline personality disorder patients with versus without a history of suicide attempt. Psychiatry Res. 2016;246:261–6.
71. Rodriguez-Seijas C, Morgan TA, Zimmerman M. Is there a bias in the diagnosis of borderline personality disorder among lesbian, gay, and bisexual patients? Assessment. 2021;28(3):724–38. https://doi.org/10.1177/1073191120961833. Epub 2020 Sep 28. PMID: 32981328
72. Rodriguez-Seijas C, Warren M, Vupputuri P, Hawthorne S. Bias in the diagnosis of borderline personality disorder among sexual- and gender-minority persons: results from a vignette-based experiment. Clin Psychol Sci. 2024;13(2):388–406.
73. Denning DM, Newlands RT, Gonzales A, Benuto LT. Borderline personality disorder symptoms in a community sample of sexually and gender diverse adults. J Personal Disord. 2022;36(6):701–16.

24 Substance Use Disorders

Francina Fonseca, Silvia Martinez, and Alba Llimona

24.1 Introduction

Substance use disorders (SUDs) are multifactorial, chronic medical conditions shaped by the interplay of genetic predispositions, environmental exposures, and sociocultural determinants. Women exhibit unique epidemiological patterns, disease trajectories, and therapeutic responses in the context of SUDs. According to the World Drug Report 2024 (UNODC, World Drug Report 2024. United Nations publication, Vienna, 2024), although the overall prevalence of SUDs remains lower among women compared to men, women with SUDs demonstrate heightened vulnerability. Notably, they exhibit increased rates of psychiatric comorbidities, heightened exposure to intimate partner violence, and greater risks to sexual and reproductive health. Furthermore, substance-dependent mothers are disproportionately at risk of child custody loss and the accumulation of adverse life experiences. Despite representing approximately one-third of the global population of individuals who use drugs, women comprise only one-fifth—or fewer—of those receiving treatment services for SUDs (UNODC, World Drug Report 2024. United Nations publication, Vienna, 2024). In general, women throughout their lifetime face more

F. Fonseca (✉)
Mental Health Institute, Hospital del Mar Research Institute, Barcelona, Spain
e-mail: mffonseca@hmar.cat

S. Martinez
CAS Barceloneta and CAS Fòrum, Mental Health Institute—Hospital del Mar, Barcelona, Spain
e-mail: silvia.martinez.lopez@hmar.cat

A. Llimona
CAS Fòrum, Mental Health Institute—Hospital del Mar., Barcelona, Spain
e-mail: allimona@hmar.cat

M. López-Atanes, M. Sáenz-Herrero (eds.), *Applying the Gender Perspective in Psychiatry and Psychotherapy*, https://doi.org/10.1007/978-3-032-17883-1_24

barriers to accessing services, and this issue is more prominent in addictive disorders; such barriers include the higher stigma attached to substance use among women, the lack of childcare, the absence of gender-sensitive protocols and treatments, and the lack of family support, among others.

Sexual (e.g., bisexual, gay, lesbian, queer) and gender (e.g., transgender, nonbinary, gender-expansive) minority individuals (SGMI) exhibit disproportionately elevated rates of alcohol and other SUDs relative to their heterosexual and cisgender counterparts (Batchelder et al. [2] LGBT Health 8(4):290–299, 2021. Schuler et al. [3] Drug Alcohol Depend. 189:139–146, 2018).

This chapter aims to present an overview of how sex and gender may influence the epidemiology, clinical manifestations, social determinants, and response to treatment in women with SUD and in sexual/gender minority populations.

24.2 Epidemiology of SUD

Historically, men have exhibited higher prevalence rates of substance use, abuse, and dependence compared to women [4–6], with women representing approximately one-quarter of individuals who have used a drug in the past year. Conversely, in the case of nonmedical use of pharmaceutical substances such as sedatives, tranquilizers, opioid analgesics, and stimulants, the proportion of women engaging in these practices can be considerably higher, and in certain instances, may approach parity with men. However, this proportion varies across different substances and geographical regions. For instance, in Asia, only 9% of cannabis users are women, whereas in North America, women constitute 45% of cannabis users. Additionally, cocaine use has risen more substantially among women in countries such as Argentina and Bolivia [1].

With respect to alcohol consumption, while men have traditionally consumed alcohol in greater quantities, with higher frequency and more hazardous drinking patterns, recent trends suggest that these gender differences are diminishing—especially among younger cohorts, where women are initiating alcohol use at earlier ages [7, 8].

Regarding opioids, recent data from the United States reveal that heroin use is increasing more rapidly among women than men, and the decline in nonmedical prescription opioid use is occurring at a slower rate in women. Furthermore, women are at higher risk for nonmedical use of prescription opioids compared to heroin [9]. Women are also more likely than men to initiate opioid use through legally prescribed medications for pain management [10].

The observed gender differences in substance use prevalence have been largely attributed to sociocultural (gender-related) rather than biological (sex-related) factors. Historically, men have had greater access to substances across many societies. When access to substances is controlled for in studies, the likelihood of substance use between men and women appears to be similar [11].

Although women typically initiate substance use later than men, they tend to escalate their use of alcohol, cannabis, cocaine, and opioids more rapidly once initiated. This phenomenon, known as the "telescoping effect," describes an accelerated trajectory from first use to the development of a substance use disorder and entry into treatment [12, 13]. Consequently, women often present to treatment services with more severe medical, psychological, behavioral, and social issues. However, it is important to note that some studies have not replicated the telescoping effect [14, 15], which may be due to methodological differences. The effect has been more consistently observed in treatment-seeking populations, suggesting that it may be more pronounced in individuals with more severe substance use profiles [16].

In terms of the sexual and gender minority individual (SGMI) population, data from a nationally representative sample in the United States ($N = 36{,}309$) demonstrated that lesbian, gay, and bisexual individuals were approximately twice as likely as heterosexual individuals to meet diagnostic criteria for alcohol use disorder (AUD), with 21.5% of sexual minority individuals and 12.8% of heterosexual individuals meeting criteria for AUD within the past year [17]. Similarly, national data have shown that SGMI adults have nearly double the likelihood of meeting criteria for any substance use disorder (SUD) compared to heterosexual adults [18]. In addition, large-scale analyses of gender minority populations have revealed significantly higher prevalence of AUD and other SUDs among transgender individuals compared to cisgender individuals. One study involving 15,637 transgender and 46,911 cisgender adults found that transgender individuals had significantly higher odds of receiving an AUD diagnosis [19]. Furthermore, the analysis of approximately nine million electronic health records from the US Department of Veterans Affairs indicated that transgender patients were more likely than cisgender patients to be diagnosed with any SUD [20].

The motivations for initiating substance use also differ by gender. Females are more likely to begin using substances as a coping mechanism for negative affective states such as depression and anxiety [21], whereas males are more often driven by peer influence or sensation-seeking behaviors [22]. Increased exposure among women to adverse life events—including trauma and intimate partner violence—has been associated with both the accelerated development of substance use disorders and the decreasing gender gap in substance use prevalence [23].

Conversely, in the SMGI population, the increased prevalence of SUD is commonly attributed to minority stress—a framework positing that individuals from stigmatized and marginalized social groups experience chronic stress due to societal prejudice, discrimination, and structural inequities, which in turn contribute to adverse health outcomes, including increased vulnerability to substance use disorders [24].

24.3 Gender-Related Social Determinants

Women with SUDs are disproportionately affected by adverse environmental and familial conditions compared to men. They are more likely to originate from households with a familial history of substance use, indicating both genetic vulnerability and increased environmental stressors. Family disruption is more commonly reported among women with SUDs, and many engage in intimate relationships with partners who also misuse substances. These partners often initiate women into substance use, with some women being coerced or pressured into drug use within the context of the relationship. In certain cases, substance-using partners facilitate or exploit women's drug dependence through involvement in sex work. Women in such contexts experience significantly higher rates of intimate partner violence (IPV) [25].

One study investigated the prevalence and types of traumatic experiences among individuals undergoing medication for opioid use disorder (MOUD), with a focus on variations across gender, posttraumatic stress disorder (PTSD) status, and the presence of chronic pain. The cross-sectional analysis included 303 participants (157 women, 144 men, two nonbinary) stabilized on MOUD. Findings revealed a high incidence of lifetime trauma within this population. Gender-specific differences were evident: women reported higher rates of intimate partner violence (85% vs 73%) and adult sexual assault (57% vs 13%), whereas men reported more physical assaults (81% vs 61%) and witnessed trauma (66% vs 48%). Both genders experienced significant childhood physical abuse and exposure to intimate partner violence during childhood, with comparable rates of adult accidents. Notably, 41% of participants screened positive for PTSD, and 57% reported chronic pain. The number of traumatic events was a significant predictor of both PTSD symptom severity and diagnostic status. Additionally, individuals with chronic pain reported significantly more childhood traumatic events (85% vs 75%) compared to those without chronic pain [26].

The co-occurrence of SUD and IPV is strongly associated with elevated rates of psychiatric comorbidities in women, including mood, anxiety, and trauma-related disorders [25]. In addition to these mental health implications, women with SUDs face several sex-specific medical complications related to substance use, including infertility, spontaneous abortion, vaginal infections, and preterm birth. These outcomes further exacerbate the physical and psychological burden of addiction among women.

From a socio-environmental perspective, women with SUDs are more likely to experience structural and familial instability, including growing up in disrupted family environments with other individuals who misuse substances. Relationships with drug-using partners and engagement in transactional sex significantly increase their vulnerability to acquiring infectious diseases such as human immunodeficiency virus (HIV) and hepatitis C virus (HCV). According to the World Health Organization, the estimated lifetime prevalence of IPV among women with SUDs ranges from 40% to 70%, markedly higher than the 17–35% prevalence in the general female population [27]. There is a bidirectional relationship between alcohol use disorder and exposure to physical or sexual IPV. Substance use is associated with an increased risk of IPV victimization, and couples in which one or both partners misuse substances exhibit a threefold increase in the likelihood of IPV perpetration [28, 29].

Another environmental aspect related to differences in alcohol use between gender is the different roles in society. Both women and men generally exhibit a decline in alcohol consumption during their mid-20 s, a developmental process commonly referred to as "maturing out." This normative reduction is largely attributed to sociocultural factors, particularly major role transitions such as entering into marriage, advancing in one's career, and becoming a parent [30]. Historically, traditional gender roles—especially those assigning women primary caregiving responsibilities—have contributed to lower alcohol consumption among women and higher consumption among men. For instance, women with childcare obligations may have reduced opportunities to engage in drinking, remain intoxicated, or recover from alcohol use episodes [31]. In addition, societal norms have historically imposed greater stigma on alcohol use among women compared to men [32]. However, evolving gender norms over recent decades appear to be contributing to a convergence in alcohol use patterns between men and women. Factors implicated in this narrowing gender gap include increased educational attainment and labor force participation among women, as well as delayed marriage and childbearing [33].

In the SMGI population, reported experiences of discrimination were positively associated with higher scores on the alcohol use disorders identification test (AUDIT) and with a greater number of self-reported alcohol-related harms in this sample. The relationship between discrimination and alcohol consumption was mediated by coping-related drinking motives and drinking to alleviate dysphoria. Furthermore, the association between discrimination and alcohol-related harms was mediated not only by coping motives and drinking to manage dysphoria but also by drinking in the context of sexual activity.

This highlights the need for a more comprehensive understanding of strategies to reduce discrimination toward these communities. Moreover, addressing maladaptive coping motives for alcohol use and promoting healthier alternative coping mechanisms may be critical for reducing alcohol-related harms in these populations [34].

Another example is the use of cannabis in the nonbinary population, where it is used intentionally and strategically to support mental health, psychosocial well-being, identity development, and self-expression [35]. These insights point to the need for more inclusive and contextually informed approaches to care that account for the complex roles drugs may play in the lives of marginalized gender-diverse populations.

Minority stress theory posits that sexual minority individuals experience elevated levels of chronic stress due to discrimination and stigmatization based on their sexual orientation. This chronic stress has been linked to poor mental health outcomes, including psychological distress [36], as well as increased risk for problematic alcohol and drug use [37, 38].

24.4 Clinical Presentation, Subjective Drug Effects, and Comorbidities in SUD

Women entering substance use treatment programs often present with a more severe clinical profile than men, characterized by a greater burden of social, medical, psychological, and psychiatric comorbidities. Despite typically initiating substance use at a later age, using smaller quantities, and for shorter durations than men, women frequently experience a more rapid progression in the severity of use and associated functional decline— previously described "telescoping phenomenon."

Sex appears to be a significant modulating factor in the subjective experience of drug effects and the development of substance use and mental health disorders [39]. However, findings remain inconsistent across studies. Some research reports no significant sex-based differences in subjective drug effects, while others suggest heightened effects in men or, conversely, in women [11]. The majority of studies are based on sex and gender has scarcely studied.

Emerging evidence suggests that women may be more susceptible to craving and relapse—critical phases in the addiction cycle—and tend to exhibit more pronounced physiological withdrawal symptoms [40, 41], along with more intense substance-related effects [42] than men. Although substance use disorders are associated with elevated risk for psychiatric comorbidities in both sexes, the nature of these comorbidities differs: women more commonly present with co-occurring depression and anxiety disorders, whereas men exhibit higher rates of antisocial personality disorder [42–44].

Sex differences are also observed in the withdrawal symptomatology during detoxification, with women and men exhibiting distinct physiological and psychological profiles [45]. In the context of alcohol use, women reach higher blood alcohol concentrations and become intoxicated with lower quantities of alcohol than men, even when blood alcohol levels are comparable—reflecting lower tolerance and possible differences in alcohol metabolism [46]. These findings support the hypothesis that ovarian steroid hormones may influence the behavioral and neurochemical effects of substances [47]. Women also demonstrate a heightened withdrawal response during abstinence and are more likely to relapse in response to drug-related cues compared to men. These findings suggest potential sex-based differences in stress reactivity and vulnerability to relapse [48].

Regarding specific substances, women with cocaine use disorder progress more rapidly to dependence and report lower levels of both euphoria and dysphoria compared to men during use [49]. In the case of nicotine, while the likelihood of developing dependence is similar across sexes, women typically consume cigarettes with lower nicotine content, smoke fewer cigarettes per day, and inhale less deeply. Despite this, women report greater positive mood enhancement following nicotine consumption and experience more pronounced mood deterioration during abstinence, relative to men [50].

24.5 Psychiatric Comorbidity (Dual Diagnosis) in Women and Nonbinary Populations with SUD

Extensive evidence indicates that women with SUDs present with higher rates of comorbid psychiatric disorders compared to their male counterparts, as well as in comparison to women without SUDs [7, 51]. These co-occurring psychiatric conditions—most commonly mood and anxiety disorders—are closely associated with the onset, maintenance, and severity of substance use. The risk of psychiatric comorbidity is further elevated in women with a history of IPV [25].

The coexistence of SUD with psychiatric disorders such as depression or anxiety is linked to a more severe clinical trajectory for both conditions. This includes heightened symptom burden, increased frequency of suicide attempts, and greater likelihood of psychiatric hospitalizations [52, 53]. In women with SUD, depressive symptoms are of particular clinical relevance, as they are associated with increased cravings and higher relapse rates, particularly in the context of alcohol use disorders [54, 55]. Furthermore, the severity of depressive episodes has been inversely associated with treatment adherence and response, indicating that more severe depressive symptoms correlate with lower compliance and reduced therapeutic efficacy [56, 57].

As women with SUDs also exhibit high rates of trauma exposure, frequently in the form of IPV, sexual assault, and childhood abuse, this contributes to a disproportionately high prevalence of posttraumatic stress disorder (PTSD). This comorbidity further complicates the course and treatment of SUD. Tirado-Muñoz et al. (2018) reported that psychiatric comorbidities are highly prevalent among women who inject drugs, with particularly elevated rates of PTSD, depression, and anxiety. In that study, 70% of women who inject drugs and reported IPV victimization were nearly twice as likely to meet diagnostic criteria for PTSD compared to those without IPV exposure (odds ratio = 1.95, 95% CI: 1.10–3.48) [25]. These findings underscore the necessity for integrated, trauma-informed approaches to treatment that address both substance use and co-occurring psychiatric conditions in women, particularly those exposed to interpersonal violence.

Also, people of SMGI groups encounter a range of minority stressors, such as gender discrimination, limited access to gender-affirming care, social rejection, and violence, which contribute to disproportionately high rates of mental health challenges, including depression and suicide [58, 59].

24.6 Perceptions and Attitudes of the Practitioner and the Patient: Stigma

Women with SUDs often encounter significant challenges in accessing treatment due to a combination of systemic, structural, and individual-level barriers. These include institutional limitations, negative provider attitudes, and personal obstacles that collectively hinder engagement with treatment services [60]. Stigmatization associated with addiction constitutes a major impediment to care, as it amplifies both structural constraints and internalized stigma, further deterring individuals from seeking help [61].

Notably, women with SUDs are subject to more pronounced stigma compared to men. They are more frequently subjected to negative stereotypes, denigrating language, and report higher levels of perceived and internalized stigma in both societal and clinical contexts [62–64].

Also, MSGI experience stigma from health workers. Overall, trans individuals face a great deal of stigma, discrimination, and violence compared to cisgender individuals [65]. For instance, 54% of all trans individuals in the European Union have reported discriminatory experiences, with 15% experiencing violence within the last 12 months (anterior). Stigma and discrimination against trans individuals are also prevalent within the healthcare system. Physicians are known to have negative attitudes toward this community, with transphobia playing an important role in the provision of healthcare services. As a result, trans individuals tend to avoid healthcare services [66].

24.7 Incorporating the Gender Perspective in Treatment

24.7.1 Access to Treatment

Women face a range of psychosocial obstacles to seeking treatment. These include the societal expectations associated with motherhood, moral judgments related to maternal substance use, internalized guilt, stigma, pregnancy-related challenges, and lack of familial or community support [67]. These factors collectively contribute to the underutilization of treatment services by women and highlight the need for gender-responsive and trauma-informed approaches to care.

Epidemiological data consistently indicate that women are less likely than men to initiate treatment for substance use problems [68]. A multitude of gender-specific factors contribute to this disparity. Childcare responsibilities are a significant barrier; women often require accessible and affordable childcare services and express greater concern over child-related issues than men. Pregnancy-related concerns also inhibit access, including the scarcity of specialized services for pregnant women, fear of legal consequences or loss of child custody, and apprehension about potential stigmatization by healthcare providers. Additional barriers include lack of support or active resistance from family members, intimate involvement with substance-using partners, heightened vulnerability to physical and sexual violence, inadequate health insurance coverage, limited social support networks, and socioeconomic challenges such as poverty and lack of transportation to treatment facilities. Psychiatric comorbidities further complicate treatment engagement and outcomes. Furthermore, the scarcity of gender-responsive and trauma-informed treatment protocols represents a critical gap in care, contributing to the underutilization of services by women with SUDs.

Traditional gender roles have also been identified as significant impediments to treatment access for women with SUD. Commonly reported barriers include childcare responsibilities, pregnancy-related concerns (e.g., limited availability of specialized services for pregnant individuals, fear of legal consequences, and apprehension about potential loss of child custody following childbirth), opposition or lack of support from family members or intimate partners, and insufficient social support networks [69]. Empirical data indicate that women are 47% less likely than men to utilize any form of alcohol-related treatment services [70]. Moreover, when women with AUD do seek help, they are more likely to do so through primary healthcare providers rather than through specialized AUD treatment facilities [70].

In addition, for SGMI people, some programs, such as alcoholics anonymous (AA), offer LGBTQ-specific meetings designed to create a supportive environment for SGMI who may prefer to engage with others who share similar identities and lived experiences [71]. Empirical evidence indicates that participation in 12-Step programs can yield meaningful benefits for SGMI, including the development of social and community support networks, increased feelings of belonging, and the acquisition of skills conducive to sustained sobriety. Nonetheless, barriers to participation have also been reported. For example, some SGMI participants have articulated discomfort with the religious or spiritual components of 12-Step programming, which may conflict with their personal identities or beliefs. Additionally, instances of discrimination or marginalization based on sexual orientation or gender identity within these groups have been reported, further impeding engagement for some SGMI individuals [72].

These findings highlight the necessity for comprehensive, gender-sensitive treatment models that address the unique sociocultural, psychological, and medical needs of women with substance use disorders. Treatment programs that integrate childcare services, prenatal care, mental health support for comorbid psychiatric conditions, and ancillary social services have been shown to effectively mitigate many of the barriers faced by women in accessing AUD treatment [73].

24.7.2 Treatment Response

Despite these challenges, women who engage in specialized treatment programs often achieve superior outcomes compared to men [74] and demonstrate greater willingness to receive information and engage with the treatment process [74]. This has been particularly demonstrated in the context of alcohol use disorders (AUDs) [75]. While the overall time to relapse does not significantly differ between sexes, women tend to experience a longer latency before resuming heavy drinking compared to men. The underlying motivations for relapse also differ by gender: women are more likely to relapse in response to negative affective states, whereas men more commonly relapse due to social or peer-related influences [7]. On the other hand, regarding pharmacological treatment for AUDs, no consistent sex-based differences have been observed in the efficacy of naltrexone or acamprosate. Similarly, in the context of prescription opioid use disorder, studies have not reported significant differences in treatment response between men and women [10].

In contrast, treatment outcomes for nicotine dependence show a less favorable response in women compared to men [76]. However, the partial nicotinic receptor agonist varenicline appears to offer greater therapeutic benefits in women in some studies, suggesting potential sex-specific pharmacodynamic effects [77, 78].

With respect to psychosocial interventions, such as cognitive-behavioral therapy (CBT) and contingency management, outcomes are generally comparable between men and women [79–81]. Likewise, treatment retention rates do not significantly differ by gender [82].

Addressing the unique clinical needs of women with AUD has led to the development of gender-responsive interventions. Research focused on AUD in women has informed the creation of female-specific and women-only treatment programs. One such intervention, female-specific cognitive behavioral therapy (FS-CBT), has demonstrated efficacy in reducing alcohol use, alleviating internalizing symptoms (e.g., anxiety and depression), and improving interpersonal functioning in women with AUD [83]. These programs are designed with content, language, and examples that are specifically tailored to women's experiences. They also include targeted modules that emphasize social support, interpersonal relationships, self-efficacy, coping mechanisms for managing negative affect and mood disturbances, and psychoeducation on the intersection of alcohol use and women's health [84]. These findings highlight the importance of incorporating sex- and gender-sensitive considerations in both pharmacological and psychological interventions for SUDs, while also emphasizing the need for further research into individualized and evidence-based treatment strategies.

Similarly, for women, SGMI individuals would have good outcomes if engaged in treatment. For instance, a subanalysis in the PRIDE Study, a large-scale, national, longitudinal investigation of health outcomes among sexual and gender minority individuals (SGMI). Participants completed supplemental measures assessing alcohol and other substance use disorders, as well as involvement in 12-Step programs. Higher levels of 12-Step participation were significantly associated with fewer past-year AUD and SUD symptoms. Among those with AUD, gay and queer individuals were more likely to report lifetime participation in 12-Step programs compared to other groups [85].

24.8 Conclusions

The most pertinent data indicate an increasing prevalence of substance use among females, with the gender gap potentially narrowing. The motivations for initiating and continuing substance use differ between men and women. Women typically exhibit a more rapid progression from substance use to addiction. The consequences of substance use are more severe for women, including pregnancy-related complications and exacerbated medical issues. Additionally, psychiatric comorbidities, such as depression and PTSD, are more prevalent among women than men. These comorbidities further elevate the risk of HCV and HIV infections in women who use drugs. The treatment response also varies between genders, with women experiencing heightened cravings and a greater propensity for relapse. Socially, women encounter greater stigma, and a higher prevalence of intimate partner violence has been consistently reported among women with SUD, contributing to an increased risk for psychiatric comorbidity. However, research specifically focusing on women who use drugs remains scarce, and treatments are not typically tailored to gender-specific needs.

Consequently, women are at an elevated risk for a range of medical, psychiatric, and psychosocial complications, which must be considered when developing pharmacological and/or behavioral interventions. These interventions may differ significantly from those most effective for men. Therefore, ensuring access to appropriate treatment for women with substance use disorders and incorporating a gender-sensitive perspective in both treatment and research is imperative.

References

1. UNODC. World drug report 2024. United Nations publication; 2024.
2. Batchelder AW, Stanton AM, Kirakosian N, King D, Grasso C, Potter J, Mayer KH, O'Cleirigh C. Mental health and substance use diagnoses and treatment disparities by sexual orientation and gender in a community health center sample. LGBT Health. 2021;8(4):290–9. https://doi.org/10.1089/lgbt.2020.0293. PMID: 34080895; PMCID: PMC8213009
3. Schuler MS, Rice CE, Evans-Polce RJ, Collins RL. Disparities in substance use behaviors and disorders among adult sexual minorities by age, gender, and sexual identity. Drug Alcohol Depend. 2018;189:139–46. https://doi.org/10.1016/j.drugalcdep.2018.05.008. Epub 2018 Jun 19. PMID: 29944989; PMCID: PMC6083846
4. Regier DA, Farmer ME, Rae DS, Locke BZ, Keith SJ, Judd LL, Goodwin FK. Comorbidity of mental disorders with alcohol and other drug abuse. Results from the epidemiologic catchment area (ECA) study. JAMA. 1990;264(19):2511–8.
5. Compton WM, Thomas YF, Stinson FS, Grant BF. Prevalence, correlates, disability, and comorbidity of DSM-IV drug abuse and dependence in the United States: results from the national epidemiologic survey on alcohol and related conditions. Arch Gen Psychiatry. 2007;64(5):566–76. https://doi.org/10.1001/archpsyc.64.5.566.
6. Rehm J, Shield KD. Global burden of disease and the impact of mental and addictive disorders. Curr Psychiatry Rep. 2019;21(2):10. https://doi.org/10.1007/s11920-019-0997-0.
7. Erol A, Karpyak VM. Sex and gender-related differences in alcohol use and its consequences: contemporary knowledge and future research considerations. Drug Alcohol Depend. 2015;156:1–13. https://doi.org/10.1016/j.drugalcdep.2015.08.023.
8. Ait-Daoud N, Blevins D, Khanna S, Sharma S, Holstege CP. Women and addiction. Psychiatr Clin North Am. 2017;40:285–97. https://doi.org/10.1016/j.psc.2017.01.005.
9. Marsh JC, Park K, Lin YA, Bersamira C. Gender differences in trends for heroin use and nonmedical prescription opioid use, 2007–2014. J Subst Abus Treat. 2018;87:79–85.
10. McHugh RK, Devito EE, Dodd D, Carroll KM, Potter JS, Greenfield SF, Weiss RD. Gender differences in a clinical trial for prescription opioid dependence. J Subst Abus Treat. 2013;45(1):38–43. https://doi.org/10.1016/j.jsat.2012.12.007.
11. McHugh RK, Votaw VR, Sugarman DE, Greenfield SF. Sex and gender differences in substance use disorders. Psychol Rev. 2018;66:12–23. https://doi.org/10.1016/j.cpr.2017.10.012.

12. Brady KT, Randall CL. Gender differences in substance use disorders. Psychiatr Clin North Am. 1999;22:241–52. https://doi.org/10.1016/S0193-953X(05)70074-5.
13. Greenfield SF, Back SE, Lawson K, Brady KT. Substance abuse in women. Psychiatr Clin North Am. 2010a;33:339–55. https://doi.org/10.1016/j.psc.2010.01.004.
14. Keyes KM, Martins SS, Blanco C, Hasin DS. Telescoping and gender differences in alcohol dependence: new evidence from two national surveys. Am J Psychiatry. 2010;167(8):969–76. https://doi.org/10.1176/appi.ajp.2009.09081161.
15. Johnson PB, Richter L, Kleber HD, McLellan AT, Carise D. Telescoping of drinking-related behaviors: gender, racial/ethnic, and age comparisons. Subst Use Misuse. 2005;40(8):1139–51. https://doi.org/10.1081/ja-200042281.
16. Kirsch DE, Belnap MA, Kady A, Ray LA. A narrative review on alcohol use in women: insight into the telescoping hypothesis from a biopsychosocial perspective. Am J Drug Alcohol Abuse. 2025;51(1):14–30. https://doi.org/10.1080/00952990.2024.2419540. Epub 2025 Jan 27
17. Boyd CJ, Veliz PT, Stephenson R, Hughes TL, McCabe SE. Severity of alcohol, tobacco, and drug use disorders among sexual minority individuals and their "not sure"l counterparts. LGBT Health. 2019;6(1):15–22. https://doi.org/10.1089/lgbt.2018.0122. Epub 2019 Jan 14. PMID: 30638419; PMCID: PMC6352513
18. Evans-Polce RJ, Kcomt L, Veliz PT, Boyd CJ, McCabe SE. Alcohol, tobacco, and comorbid psychiatric disorders and associations with sexual identity and stress-related correlates. Am J Psychiatry. 2020;177(11):1073–81. https://doi.org/10.1176/appi.ajp.2020.20010005. Epub 2020 Sep 11. PMID: 32911997; PMCID: PMC7606786
19. Hughto JMW, Restar AJ, Wolfe HL, Gordon LK, Reisner SL, Biello KB, Cahill SR, Mimiaga MJ. Opioid pain medication misuse, concomitant substance misuse, and the unmet behavioral health treatment needs of transgender and gender diverse adults. Drug Alcohol Depend. 2021;222:108674. https://doi.org/10.1016/j.drugalcdep.2021.108674. Epub 2021 Mar 18. PMID: 33773869; PMCID: PMC8058310
20. Frost MC, Blosnich JR, Lehavot K, Chen JA, Rubinsky AD, Glass JE, Williams EC. Disparities in documented drug use disorders between transgender and cisgender U.S. Veterans Health Administration Patients. J Addict Med. 2021;15(4):334–40. https://doi.org/10.1097/ADM.0000000000000769. PMID: 33252409; PMCID: PMC8384140
21. Kuntsche E, Muller S. Why do young people start drinking? Motives for first-time alcohol consumption and links to risky drinking in early adolescence. Eur Addict Res. 2012;18:34–9.
22. Haas AL, Peters RH. Development of substance abuse problems among drug involved offenders. Evid Telesc Eff J Subst Abus. 2000;12:241–53.
23. Wilson HW, Widom CS. A prospective examination of the path from child abuse and neglect to illicit drug use in middle adulthood: the potential mediating role of four risk factors. J Youth Adolesc. 2009;38:340–54.
24. Meyer IH, Bayer R. School-based gay-affirmative interventions: first amendment and ethical concerns. Am J Public Health. 2013;103(10):1764–71. https://doi.org/10.2105/AJPH.2013.301385. Epub 2013 Aug 15. PMID: 23948002; PMCID: PMC3780740
25. Tirado-Muñoz J, Gilchrist G, Fischer G, Taylor A, Moskalewicz J, Giammarchi C, Köchl B, Munro A, Dąbrowska K, Shaw A, Di Furia L, Leeb I, Hopf C, Torrens M. Psychiatric comorbidity and intimate partner violence among women who inject drugs in Europe: a cross-sectional study. Arch Womens Ment Health. 2018;21(3):259–69. https://doi.org/10.1007/s00737-017-0800-3.
26. Rodríguez MN, Colgan DD, Leyde S, Pike K, Merrill JO, Price CJ. Trauma exposure across the lifespan among individuals engaged in treatment with medication for opioid use disorder: differences by gender, PTSD status, and chronic pain. Subst Abuse Treat Prev Policy. 2024;19(1):25. https://doi.org/10.1186/s13011-024-00608-8. PMID: 38702783; PMCID: PMC11067259
27. WHO. https://apps.who.int/adolescent/second-decade/section/section_4/level4_4.php
28. Devries KM, Child JC, Bacchus LJ, et al. Intimate partner violence victimization and alcohol consumption in women: a systematic review and meta-analysis. Addiction. 2014;109:379–91.

29. Moore TM, Stuart GL, Meehan JC, Rhatigan DL, Hellmuth JC, Keen SM. Drug abuse and aggression between intimate partners: a meta-analytic review. Clin Psychol Rev. 2008;28:247–74.
30. Kendler KS, Larsson Lönn S, Salvatore JE, Sundquist J, Sundquist K. The impact of parenthood on risk of registration for alcohol use disorder in married individuals: a Swedish population-based analysis. Psychol Med. 2019;49:2141–8. https://doi.org/10.1017/S0033291718002969.
31. O'Malley PM. Maturing out of problematic alcohol use. Alcohol Res Health. 2004;28:202–4.
32. de Visser RO, McDonnell EJ. That's OK. He's a guy': a mixed-methods study of gender double-standards for alcohol use. Psychol Health. 2012;27:618–39. https://doi.org/10.1080/08870446.2011.617444.
33. Kuntsche S, Knibbe RA, Kuntsche E, Gmel G. Housewife or working mum-each to her own? The relevance of societal factors in the association between social roles and alcohol use among mothers in 16 industrialized countries. Addiction. 2011;106:1925–32. https://doi.org/10.1111/j.1360-0443.2011.03507.x.
34. Davies EL, Ezquerra-Romano I, Thayne B, Holloway Z, Bayliss J, O'Callaghan S, Connolly DJ. Discrimination, gender dysphoria, drinking to cope, and alcohol harms in the UK trans and non-binary community. Alcohol Alcohol. 2024;59(1):agad060. https://doi.org/10.1093/alcalc/agad060.
35. Barborini C, Goodyear T, Kia H, Gilbert M, Ferlatte O, Knight R. "To smoke feels gender": exploring the transformative and emancipatory capacities of cannabis among transgender, non-binary and gender non-conforming (TGNC) youth. Int J Drug Policy. 2024;131:104536. https://doi.org/10.1016/j.drugpo.2024.104536. Epub 2024 Aug 13
36. Livingston NA, Christianson N, Cochran BN. Minority stress, psychological distress, and alcohol misuse among sexual minority young adults: a resiliency-based conditional process analysis. Addict Behav. 2016;63:125–31. https://doi.org/10.1016/j.addbeh.2016.07.011. Epub 2016 Jul 21
37. Hughes T. Alcohol-related problems among sexual minority women. Alcohol Treat Q. 2011;29(4):403–35. https://doi.org/10.1080/07347324.2011.608336. Epub 2011 Oct 12. PMID: 22470226; PMCID: PMC3315841
38. Lehavot K, Simoni JM. Victimization, smoking, and chronic physical health problems among sexual minority women. Ann Behav Med. 2011;42(2):269–76. https://doi.org/10.1007/s12160-011-9289-6. PMID: 21735343; PMCID: PMC4083397
39. Zagni E, Simoni L, Colombo D. Sex and gender differences in central nervous system-related disorders. Neurosci J. 2016;2016:2827090. https://doi.org/10.1155/2016/2827090.
40. Becker JB, Koob GF. Sex differences in animal models: focus on addiction. Pharmacol Rev. 2016;68:242–63. https://doi.org/10.1124/pr.115.011163.
41. Copersino ML, Boyd SJ, Tashkin DP, Huestis MA, Heishman SJ, Dermand JC, Simmons MS, Gorelick DA. Sociodemographic characteristics of cannabis smokers and the experience of cannabis withdrawal. Am J Drug Alcohol Abuse. 2020;36:311–9. https://doi.org/10.3109/00952990.2010.503825.
42. Cooper ZD, Haney M. Investigation of sex-dependent effects of cannabis in daily cannabis smokers. Drug Alcohol Depend. 2014;136:85–91. https://doi.org/10.1016/j.drugalcdep.2013.12.013.
43. Colon-Perez LM, Pino JA, Saha K, Pompilus M, Kaplitz S, Choudhury N, Jagnarine DA, Geste JR, Levin BA, Wilks I, et al. Functional connectivity, behavioral and dopaminergic alterations 24 hours following acute exposure to synthetic bath salt drug methylenedioxypyrovalerone. Neuropharmacol. 2018;137:178–93. https://doi.org/10.1016/j.neuropharm.2018.04.031.
44. NIDA. Drug facts: substance use in women | National Institute on Drug Abuse (NIDA). DrugFacts; 2020.
45. Sanvisens A, Zuluaga P, Short A, Rubio G, Gual A, Torrens M, Fuster D, Bolao F, Rodríguez de Fonseca F, Muga R, CohRTA study*. Sex-specific associations of alcohol withdrawal in patients admitted for the treatment of alcohol use disorder. J Addict Med. 2020:4. https://doi.org/10.1097/ADM.0000000000000704.

46. Calafat A, Fernández-Hermida JR, Becoña E, Juan M, Duch M, Fernández del Rio E, et al. Blood alcohol level tests in nightlife recreational settings as a preventive tool. Actas Esp Psiquiatr. 2013;41:10–6.
47. Newman JL, Mello NK. Neuroactive gonadal steroid hormones and drug addiction in women. In: Brady KT, Back SE, Greenfield SF, editors. Women and addiction: a comprehensive handbook. New York: Guilford Press; 2009. p. 35–64.
48. Back SE, Waldrop AE, Saladin ME, Yeatts SD, Simpson A, McRae AL, Upadhyaya HP, Contini Sisson R, Spratt EG, Allen J, Kreek MJ, Brady KT. Effects of gender and cigarette smoking on reactivity to psychological and pharmacological stress provocation. Psychoneuroendocrinology. 2008;3(5):560–8.
49. Becker JB, Hu M. Sex differences in drug abuse. Front Neuroendocrinol. 2008;29:36–47.
50. Shiffman S, Paton SM. Individual differences in smoking: gender and nicotine addiction. Nicotine Tob Res. 1999;1(2):S153–S157; discussion S165-6. https://doi.org/10.1080/14622299050011991 2008;33(5):560-8, https://doi.org/10.1016/j.psyneuen.2008.01.012.
51. Taghizadeh N, Vonk JM, Boezen HM. Lifetime smoking history and cause-specific mortality in a cohort study with 43 years of follow-up. PLoS One. 2016;11(4):e0153310. https://doi.org/10.1371/journal.pone.0153310. eCollection 2016.
52. Haro JM, Palacín C, Vilagut G, Martínez M, Bernal M, Luque I, Codony M, Dolz M, Alonso J, Grupo ESEMeD-España. Prevalence of mental disorders and associated factors: results from the ESEMeD-Spain study. Med Clin (Barc). 2006;126(12):445–51. https://doi.org/10.1157/13086324.
53. Torrens M, Gilchrist G, Domingo-Salvany A, psyCoBarcelona Group. Psychiatric comorbidity in illicit drug users: substance-induced versus independent disorders. Drug Alcohol Depend. 2011;113(2–3):147–56. https://doi.org/10.1016/j.drugalcdep.2010.07.013.
54. Abulseoud OA, Karpyak VM, Schneekloth T, Hall-Flavin DK, Loukianova LL, Geske JR, et al. A retrospective study of gender differences in depressive symptoms and risk of relapse in patients with alcohol dependence. Am J Addict. 2013;22:437–42. https://doi.org/10.1111/j.1521-0391.2013.12021.x.
55. Zilberman ML, Tavares H, Hodgins DC, el-Guebaly N. The impact of gender, depression, and personality on craving. J Addict Dis. 2007;26:79–84. https://doi.org/10.1300/J069v26n01_10.
56. Gjestad R, Franck J, Hagtvet KA, Haver B. Level and change in alcohol consumption, depression and dysfunctional attitudes among females treated for alcohol addiction. Alcohol. 2011;46:292–300. https://doi.org/10.1093/alcalc/agr018.
57. Merrill JE, Reid AE, Carey MP, Carey KB. Gender and depression moderate response to brief motivational intervention for alcohol misuse among college students. J Consult Clin Psychol. 2014;82:984–92. https://doi.org/10.1037/a0037039.
58. Pattison R, Puyat JH, Giesbrecht A, Zenone M, Mathias S, Barbic S. Examining mental health differences between transgender, gender nonconforming, and cisgender young people in British Columbia. Front Psychol. 2021;12:720681. https://doi.org/10.3389/fpsyt.2021.720681. PMID: 34658957; PMCID: PMC8511444
59. Veale JF, Watson RJ, Peter T, Saewyc EM. Mental health disparities among Canadian transgender youth. J Adolesc Health. 2017;60(1):44–9. https://doi.org/10.1016/j.jadohealth.2016.09.014. PMID: 28007056; PMCID: PMC5630273
60. Gilchrist G, Fonseca F, Torrens M. Access to treatment for people with alcohol and other substance abuse problems. Adicciones. 2011a;23(4):343–8.
61. Volkow ND. It's time for addiction science to supersede stigma. 2008. https://www.sciencenews.org/article/it%E2%80%99s-time-addiction-science-supersede-stigma Published October 24, 2008.
62. Spooner C, Saktiawati MA, Lazuardi E, Worth H, Subronto W, Padmawati RS. Impacts of stigma on HIV risk for women who inject drugs in Java: a qualitative study. Int J Drug Policy. 2015;26:1244–50.
63. Terplan M, Kennedy-Hendricks A, Chislom MS. Prenatal substance use: exploring assumptions of maternal unfitness. Subst Abuse Res Treat. 2015;9:1–4.

64. Verissimo ADO, Grella CE. Influence of gender and race/ethnicity on perceived barriers to help seeking for alcohol or drug problems. J Subst Abus Treat. 2017;75:54–61. https://doi.org/10.1016/j.jsat.2016.12.013.
65. European Union Agency for Fundamental Rights. Being trans in the European Union—comparative analysis of EU LGBT survey data. 2014 [cited 2022 09.08.2022]; Available from: https://fra.europa.eu/sites/default/files/fra-2014-being-trans-eu-comparative-0_en.pdf.
66. von der Warth R, Metzner G, Körner M, Farin-Glattacker E. Exploring communication preferences of trans and gender diverse individuals-a qualitative study. PLoS One. 2023;18(8):e0284959. https://doi.org/10.1371/journal.pone.0284959. PMID: 37611052; PMCID: PMC10446207
67. Gilchrist G, Blázquez A, Torrens M. Exploring the relationship between intimate partner violence, childhood abuse and psychiatric disorders among female drug users in Barcelona. Adv Dual Diagn. 2012;5(2):46–58. https://doi.org/10.1108/17570971211241895.
68. Greenfield SF, Brooks AJ, Gordon SM, Green CA, Kropp F, McHugh RK, Miele GM. Substance abuse treatment entry, retention, and outcome in women: a review of the literature. Drug Alcohol Depend. 2007;86(1):1–21. https://doi.org/10.1016/j.drugalcdep.2006.05.012.
69. Frazer Z, McConnell K, Jansson LM. Treatment for substance use disorders in pregnant women: motivators and barriers drug alcohol depend. Drug Alcohol Depend. 2019;205:107652. https://doi.org/10.1016/j.drugalcdep.2019.107652.
70. Gilbert PA, Pro G, Zemore SE, Mulia N, Brown G. Gender differences in use of alcohol treatment services and reasons for nonuse in a national sample. Alcohol Clin Exp Res. 2019;43:722–31. https://doi.org/10.1111/acer.13965.
71. Alcoholics Anonymous World Services, Inc., 2018.
72. McGeough BL, Paceley M, Zemore SE, Lunn MR, Obedin-Maliver J, Lubensky ME, Flentje A. Understanding the social and community support experiences of sexual and gender minority individuals in 12-Step programs. J Gay Lesbian Soc Serv. 2023;35(4):398–419. https://doi.org/10.1080/10538720.2023.2172759. Epub 2023 Jan 25. PMID: 38152636; PMCID: PMC10752627
73. McCrady BS, Epstein EE, Fokas KF. Treatment interventions for women with alcohol use disorder. Alcohol Res. 2020;40:08. https://doi.org/10.35946/arcr.v40.2.08.25.
74. Bravo F, Gual A, Lligoña A, Colom J. Gender differences in the long-term outcome of alcohol dependence treatments: an analysis of twenty-year prospective follow up. Drug Alcohol Rev. 2013;32:381–8. https://doi.org/10.1111/dar.12023.
75. Greenfield SF, Pettinati HM, O'Malley S, Randall PK, Randall CL. Gender differences in alcohol treatment: an analysis of outcome from the COMBINE study. Alcohol Clin Exp Res. 2010b;34(10):1803–12. https://doi.org/10.1111/j.1530-0277.2010.01267.x.
76. Smith PH, Kasza KA, Hyland A, Fong GT, Borland R, Brady K, McKee SA. Gender differences in medication use and cigarette smoking cessation: results from the International Tobacco Control Four Country Survey. Nicotine Tob Res. 2015;17(4):463–72. https://doi.org/10.1093/ntr/ntu212.
77. McKee SA, Smith PH, Kaufman M, Mazure CM, Weinberger AH. Sex differences in Varenicline efficacy for smoking cessation: a meta-analysis. Nicotine Tob Res. 2016;18(5):1002–11. https://doi.org/10.1093/ntr/ntv207.
78. Smith PH, Weinberger AH, Zhang J, Emme E, Mazure CM, McKee SA. Sex differences in smoking cessation pharmacotherapy comparative efficacy: a network meta-analysis. Nicotine Tob Res. 2017;19(3):273–81. https://doi.org/10.1093/ntr/ntw144.
79. Burch AE, Rash CJ, Petry NM. Sex effects in cocaine-using methadone patients randomized to contingency management interventions. Exp Clin Psychopharmacol. 2015;23(4):284–90. https://doi.org/10.1037/pha0000034.
80. Campbell AN, Nunes EV, Pavlicova M, Hatch-Maillette M, Hu MC, Bailey GL, Greenfield SF. Gender-based outcomes and acceptability of a computer-assisted psychosocial intervention for substance use disorders. J Subst Abus Treat. 2015;53:9–15. https://doi.org/10.1016/j.jsat.2014.12.006.

81. DeVito EE, Babuscio TA, Nich C, Ball SA, Carroll KM. Gender differences in clinical outcomes for cocaine dependence: randomized clinical trials of behavioral therapy and disulfiram. Drug Alcohol Depend. 2014;145:156–67. https://doi.org/10.1016/j.drugalcdep.2014.10.007.
82. Korte JE, Rosa CL, Wakim PG, Perl HI. Addiction treatment trials: how gender, race/ethnicity, and age relate to ongoing participation and retention in clinical trials. Subst Abus Rehabil. 2011;2:205–18. https://doi.org/10.2147/sar.s23796.
83. Epstein EE, McCrady BS, Hallgren KA, Gaba A, Cook S, Jensen N, Hildebrandt T, Holzhauer CG, Litt MD. Individual versus group female-specific cognitive behavior therapy for alcohol use disorder. J Subst Abus Treat. 2018;88:27–43. https://doi.org/10.1016/j.jsat.2018.02.003.
84. Epstein EE, McCrady BS, Hallgren KA, Cook S, Jensen NK, Hildebrandt T. A randomized trial of female-specific cognitive behavior therapy for alcohol dependent women. Phychol Addict Behav. 2018;32:1–15. https://doi.org/10.1037/adb0000330.
85. McGeough BL, Zemore SE, Dastur Z, Neilands TB, Lisha NE, Lunn MR, Obedin-Maliver J, Lubensky ME, Flentje A. Levels and outcomes of 12-step participation among sexual and gender minority subgroups. J Subst Use Addict Treat. 2024;167:209519. https://doi.org/10.1016/j.josat.2024.209519. Epub 2024 Sep 10. PMID: 39260805; PMCID: PMC11583376

25 Psychosomatic and Dysmorphophobia

García-Albea Julia, Navas Marta, Mayor Federico, and Fernández Marina

25.1 Introduction

Somatoform disorders, now classified under somatic symptom disorders (SSD) in the DSM V, are characterized by persistent physical symptoms without an identifiable medical cause, accompanied by excessive concern that leads to frequent medical consultations. In this edition, the DSM-5 categorizes several subtypes within this group, including somatic symptom disorder, illness anxiety disorder, conversion disorder, and factitious disorder. These disorders are often among the primary reasons for primary care visits, highlighting the limitations of the dualistic mind–body model, which fails to adequately address the interaction between physical symptoms and underlying psychological factors [1].

In this context, the diagnosis of these disorders is influenced by complex variables, including gender differences, which impact both the prevalence and clinical presentation of symptoms. One of the most significant findings is the higher prevalence of SSD in women, suggesting a gender bias in diagnosis [2]. Women not only exhibit somatic symptoms more frequently but also demonstrate greater sensitivity to pain, which is modulated by hormonal factors affecting pain perception [3]. However, scientific literature has historically focused more on men, limiting a proper understanding of gender differences in somatization and pain perception [4].

At the sociocultural level, women, subjected to pressures from caregiving roles and multiple family and work responsibilities, are more likely to somatize, while men, socialized to avoid vulnerability, tend to downplay their symptoms, which

G.-A. Julia (✉) · N. Marta · M. Federico
Hospital Clínico San Carlos, Madrid, Spain

F. Marina
Hospital Universitario Infanta Leonor, Madrid, Spain

M. López-Atanes, M. Sáenz-Herrero (eds.), *Applying the Gender Perspective in Psychiatry and Psychotherapy*, https://doi.org/10.1007/978-3-032-17883-1_25

complicates diagnosis [5]. This chapter explores how these gender dynamics affect the prevalence, diagnosis, and treatment of somatoform disorders, emphasizing the need for more sensitive and balanced clinical approaches.

25.2 Somatization and Gender

Somatic symptom disorders, formerly known as somatoform disorders, are significantly more prevalent in women, with rates up to ten times higher than in men, except for illness anxiety disorder and body dysmorphic disorder, previously included under SSD [3].

Somatization, understood as the manifestation of psychological distress through physical symptoms, is notably prevalent among women and is influenced by both biological factors and sociocultural constructs related to gender [6]. The tendency of SSD to be diagnosed more frequently in women than in men may be linked to gender stereotypes that affect symptom expression and the diagnostic and therapeutic approaches in medical contexts [7]. In many cases, this tendency to somatize in women reflects the complexity of human psychology alongside socially imposed roles and expectations, which may predispose women to express emotional distress through physical symptoms [7].

The distinction between sex (biological) and gender (social construct) is fundamental to understanding these patterns, as women's socialization often directs them to prioritize others' care over their physical and emotional well-being, contributing to a greater predisposition to somatic symptoms [2]. This perspective explains why women not only experience but also seek treatment for physical symptoms more than men, underscoring the need for psychiatric approaches to consider the complex interactions between gender and somatization to avoid diagnostic biases and provide more precise and equitable care [7].

Gender differences in somatic symptom disorders have been widely studied, with one of the most researched theories pointing to biological variations, particularly those related to female sex hormones such as estrogen and progesterone [6]. Women experience significant hormonal fluctuations throughout their lives due to menstruation, pregnancy, and menopause, which can influence pain perception and increase vulnerability to developing SSD [2]. Studies on pain sensitivity suggest that these hormones may play a key role in how women experience and communicate physical symptoms, contributing to a higher prevalence of these disorders than men [7].

Additionally, certain chronic medical syndromes, such as fibromyalgia and irritable bowel syndrome, predominantly affect women and are associated with SSD. These conditions are characterized by symptoms like widespread pain and digestive disturbances, often without a clear medical explanation, but causing considerable suffering [2]. While they have biological components, these conditions are also shaped by social and cultural factors. Their impact is often underestimated or misunderstood due to stereotypes about women's health, which can once again affect the perception and treatment of these disorders in the medical field [7].

Although diagnostic criteria in the DSM-III and DSM-IV aimed to be gender-neutral, they included symptoms specific to women, such as menstrual irregularities or pregnancy-related symptoms, and male-specific symptoms, such as sexual dysfunctions [8]. This led to criticism because, despite these inclusions, the criteria were insufficient to ensure true gender neutrality. In response, the DSM-5 shifted focus away from sex-specific symptoms to emphasize the psychological components of somatic symptoms, such as thoughts, feelings, and behaviors related to physical sensations [1].

However, recent studies suggest that even with these changes, factors influencing somatization remain gender-specific. Women, for instance, often present somatic symptoms with greater frequency and intensity than men, which can be attributed to biological, social, and cultural factors [4, 5]. Research in this field indicates that the interaction of these elements not only affects prevalence but may also lead to biased diagnoses when criteria do not align with each gender's specific experiences. Cloninger et al., after analyzing the DSM-III, suggested that adjusting diagnostic thresholds could balance prevalence rates between genders but warned that this could mask a higher real frequency in women due to their greater predisposition to somatize symptoms [9].

25.3 Somatization and Related Disorders

When analyzing various somatization disorders, considering predisposing, precipitating, and perpetuating factors can help identify the origin of symptoms and guide treatment. Some of these factors include personality traits such as histrionism in women or antisocial traits in men, lifestyle or personal beliefs, and psychological variables such as anxiety, depression, neuroticism, or alexithymia [10–12]. Additionally, in women, specific factors related to their often subordinate social roles in many cultures, the balancing of work and family, as well as personal histories of violence or abuse, can play a role. However, multiple protective factors associated with gender have also been described, such as empowerment through autonomy, supportive environments, self-acceptance, or access to specific resources [12–14].

25.4 Somatic Symptom Disorder

Somatic symptom disorder is characterized by subjective somatic complaints affecting various bodily systems, for which no underlying medical cause has been identified. Recent updates to international diagnostic classifications broaden the scope to include not only medically unexplained symptoms but also physical symptoms explainable by a medical diagnosis and accompanied by disproportionate worry or distress [15].

From Briquet's initial 1850 descriptions of pain and sexual symptoms in young women [16], this disorder has been strongly associated with female sex and gender.

Comparative epidemiological studies confirm this gender disparity, with prevalence rates ranging from 0.2% to 3% in women compared to 0.2% in men [17]. Following the removal of diagnostic biases in current classifications, the gender prevalence gap has narrowed [18].

Recent studies in primary care settings indicate that women more frequently and promptly seek consultations for somatic symptoms, which are often nonspecific or prodromal. However, the frequency of follow-up diagnostic tests (such as comprehensive physical examinations, diagnostic testing, or specialist referrals) is lower than in men, and a component of somatization is more readily assumed in women's somatic complaints [19].

25.5 Pain Disorder

Pain disorder is diagnostically defined by chronic pain without an underlying medical explanation [20], in which psychological factors play a crucial role in its onset, intensity, or persistence [1].

Several factors are associated with chronic pain, such as advanced age, low socioeconomic status, the presence of physical comorbidities, and female sex. Studies on chronic pain syndromes, such as low back pain, fibromyalgia, migraines, or irritable bowel syndrome, indicate a significantly higher incidence in women than in men [21], as well as a generally longer duration of symptoms over time [22].

While numerous neurobiological or behavioral explanations for this divergence have been proposed, social or gender-specific factors are often overlooked. For example, aspects such as the gendered organization of family caregiving, experiences of violence and trauma, social marginalization, intergenerational poverty, or the minimization of women's health concerns modify and amplify the experience of pain. Thus, a complementary socio-health approach is needed, one that considers these factors not only in the appearance and persistence of pain but also as potential elements for its resolution [23].

25.6 Conversion Disorder or Functional Somatic Symptom Disorder

Conversion disorder, historically termed hysterical conversion neurosis and now conceptualized as a functional neurological symptom disorder, encompasses a heterogeneous set of clinical manifestations (including motor, sensory, seizure-like, or consciousness-altering symptoms) that mimic neurological conditions [15]. A characteristic "la belle indifférence" toward symptoms is often noted [17].

Traditionally, the emergence of these symptoms was viewed as a psychological defense against extreme psychosocial stressors, with the primary gain being the reduction of intrapsychic pain [24, 25]. Current understanding focuses on the interaction of psychological and cognitive factors (biased attention processing, alexithymia, dissociation, catastrophizing tendencies, or aberrant predictive processing), biological factors (general pain mechanisms, somatosensory amplification, sex hormones), and social factors (low socioeconomic status, rural environments) [26].

The diagnosis of this disorder is more frequent in women than in men, with proportions ranging from 2:1 to 10:1 [17]. Recent studies suggest no significant differences in the semiological expression of the disorder between genders, but risk factors differ, with women reporting much higher rates of physical or sexual abuse history (33–77% depending on the study) [27]. A higher prevalence of this disorder is also noted in transgender individuals and sexual minorities, potentially linked to adverse life experiences, chronic stress, or stigma in healthcare settings [27]. Another potential factor is diagnostic bias among healthcare professionals, with a greater tendency to assume somatization or factitious disorder in women than in men [28].

25.7 Illness Anxiety Disorder

Illness anxiety disorder, formerly hypochondria, is characterized by persistent worry about having a severe illness, based on a misinterpretation of bodily signs and symptoms [17]. Psychopathologically, three key elements are defined: conviction of illness, fear of illness, and close monitoring of symptoms [29]. These contribute to significant functional deterioration, reduced quality of life, and frequent healthcare utilization, which only temporarily alleviates symptoms [15].

Although higher levels of health-related anxiety have been reported in women than in men [30], no clear epidemiological difference exists in the occurrence of illness anxiety disorder between genders, with an estimated prevalence of 3–9% [17]. However, comorbid psychopathology rates in illness anxiety disorder are high, with anxiety, depressive, and personality disorders appearing in up to 80% of cases [31, 32].

Gender bias in medicine plays a key role in how illness anxiety disorder is diagnosed and treated in women, contributing to the delegitimization of their health concerns and unequal access to adequate care. In many medical contexts, women are more often diagnosed with emotional disorders, such as anxiety or depression, even when symptoms may be related to physical problems. This phenomenon is also evident in the treatment of illness anxiety disorder, where gender stereotypes can influence the perception of women's symptoms. Women are often assumed to be more emotional or prone to hypochondria, leading doctors to minimize or dismiss their symptoms without proper evaluation, negatively impacting their health and quality of life.

25.8 Body Dysmorphic Disorder

Body dysmorphic disorder (BDD) is defined as a distressing or impairing preoccupation with an imagined or slight feature of physical appearance that causes significant discomfort or is associated with severe interference in the life of the patient

[33].The nuclear phenomenology of this disorder is no longer included in the somatomorphic disorders chapter, due to the fact that most patients with BDD have BDD-related compulsive behaviors, which were not truly reflected in DSM-IV. The disorder has been relocated to the obsessive-compulsive disorder and related disorders section in the DSM-V [33].

Currently, concerns with beauty, physical appearance, and body image have become elements that generate large consumption in an industry that moves billions of euros a year. At present, beauty is a rising value, which is intimately related to social success, firstly burdening women, and nowadays involving men as well. Great importance is granted to beauty since body image is closely related to one's professional and personal satisfaction, having increased exponentially with the use of social networks, especially Instagram [34].

On many occasions, they undergo aggressive (surgical, cosmetic, dermatological, capillary, etc.) treatments repeatedly and with irrational demands that may worsen the disorder, causing the emergence of more intense concerns [35]. Instagram is known as a self-promotion showcase where users often upload photographs that emphasize their physical attractiveness. This behavior offers the opportunity for comparing one's appearance with models or peers who also share their idealized pictures of themselves [36]. Several studies have found a significant relationship between more social network activity (sharing, seeing, & commenting) and body image impairment [37]. Therefore, these pathological concerns may probably be activated about others paying special attention to the perceived defect, making comments, laughing at them, or simply not showing their approval with "likes," which could seriously reinforce DC symptomatology [36].

BDD is more common than OCD, with a current prevalence of nearly 2–3% of the general population [38]. The age of the patients varies between 15 and 40 years old, and there is an overrepresentation of single people and those without partners [39]. Dysmorphic concerns seem to be more frequent in women [40].

The most common symptoms refer to imaginary defects or defects of little importance on the face or head, such as hair thinning, acne, wrinkles, scars, vascular signs, paleness or redness of the skin, swelling, facial asymmetry or disproportion, and excess hair on the face [41].

According to a gender study, men were more likely than women to be excessively concerned with the appearance of their genitals. They were also more likely to obsess about their body build (90% of whom thought they were too small and/or inadequately muscular). However, women were more likely to obsess about the appearance of their skin, stomach, weight, breasts/chest, buttocks, thighs, legs, hips, and toes, and were more prone to focus on hips and weight, scratching their skin and showing safety behaviors such as hiding behind makeup [42–44]. These findings seem to bear out what some studies based on evolutionary theories have been suggesting for many years: facial appearance in women could be unconsciously related to fertility and youth, attributes extremely valued by men in choosing an adequate partner (able to continue the lineage).

Muscle dysmorphia in men appears to be a BDD specifier in the DSM-V, and is defined as a preoccupation with the inaccurate belief that their body builds is too small or insufficiently muscular [45]. Taking a glance at these evolutive theories, their theoretical strength seems to be linked to protectiveness and caring, qualities valued historically by women, and also enhancing men's feelings of self-esteem, control, and lustiness. (David Buss).

These findings do not seem to be a coincidence when we observe dysmorphic concerns linked to gender.

People with this disorder, who stubbornly adhere to an appreciation not shared by the majority of people, are afraid that others will realize the alleged physical defect, and showing feelings of guilt and shame, constantly worrying, feeling overvalued or delusional, avoiding social situations and showing their bodies, they have rituals, and they request repeated medical and cosmetic treatments [46]. Senín Calderon et al. [36] suggested that Instagram use is closely related to dysmorphic concerns through three main subjects: appearance-related comparisons, ideas of reference related to laughing and commenting, and adaptive emotion regulation difficulties, regardless of gender. A relationship between Instagram use and DC has been shown, according to the social comparison theory supported by Festinger in 1954, based on appearance-related comparisons [47].

The avoidance of their usual activities can lead to extreme social isolation. In some cases, individuals leave their homes only at night (when they cannot be seen) or remain in them for a long time, sometimes even years.

Dysmorphic body disorder may be associated with a major depressive disorder, a delusional disorder, social phobia, and an obsessive-compulsive disorder [48, 49].

A similarly high proportion of men and women have experienced lifetime suicidal ideation, have attempted suicide, and have experienced high levels of functional impairment and poor quality of life [42], regardless of gender. However, men are more likely to have a substance use disorder, and women are more likely to have an eating disorder.

Lastly, BDD should not be diagnosed if the diagnostic criteria for gender dysphoria are met, if appearance concerns focus only on secondary sex characteristics, genitals, or other aspects of appearance that reflect one's natal sex, or if other diagnostic criteria for gender dysphoria are met [50].

References

1. American Psychiatric Association. Diagnostic and statistical manual of mental disorders. 5th ed. Arlington: American Psychiatric Publishing; 2013.
2. Tyrer P, Reed G, Crawford M. Somatic symptom disorder: a review of the literature. Psychosomatics. 2015;56(5):465–72.
3. Kuehner C. Why is depression more common among women than among men? Lancet Psychiatry. 2017;4(2):146–58.
4. Barsky AJ, Borus JF. Somatization and medicalization in the era of managed care. JAMA. 1995;274(24):1931–4.
5. Piccinelli M, Wilkinson G. Gender differences in depression: critical review. Br J Psychiatry. 2000;177(6):486–92.
6. Roth T, Choy E, Keane TM, et al. The role of gender in the expression and treatment of pain. J Pain Symptom Manag. 2011;42(2):281–91.

7. Brennan F, Cousins M, Carr DB. Somatic symptom disorder and gender differences. J Pain Symptom Manag. 2013;45(4):765–77.
8. American Psychiatric Association. Diagnostic and statistical manual of mental disorders. 4th ed. Washington, DC: American Psychiatric Publishing; 2000.
9. Cloninger CR, Martin RL, Guze SB. Diagnosis and clinical implications of somatization. JAMA. 1985;253(11):1603–7.
10. Kellner R, Abbott P, Winslow WW, Pathak D. Anxiety, depression, and somatization in DSM-III hypochondriasis. Psychosomatics. 1989;30(1):57–64.
11. Claraco LM, Monreal A, García J. Manejo del paciente somatizador en atención primaria. Form Méd Cont. 1999;6(8):536–43.
12. Brambila-Tapia AJL, Saldaña-Cruz AM, Meléndez-Monreal KC, Esparza-Guerrero Y, Martínez-Hernández A, Rosales-Torres BG, et al. Association of personal, behavioral and positive psychological variables with somatization and number of diseases in Mexican general population: the influence of gender. Psychol Health Med [Internet]. 2023;28(4):995–1003.
13. Romito P. Work and health in mothers of young children. Int J Health Serv. 1994;24(4):607–28.
14. Hankin JR. Gender and Mental Illness. Resea Com Ment Health. 1990;6:183–201.
15. Boland R, Verduin ML. Trastorno de síntomas somáticos y trastornos relacionados. In: Ruiz P, editor. Kaplan & Sadock Sinopsis de Psiquiatria. 12th ed. Barcelona: Wolters Kluwer; 2022. p. 451–68.
16. Simon GE, Gureje O. Stability of somatization disorder and somatization symptoms among primary care patients. Arch Gen Psychiatry. 1999;56(1):90–5.
17. Yutzy SH, Parish BS. Trastornos somatomorfos. In: Hales RE, Yudofsky SC, Gabbard GO. Tratado de Psiquiatría Clínica. 5th ed. Barcelona: Elsevier España; 2009. p. 577–608.
18. Löwe B, Levenson J, Depping M, Hüsing P, Kohlmann S, Lehmann M, et al. Somatic symptom disorder: a scoping review on the empirical evidence of a new diagnosis. Psychol Med [Internet]. 2022;52(4):632–48.
19. Ballering AV, Muijres D, Uijen AA, Rosmalen JGM, olde Hartman TC. Sex differences in the trajectories to diagnosis of patients presenting with common somatic symptoms in primary care: an observational cohort study. J Psychosom Res [Internet]. 2021;149(110589):110589.
20. García P, Magarito M. Guía de la clasificación de bolsillo CIE-10: clasificación de los trastornos mentales y del comportamiento. Interne; 2000.
21. Li JXL, Wang X, Henry A, Anderson CS, Hammond N, Harris K, et al. Sex differences in pain expressed by patients across diverse disease states: individual patient data meta-analysis of 33,957 participants in 10 randomized controlled trials. Pain [Internet]. 2023;164(8):1666–76.
22. Mohan I, Lawson-Smith C, Coall DA, Van der Watt G, Janca A. Somatoform disorders in patients with chronic pain. Australas Psychiatry [Internet]. 2014;22(1):66–70.
23. Rice K, Connoy L, Webster F. Gendered worlds of pain: women, marginalization, and chronic pain. J Pain [Internet]. 2024;25(11):104626.
24. Vaillant GE. Theoretical hierarchy of adaptive ego mechanisms: a 30-yearfollow-up of 30 men selected for psychological health. Arch Gen Psychiatry. 1971;24:107–18.
25. Lazare A. Current concepts in psychiatry. Conversion symptoms. N Engl J Med. 1981;305:745–8.
26. Lerario MP, Fusunyan M, Stave CD, Roldán V, Keuroghlian AS, Turban J, et al. Functional neurological disorder and functional somatic syndromes among sexual and gender minority people: a scoping review. J Psychosom Res [Internet]. 2023;174(111491):111491.
27. Ertan D, Aybek S, LaFrance WC Jr, Kanemoto K, Tarrada A, Maillard L, et al. Functional (psychogenic non-epileptic/dissociative) seizures: why and how? J Neurol Neurosurg Psychiatry [Internet]. 2022;93(2):144–57.
28. Kanaan RA, Armstrong D, Wessely SC. Neurologists' understanding and management of conversion disorder. J Neurol Neurosurg Psychiatry [Internet]. 2011;82(9):961–6.
29. Scarella TM, Boland RJ, Barsky AJ. Illness anxiety disorder: psychopathology, epidemiology, clinical characteristics, and treatment. Psychosom Med [Internet]. 2019;81(5):398–407.
30. Lebel S, Mutsaers B, Tomei C, Leclair CS, Jones G, Petricone-Westwood D, et al. Health anxiety and illness-related fears across diverse chronic illnesses: a systematic review on

conceptualization, measurement, prevalence, course, and correlates. PLoS One [Internet]. 2020;15(7):e0234124.
31. Barsky AJ, Wyshak G, Klerman GL. Psychiatric comorbidity in DSM-III R hypochondriasis. Arch Gen Psychiatry. 1992;49:101–8.
32. Tyrer P, Fowler-Dixon R, Ferguson B, Kelemen A. A plea for the diagnosis of hypochondriacal personality disorder. J Psychosom Res. 1990;34(6):637–42.
33. Phillips K, Wilhelm S, Koran L, Didie E, Fallon B, Feusner J, Stein D. Body dismorphic disoder: some key issues for DSM-V. Depress Anxiety. 2010;27(6):573–91.
34. Statista. Distribution of Instagram users worldwide as of January 2020, by gender. 2020.
35. Hollander E, Cohen LJ, Simeon D. Body dysmorphic disorder. Psychiatr Ann. 1993;23:359–64.
36. Senín Calderón C, Perona-Garcelán S, Rodríguez Testal Juan F. The dark side of Instagram: predictor model of dysmorphic concerns. Int J Clin Health Psychol. 2020;20:253–61.
37. Fardouly J, Pinkus RT, Vartanian LR. The impact of appearance comparisons made through social media, traditional media, and in person in women's everyday lives. Body Image. 2017;20:31–9.
38. Fishbain DA. Dysmorphophobia misdiagnosed as obsessive-compulsive disorder. Psychosomatics. 1991;32(4):469.
39. Phillips KA. Body dysmorphic disorder clinical aspects and treatment strategies. Bull Menn Clin. 1998;62:33–48.
40. Pascual-Vera B, Akin B, Belloch A, Bottesi G, Clark DA, Doron G, Fernández-Alvarez H, et al. The cross-cultural expression and transdiagnostic nature of unwanted mental intrusions. Int J Clin Health Psychol. 2019;19:85–96.
41. Phillips KA, McElroy SL. Insight, overvalued ideation, and delusional thinking in body dysmorphic disorder: theoretical and treatment implications. J Nerv Ment Dis. 1993;181:699–702.
42. Phillips K, Menarda W, Faya C. Gender similarities and differences in 200 individuals with body dysmorphic disorder. Compr Psychiatry. 2006;47(2):77–87.
43. Malcolm A, Pikoos T, Castle D, Rossell S. An update on gender differences in major symptom phenomenology among adults with body dysmorphic disorder. Psychiatry Res. 2021;295:113619.
44. Phillips KA, Diaz S. Gender differences in body dysmorphic disorder. J Nerv Ment Dis. 1997;185:570–7.
45. Pope CG, Pope HG, Menard W. Clinical features of muscle dysmorphia among males with body dysmorphic disorder. Body Image. 2005;2:395–400.
46. Neziroglu R, Yaryura-Tobias JA. A review of cognitive behavioral and pharmacological treatment of body dysmorphic disorder. Behav Modif. 1997;21:324–40.
47. Festinger L. A theory of social comparison processes. Hum Relat. 1954;7:117–40.
48. Hollander E, Neville D, Frenkel M, Josephson S, Liebowitz MR. Body dysmorphic disorder. Diagnostic issues and related disorders. Psychosomatics. 1992;33(2):156–65.
49. Vitiello B, De Leon J. Dysmorphophobia misdiagnosed as obsessive-compulsive disorder. Psychosomatics. 1990;31:220–2.
50. Phillips K, Kelly M. Body dysmorphic disorder: clinical overview and relationship to obsessive-compulsive disorder. Focus. 2021;19:413–29.

Dissociative Disorders

26

Agueda-Rojo Pantoja, María Pérez Martín,
Carmen Garrido Fernández, and Margarita Sáenz-Herrero

26.1 Introduction

Modern-day psychopathology keeps dissociation and dissociative symptoms within the bounds of the psychopathology of consciousness. It defines dissociation as a restriction of the field of consciousness, which denotes a disruption in the normal and continuous flow of ideas, thoughts, perceptions, etc. That brings about a split between cognitive, perceptive, and behavioral elements, with the behavior adopting automatic modes [1]. The processes involving a restriction of consciousness have the following psychopathological elements: drop in the levels of alertness and attention, spatial and temporal disorientation, automatic behavior, post-critical amnesia, absent delirium, and partially preserved sensory reactivity. Other symptoms that are considered dissociative are the dissolution of the self or split personality, dissociative amnesia, depersonalization, derealization, auditory hallucinations [2], trance states [3], and somatoform symptoms.

We owe the term dissociation to Pierre Janet, since its genesis can be found in his désagrégation psychologique [4] and also to the reformers of eighteenth-century associationism, such as Maine de Biran and Herbart, because they provided Janet with a conceptual framework, which was later elaborated upon by Sigmund Freud. Moving on to the fin-de-siècle spirit, we find that the artists in Paris were familiar with Charcot's theories about nervous diseases.

A.-R. Pantoja
Psychiatrist University Hospital Complex, Vigo, Spain

M. P. Martín · C. G. Fernández · M. Sáenz-Herrero (✉)
Psychiatrist Cruces University Hospital, Bilbao, Spain

University of the Basque Country, Santsoena, Spain
e-mail: margarita.saenzherrero@osakidetza.eus

M. López-Atanes, M. Sáenz-Herrero (eds.), *Applying the Gender Perspective in Psychiatry and Psychotherapy*, https://doi.org/10.1007/978-3-032-17883-1_26

Neurasthenia, which was believed to be primarily caused by the fast-paced urban lifestyle, became a trendy condition. Psychiatry exerted a significant influence on the cultural zeitgeist of the time, and there is a notable overlap between the individuals depicted by psychiatrists and the characters represented by novelists and playwrights.

Ellenberger [5] cites similarities between Janet's Irene (1907) and Zola's Pauline, from his work La joie de vivre, between Hofmannsthal's Electra and de Breuer's Anna O; between Freud's Dora and the characters in the short stories by Schnitzler. In this cultural-historical context, we can find a predilection for hysteria as the diagnosis for women of the day.

In 1875 Eugène Azam spoke for the first time of the "French split personality," embodied by Félida. He first described the case as "temporal amnesia," later calling it "double awareness" and finally "split personality."

An interesting issue for debate is whether the apparent proliferation of dissociative disorders among women in the past was an epidemiological reality or simply a reflection of the cultural trends of the time. Two centuries later, the prevalence of these disorders seems to be greater in the United States than in Europe. Recent studies, as referenced in the bibliography, reveal contradictory findings about the prevalence of dissociative disorders among sexes, challenging the assumption that women are more susceptible to these conditions.

However, dissociation is not confined to the phenomenon of split personality, now recognized as dissociative identity disorder. It also underpins a range of mental health disorders with diverse psychological and physical manifestations. Dissociation encompasses not only dissociative amnesia, depersonalization, derealization, and fragmented identity but, as noted by Pierre Janet and other psychiatrists during World War I, also reflects a deficient integration of somatomorphic components. Various authors have suggested using the term "psychological dissociation" rather than "somatomorphic dissociation" to highlight that many somatic symptoms are rooted in dissociative mechanisms.

The high prevalence of mental disorders among women in the nineteenth century should be viewed as a cultural bias of the era. Women were perceived as fragile and primarily defined by their roles as mothers, with many likely suffering under oppressive societal conditions. However, physicians rarely consider social determinants as potential causes of these disorders. Discrimination played a crucial role in the treatment of conditions often considered exclusive to women, with stress being cited as an exacerbating factor due to the perception that women were more delicate and emotionally sensitive.

The question of whether dissociative disorders are more prevalent among women than men remains to be definitively answered. We aim to analyze all available data to determine whether these disorders are more common in one sex than the other. It is essential to interpret the statistical data associated with different disorders and to ascertain whether the observed patterns are driven by factors unique to women or influenced by cultural determinants.

26.2 Janet and Systematic Anesthesias

There is little doubt that the term "dissociation" originated with Pierre Janet, specifically in his concept of *désagrégation*, within a very specific historical context—the French fin-de-siècle. Sigmund Freud also warrants mention, as it is around this time that references to the idea of dissociation begin to appear in his work. Freud would soon abandon this concept in favor of repression, shifting his theories toward a new direction, leaving hypnosis behind and embracing the emerging ideas of psychoanalysis. Although both authors held conflicting views regarding the origin of dissociation, their studies often overlapped at various points, frequently leading to similar conclusions.

Pierre Janet's work introduces several concepts (suggestion, the subconscious, the narrowing of the field of consciousness, psychological misery, and fixed ideas) that would lay the groundwork for his theory of *désagrégation psychologique*. His most significant work, *L'Automatisme psychologique* (1889), is the result of research conducted in the laboratory of the Le Havre hospital, where he elaborates on his theory of disaggregation [4].

It was through his clinical observations of patients and instances of partial catalepsies that Janet developed the notion of partial consciousness—the dissociation of the content of consciousness into separate compartments. He described women who performed actions subconsciously, that is, actions that exhibited all the characteristics of a psychological phenomenon except for one: the subject was unaware of what they were doing in the moment [4]. Psychological automatism does not direct all conscious thought but affects only a small set of phenomena, which are partially separated from the individual's overall consciousness, continuing to operate independently and in a different manner. The simplest expressions of these partial automatisms include partial catalepsies and suggestions via distraction.

According to Janet, distraction appears to divide the field of consciousness into two segments: one that remains conscious, and another that the subject seems unaware of. Distraction functions like an anesthesia, through which acts, and even hallucinations, can be suggested. While the distracted consciousness engages with other ideas, the suggested act is carried out without the subject's awareness. Through suggestion, Janet discovered that he could suppress certain sensations, producing partial blindness or deafness in the subject. Additionally, Janet posited that during conscious perception of sensations, a two-stage operation occurs. First, all sensations from various senses converge, and then there is an active synthesis, as these sensations group together and combine to form a unified perception. In the case of the "distracted hysterical" [4] subject, however, some sensations escape from consciousness during the second phase. These sensations cannot be linked to the individual's sense of self and are thus not recognized by the subject. This represents the initial concept of dissociation.

"It is undeniable that what gave hysteria coherence over a long period of time was its exclusively female nature" [13]. Up until the twentieth century, three potential origins for hysteria were considered: the uterus, the brain, and the nerves. The first option suggested that only women could suffer from the condition, but later, its origin was generally believed to be in the brain. Due to the analogy between hysteria and epileptic convulsions, it was concluded that a single organ must be responsible for the pathology, leading to the development of the concept of *hystero-epilepsy*, which was endorsed by the Charcot School. During the French fin-de-siècle, hysteria was still largely seen as a condition affecting only women. However, it was Charcot himself who demonstrated that hysteria could also afflict men [6].

The recognition of male hysteria in the nineteenth century occurred within the historical context of industrialization, particularly the rise of the railway, which symbolized the modern understanding of trauma as something that could occur randomly. The term "railway spine" was coined by John Eric Erichsen to describe symptoms that lacked a clear physical injury. Russell Reynolds later suggested that disorders such as paralysis or spasms might arise from psychological factors like ideas or emotions, a theory that resembled hysteria. This view allowed Charcot to reframe male hysteria, which had previously been associated with effeminacy, in a new light. Using hypnosis on a clearly masculine subject, Charcot demonstrated that memory, hysteria, hypnosis, and physical trauma were interconnected [7, 8].

After working for several years in Le Havre, Janet moved to La Salpêtrière and became a student of his mentor, Charcot [9]. Charcot's work on fixed ideas as central to certain neuroses served as the foundation for Janet's theory of dissociation. In *L'État mental des hystériques*, Janet explains the existence of purely somatic phenomena with psychological etiology, and Charcot is the first to link these physical symptoms to traumatic experiences. Janet argued that hysteria is a mental disorder in which cerebral stress gives rise to vague physical symptoms. A weakening of the field of consciousness prevents certain sensations and images from being perceived, leaving them beyond the reach of personal awareness. This lack of synthesis allows for the formation of parasitic ideas, which, being completely isolated from personal consciousness, manifest as physical disorders. These parasitic ideas form the basis of Janet's concept of fixed ideas, which he considered to be the cause of mental disturbances in hysterics, explaining traumatic hysteria in terms of the manifestation of these ideas.

"We know that, in individuals in a deep state of hypnosis, it is possible, through suggestion and intimidation, to implant an idea—a coherent set of associated ideas—that takes root in the mind like a parasite, becoming isolated from everything else and later manifesting in corresponding motor phenomena" [8].

For Charcot, hysteria is a disease with multiple symptoms, including contractions, paralysis, anesthesia, convulsions, hallucinations, and delirium. Beginning in 1878, he became interested in hypnosis as a means of inducing hysteria-like symptoms in his patients, asserting that both hysteria and hypnosis occurred only in individuals with weak and degenerate nervous systems.

Charcot faced criticism from Liébeault and Bernheim, who denied any connection between hypnosis and hysteria. They argued that the ability to undergo hypnosis was based on suggestibility, not mental illness. In response, Charcot proposed a psychological explanation, acknowledging that personality disorders caused by trauma could act as triggers for hysteria. This new approach allowed for the development of a therapeutic method, which was later formulated by two of Charcot's disciples, Freud and Janet [10].

At the turn of the twentieth century, the role of emotion in the development of hysteria became a controversial issue. According to Janet, past traumatic events that had been "forgotten" remained active in the subconscious, forming fixed ideas with a life of their own in a dissociated state of consciousness. From Janet's perspective, emotion triggered dissociation, narrowing the field of consciousness and enabling the formation of fixed ideas. Freud, however, argued that emotion, due to its heightened excitation, overloaded the body, which could not release the tension through the normal process of abreaction (the release of emotional tension).

26.3 Freud and Conversion

In the 1893 Preliminary Communication, Freud and Breuer extended Charcot's pathogenic formula for hystero-traumatic paralysis to all forms of hysteria. In this work, Freud outlines two psychological processes involved in traumatic neuroses. One is a dissociation mechanism, whereby a break occurs in the association between a bodily function and the rest of its psychological activity. The second is a *Clivage* (Spaltung), which maintains this separation or diversion so completely that it becomes unbridgeable, rendering these dissociated phenomena inaccessible to any form of association. For these mechanisms to activate, there must be an intense affective charge. The difference between Janet's and Freud's understanding of this dissociation lies in the former's explanation, which attributes it to a deficiency in the synthesis function or a narrowing of the field of consciousness, whereas Freud associates it with the affective charge.

For Freud, in cases of male hysteria, subjects experienced trauma—such as a railway accident—that caused them to feel intense fear. In the case of hysterical women, experiences that could be considered traumatic were found to be present in the content of their attacks. However, it was not the memory itself that was traumatic, but rather that the event occurred during a period of predisposition, which is why it became a traumatic memory. Freud proposed that this memory is unconscious, meaning it exists in a second state of consciousness [11]. He theorized that the symptomatic complex of hysteria supports the hypothesis of a dissociation of consciousness, where separate psychic groups form. However, he did not share the prevailing views at the time regarding the origin of this dissociation. While Janet considered dissociation to be a primary feature of hysteria, resulting from a genetic weakness in psychical synthesis and thus leading to degeneration in hysterical individuals, Freud rejected this hypothesis.

The split of consciousness, akin to the double consciousness observed in classic hysteria cases, is present in all forms of hysteria. The tendency to dissociate and experience altered states of consciousness, known as hypnosis, is the core phenomenon behind neurosis [12]. Hypnotic states are dreamlike and characterized by a reduction in associative thinking. Thoughts from these states are disconnected from normal associations, leading to dissociation, which is learned rather than innate [13].

It would take Freud a considerable amount of time to depart from Breuer's theories and develop his own concept of "conversion" in relation to the so-called "defense hysterias." Unlike Janet, who regarded the dissociation of consciousness as a defining feature of hysteria, Freud (1894) considered the capacity for conversion to be the hallmark of hysteria [14]. "In hysteria, the unbearable representation is rendered harmless by transforming the intensity of the stimulus into somatic excitations, a process we term conversion. Conversion may be either total or partial and affects the motor or sensory innervation most closely associated with the traumatic event. The mnemic trace does not disappear as a result but instead forms the nucleus of a second psychic group thereafter."

Freud's concept of repression first appears in his *Neuropsychosis of Defense* (1894) [14] and is subsequently developed in his *Studies on Hysteria* (1895) [12]. Freud explained that the "dissociation of the contents of consciousness (as a result of repression) is a consequence of the patient's will, set into motion by an effort of willpower, whose motivation can be determined." "I viewed the psychic split as a result of the process of repulsion, which I later termed defense, and eventually repression" [14].

With the growing importance of psychoanalysis, following the publication of *Studies on Hysteria* by Breuer and Freud, the concept of dissociation gradually lost favor and was ultimately supplanted by the model of repression. Both Freud and Janet acknowledged the significant role psychological trauma played in the formation of symptoms. However, with Freud's development of the defense mechanism concept, psychoanalytic theory distanced itself from contemporary theories of dissociation. The popularity of dissociation, once a central idea in late nineteenth and early twentieth-century psychological thought, gradually waned until it all but disappeared from scholarly discourse [15].

26.4 Dissociation and Conversion in Modern-Day Classifications

The concept of dissociation found in the work of Pierre Janet does not refer to the same idea found in the work of Sigmund Freud, as we have already seen in this brief analysis of its conceptual and historical evolution. The notions of Pierre Janet have provided a framework for modern-day diagnostic manuals, both the DSM in the United States and the ICD in Europe [16]. In the changes that were proposed for the DSM IV we can already find the term "dissociative identity disorder" (300.14) instead of "dissociative personality"; "dissociative amnesia" (300.12) instead of "psychogenic amnesia," and "dissociative fugue" (300.13) instead of psychogenic fugue. All these terms correspond with manifestations that can be explained by means of Pierre Janet's dissociation.

Classically, there have been different diagnostic visions between American and European psychiatry. The former has avoided the somatic manifestations of the dissociative disorders, in such a way that the DSM-III-R defined the fundamental feature of dissociative disorders as "a disorder or alteration in the integration of functions connected with identity, memory, or consciousness" [17]. It focused on dissociative disorders as disruptions in identity, memory, or consciousness, excluding somatic symptoms, which were classified separately (e.g., somatization, pain, or conversion disorders). In stark contrast, the International Classification of Diseases, ICD-10 does contemplate that dissociation can affect somatoform functions [18]. This diagnostic manual only deals with dissociative disorders presenting a loss of sensations or loss of, or interference with, movements. Disorders that may include further sensations such as pain are categorized as somatoform disorders, the same as somatization disorder. In ICD-10, "Dissociative disorders (conversion disorders)" are spoken of, under the assumption that they are equivalent concepts, although, as we have already seen, they refer to different concepts, according to the two different authors whom described them. In ICD-11, the term "conversion" is removed, and these disorders are grouped under "dissociative disorders." This reflects a more dissociation-centered approach, without the psychodynamic connotation of conversion [19].

As already mentioned, in the American classification, the conversion disorder can be found among somatoform disorders and is defined as "the presence of symptoms or deficit that affects motor or sensorial skills, and that suggest a neurological disorder or some other medical condition" [20]. The current DSM-5 renames conversion disorders as "Functional Neurological Symptomatic Disorder" [21], stressing the need for neurological tests ("consistency in the test is a way of proving incompatibility between the symptom and well-known medical or neurological conditions" [21]) and also implying that the presence of relevant psychological factors cannot always be proven at diagnosis, which seems to give currency to the idea they are not always be linked to psychological disorders.

The opposite occurs in the case of somatization disorder, which is now called "somatic symptom disorder" [21], clarifying that to reach this diagnosis there must be somatic symptoms and also maladaptive thoughts, feelings, and behaviors. Previously, this disorder was defined as having somatic symptoms that could not be explained medically, but in the current diagnostic framework, this criterion is consigned to conversion disorders and pseudocyesis because these are the only cases in which it is thought that it can be demonstrated that the symptoms are not consistent with medical pathophysiology. There is a substantial difference between these diagnostic criteria and previous ones, since there is a breakaway from the classic understanding of the somatization disorder (or Briquet syndrome) belonging to hysteria and therefore to psychological causation. Also, it does not specify, but somatization disorder shows a greater prevalence among women [21].

In the DSM-5, depersonalization is classified under "depersonalization/derealization disorder," an independent diagnosis within dissociative disorders, with specific criteria requiring significant distress. It adds a prevalence of the disorder of 2% and a ratio related to gender of 1:1, unlike previous manuals, which claimed they did not have any information related to this. In contrast, ICD-11 also includes it under "dissociative disorders" but takes a more flexible approach, allowing it to be part of a dissociative spectrum without requiring a separate diagnosis. While the

DSM-5 maintains more clearly defined categories, ICD-11 emphasizes the variability and continuity of dissociative symptoms [19].

There are a few references in these classifications to the number of manifestations of these disorders in one sex or another. According to Gaviria [22], this approach has been minimal in the DSM-I (1952) and DSM-II (1968) and was probably due to the lack of research concerning the relation between gender and psychopathology. In the DSM-III (1980), there was a slight increase in interest in sex/gender and in the section on conversion disorder, it is said that "there is no conclusive information" [22], but that globus hystericus is apparently more frequent in women. The DSM-III-R (1987) and DSM-IV continued to make some headway in this area, and this time there was information about variations in the expression and length of the disorders according to gender that was included in the section called "specific characteristics including culture, age, and gender" [20]. The DSM-5 continues this trend of mentioning sex differences without delving into the etiological nature of these differences.

Conversion disorders appear more frequently in women than in men in a ratio ranging between 2:1 and 10:1, and many of these women later present with somatization disorder. In the case of men, there is an association with antisocial personality disorder, in military contexts and in accidents in the workplace [20], which could be interpreted as based on a sociocultural bias. Dissociative amnesia is described in both classifications as being less common in men, with extreme cases primarily linked to combat stress [18, 20], which we believe reflects a cultural bias. In the DSM-5, there is a brief mention of dissociative amnesia being more prevalent in women. However, this reference is based on a single, small-scale US study [21] that estimated a 12-month prevalence of 1.8% (1% in men and 2.6% in women). Additionally, the DSM-5 no longer considers dissociative fugue a separate diagnostic entity but instead classifies it as a feature of dissociative amnesia.

In the DSM-5, dissociative identity disorder is presented with more information about gender differences, though no specific etiological explanations are provided. The disorder is more common in women, but data on children are lacking. It is suggested that men often deny symptoms and traumatic memories, leading to false negatives. Women tend to exhibit acute symptoms like flashbacks, amnesia, fugues, conversion symptoms, hallucinations, or self-mutilation, while men are more likely to display violent or criminal behavior. Triggers for acute episodes in men include combat, prison, or physical/sexual aggression [21].

26.5 Female Gender in Dissociative Disorders

We start from the assumption that there seem to be differences in how psychical symptoms are perceived in men and women, though this premise could be questionable according to other variables such as social class, ethnic group, or cultural environment. In our sociocultural context, women present more often a subjective perception of lower psychical well-being, worse quality of life, and worse state of health than men and tend to use health services more often [23].

Assuming traumatic events are factors of vulnerability and triggers of mental disorders, it is known that if these traumatic events take place during infancy, they are more serious. Thus, suffering from sexual abuse in infancy increases the risk of suffering from anxiety disorders. There is, moreover, a different response to a psychical trauma according to gender. In general, women suffer fewer traumatic experiences, but they are more vulnerable to them [24].

A subtype of posttraumatic stress disorder (PTSD), called "dissociative," is characterized by dissociative symptoms. Studies, including neuroimaging research, show that this disorder is linked to various types of trauma, such as childhood sexual and physical abuse and military combat. Prevalence estimates indicate that 20% of women and 8% of men with this disorder experienced childhood sexual abuse [25]. Among Vietnam veterans, 15% of men and 8% of women had PTSD 15 years after their service [26]. This study demonstrates that boys are more likely to experience physical aggression or witness violence, while girls are at higher risk for sexual assault [27].

Peritraumatic dissociation refers to alterations, disruptions, or gaps in alertness and memory that occur during or immediately after a traumatic event. It includes experiences of derealization, depersonalization, dissociative amnesia, emotional numbing or detachment, and reduced awareness of one's surroundings. From a psychological perspective, it can be seen as an adaptive response, as the individual momentarily distances themselves from a traumatic experience. However, dissociative reactions often hinder proper processing of the event, preventing the emotional integration of the traumatic memory. Peritraumatic dissociation is more prevalent in women, within the context of a society that has normalized violence against them, and has been strongly linked to a history of sexual abuse [28].

Additionally, dissociative phenomena in many women are associated with revictimization events, particularly in adolescents exposed to interpersonal violence [29]. Furthermore, research has shown that dissociative symptoms are highly prevalent among transgender individuals and are commonly linked to body dysphoria and childhood trauma, highlighting stressful, discriminatory situations experienced by these individuals due to the stigma surrounding them in a society that punishes nonconventional gender expressions. Treatment, as well as gender reassignment procedures, has been shown to reduce these dissociative symptoms [30].

We keep on linking hysteria with the female gender today. There is a widely held belief that dissociative symptoms and disorders are predominantly found in women. Empirical studies in the general population and in different clinical trials indicate that there are no differences between genders. One explanation that has been postulated to account for this apparent prevalence of dissociative disorders among women is that women resort more often to healthcare providers, while the condition is usually identified among men in law-related environments such as prisons or forensic institutions [31]. A study in New York [32] did not find any differences in gender in the distribution of dissociative disorders. There is a general belief, based on clinical observations and pointed out in the DSM-5 [21], that among clinical populations, male patients easily hide their symptoms and histories of trauma. On the other hand, Sar et al. [33]

found in a Turkish study, among high-performance university students, that the male students reported more traumas during childhood than the female students.

There are other explanations, determined culturally, that would explain a greater prevalence of dissociative disorders among women, as demonstrated by Wolfrad [34], in his study seeking the relation between dissociative experiences, anxiety features, and paranormal beliefs among a sample of students, in which these were more frequent among women, along with higher scores in dissociative experiences. Along the same lines, Pires [35] demonstrated that there was a greater psychological impact on women than on men who have suffered a car accident, but they did not find any significant differences between genders when looking at peritraumatic dissociation.

Other studies, the vast majority, demonstrate that there is a greater prevalence of dissociative and somatoform disorders among women. Nicolai [36] offers different explanations for these differences in the prevalence according to gender, and one of them is attachment disorder and abuse in childhood of these women.

Many studies have shown that dissociation plays a significant role in sleep disorders and eating disorders [37]. This relationship between dissociation and eating disorders also exhibits sex-specific patterns, with women being more likely to experience depersonalization and derealization phenomena associated with these disorders [38]. In these disorders, where many of the patients have a history of traumatic experiences, we can once again see the relationship between trauma and dissociation.

Of special interest to clinicians who treat somatizations or other somatoform disorders without a clear medical etiology are some of the results of the study ACE46 (The Adverse Childhood Experiences), in which a direct relation is found between the probability of sexual abuse in childhood and the number of medically inexplicable symptoms in adult age. Women have a 50% greater probability of having suffered five or more categories of adverse experiences in childhood. Felitti et al. [39] consider that this is key to understanding the greater propensity of women to suffer health problems such as fibromyalgia, chronic fatigue syndrome, obesity, irritable bowel syndrome, and nonmalignant pain syndromes.

Many studies find a higher prevalence of conversion disorders among women [40], although this difference can vary according to the type of disorder. Stone et al. [41] found that the proportion of women was lower in cases of psychogenic weakness syndromes than in cases of epileptic pseudocrises. When discussing conversion disorders, it is important to address pseudocrises—convulsive episodes without epileptic activity on EEG, classified as a conversion symptom. The prevalence of these pseudocrises is higher in women, and they also tend to be more severe and have a greater impact, persisting longer and with a higher tendency toward self-injury during episodes compared to men [42]. Traumatic events have been documented as predisposing, precipitating, and perpetuating factors for these pseudocrises, with sexual abuse being the most prevalent trauma among affected women [43]. It is theorized that emotional reactions to sexual trauma, relegated to the subconscious, may be expressed physically through these seizures [44], reflecting feelings of rage, fear, and helplessness in response to domination or abuse in patriarchal societies, as described by Rosenbaum [42].

Non-epileptic psychogenic crises are recognized in all studies as being more prevalent in women than in men [45, 46], which seems to be consistent with a greater prevalence in conversion disorders as well, and both are included among somatoform disorders in the DSM.

26.6 Conclusions

Dissociative symptoms are observed across various psychiatric disorders, as defined by current diagnostic classifications, such as the latest DSM and ICD-11. To fully understand the psychopathology of dissociative symptoms, it is crucial to consider the cultural and historical context in which the concept of dissociation originated, as well as the paths its evolution has followed throughout the history of psychiatry. Over time, various related concepts have emerged, introduced by different authors, including Janet, Charcot, and Sigmund Freud.

Different psychological theories have attempted to explain somatic and psychogenic symptoms—those whose medical etiology remains unknown—often drawing connections to hysteria and its associated phenomenology. This has led to considerable confusion surrounding concepts and terminology, which we have attempted to clarify as much as possible. From Pierre Janet's concept of "désagrégation psychologique" to Sigmund Freud's theory of conversion and the somatization disorder outlined in the DSM-IV, descriptive psychopathology has continually evolved.

Dissociation has traditionally been linked to hysteria, which has historically been associated with women. We have explored the cultural and historical factors behind this prevalence in the nineteenth century, when the concept first emerged, and have reminded readers of the medical references to male hysteria from that time—largely forgotten today, but an important part of Charcot's case studies and his work on traumatic hysteria. Conditions such as split personality or demonic possession were not exclusive to women; in modern psychopathology, these are clearly recognized as dissociative disorders.

Epidemiological studies suggest a higher prevalence of conversion disorders among women, but dissociative disorders do not appear in the same proportions, and the findings remain controversial. The reasons behind this statistical difference remain unclear, though it is possible that gender-related psychopathological factors may explain the greater prevalence of somatoform disorders among women. This leads us to conclude that further research is needed and that more attention should be paid to mental health care for women. Incorporating a gender perspective is essential for advancing high-quality scientific understanding.

References

1. Gastó C. Psicopatología de la conciencia. In: Vallejo Ruiloba J, editor. Introducción a la psicopatología y la psiquiatría. 6ª ed. Barcelona: Masson; 2006. p. 129–43.
2. Spiegel D, Loewenstein RJ, Lewis-Fernández R, Sar V, Simeon D, Vermetten E, et al. Dissociative disorders in DSM-5. Depress Anxiety. 2011;28(9):824–52.

3. American Psychiatric Association. Manual diagnóstico y estadístico de los trastornos mentales, texto revisado. 1ª ed. Barcelona: Masson; 2002.
4. Janet P. L'Automatisme psychologique. 1ª reimpresión. París: Odile Jacob; 1989.
5. Ellenberger H. El descubrimiento del inconsciente. 1ª reimpresión. Madrid: Gredos; 1976.
6. Bolzinger A. Freud et les Parisiens. París: Campagne Première; 2002.
7. Hacking I. L'âme réécrite. Étude sur la personnalité multiple et les sciences de la mémoire. Le Plessis Robinson: Institut Synthélabo pour le progrès de la connaissance; 1998.
8. Charcot JM. Lecciones sobre la histeria traumática. In: Pereña F, Desviat M, editors. compiladores . Madrid: Nieva; 1989.
9. Janet P. L'état mental des hystériques. 1ª reimpresión. Marseille: Laffitte Reprints; 1983.
10. Cagigas A. Charcot y las lecciones del martes. In: Charcot JM, editor. Histeria. Jaén: Del Lunar; 2003. p. 7–12.
11. Freud S. Sobre la teoría del ataque histérico. In: Freud S. Obras completas. 1. Buenos Aires: Amorrortu; 1982. p. 187–190.
12. Freud S. Sobre el mecanismo psíquico de fenómenos histéricos: comunicación preliminar. In: Freud S. Obras completas. 2. Buenos Aires: Amorrortu; 1999. p. 27–44.
13. Rojo A. El concepto dissociation en el fin-de-siècle.: P. Janet y S. Freud [Tesis doctoral]. Madrid: Universidad Complutense; 2005.
14. Freud S. Las neuropsicosis de defensa. In: Freud S. Obras completas. Vol. 1. 2ª ed. Madrid: Biblioteca Nueva; 2001. p. 169–177.
15. Pérez S, Galdón J. Los fenómenos disociativos: una revisión conceptual. Rev Psicop Psicol Clin. 2003;8(2):85–108.
16. Garrabé J. La taxonomie actuelle des troubles dissociatifs. Évol Psychiatr. 1999;64(4):717–26.
17. Nijenhuis ERS. Somatoform dissociation: phenomena, measurement, and theoretical issues. New York: Norton & Company; 2004.
18. López Ibor JJ, editor. CIE-10. Décima revisión de la clasificación internacional de las enfermedades. Trastornos mentales y del comportamiento. Descripciones clínicas y pautas para el diagnóstico. Madrid: Meditor; 1992.
19. World Health Organization (WHO). International classification of diseases. 11th ed. Geneva: WHO; 2018.
20. López Ibor JJ. DSM-IV. Manual diagnóstico y estadístico de los trastornos mentales. Barcelona: Masson; 1995.
21. American Psychiatric Association. Diagnostic and statistical manual of mental disorders, DSM-5. 5ª ed. Arlington: American Psychiatric Association; 2013.
22. Gaviria SL, Alarcón RD. Psicopatología y género: visión longitudinal e histórica a través del DSM. Rev Colomb Psiquiat. 2010;39(2):389–404.
23. Ezquiaga E. Aspectos diferenciales en los trastornos de ansiedad. In: Saiz J, editor. Salud mental y género en la práctica clínica. Madrid: Ars Medica; 2007. p. 59–78.
24. Punamäki RL, Komproe IH, Quota S, Elmasri M, De Jong JT. The role of peritraumatic dissociation and gender in the association between trauma and mental health in a Palestinian community sample. Am J Psychiatry. 2005;162:545–51.
25. Pereda N, Guilera G, Forns M, Gómez-Benito J. The prevalence of child sexual abuse in community and student samples: a meta-analysis. Clin Psychol Rev. 2009;29(4):328–38.
26. Schlenger WE, Kulka RA, Fairbank JA, Hough RL, Jordan BK, Marmar CR, et al. The prevalence of post-traumatic stress disorder in the Vietnam generation: a multimethod, multisource assessment of psychiatric disorder. J Trauma Stress. 1992;5(3):333–63.
27. Karestan CK, Roberts AL, Stone DM, Dunn EC. The epidemiology of early childhood trauma. In: Lanius RA, Vermetten E, Pain C, editors. The impact of early life trauma on health and disease. The hidden epidemic. 5ª ed. Cambridge: Cambridge University Press; 2013. p. 13–24.
28. Boisclair Demarble J, Fortin C, D'Antono B, Guay S. Gender differences in the prediction of acute stress disorder from peritraumatic dissociation and distress among victims of violent crimes. J Interpers Violence. 2020;35(5–6):1229–50.
29. Kouri NA, Simon VA, Partridge T. Dissociation as a mechanism of risk for interpersonal victimization among adolescent girls. J Interpers Violence. 2025;40(1–2):419–42.

30. Colizzi M, Costa R, Todarello O. Dissociative symptoms in individuals with gender dysphoria: is the elevated prevalence real? Psychiatry Res. 2015;226(1):173–80.
31. Spitzer C. Gender differences in dissociation. A dimensional approach. Psychopathology. 2003;36(2):65–70.
32. Johnson JG, Cohen P, Kasen S, Brook JS. Dissociative disorders among adults in the community, impaired functioning, and Axis I and II comorbidity. J Psychiatr Res. 2006;40(2):131–40.
33. Sar V, Gamze A, Kugu N, Ozturk E, Ertem-Vehid H. Axis I dissociative disorder comorbidity in borderline personality disorder and reports of childhood trauma. J Clin Psychiatry. 2006;67:1583–90.
34. Wolfradt U. Dissociative experiences, trait anxiety and paranormal beliefs. Pers Individ Differ. 1997;23(1):15–9.
35. Pires TSF. Are men more resilient than women after a road traffic accident? Psychol Health. 2012;27(1):104–5.
36. Nicolai NJ. Chronic stress, sex and gender. Tijdschr Psychiatr. 2009;51(8):569–77.
37. Cheng QL, Deng YY, Zhao G, Chen JF, Xie L, Wang L. Exploring gender differences in adolescent dissociative symptoms via a structural equation model. Biomed Environ Sci. 2023;36(8):773–8.
38. Meyer C, Waller G. Dissociation and eating psychopathology: gender differences in a nonclinical population. Int J Eat Disord. 1998;23(2):217–21.
39. Felitti VJ, Anda RF. The relationship of adverse childhood experiences to adult medical disease, psychiatric disorders and sexual behavior: implications for healthcare. In: Lanius RA, Vermetten E, Pain C, editors. The impact of early life trauma on health and disease. The hidden epidemic. 5ª ed. Cambridge: Cambridge University Press; 2013. p. 77–87.
40. Carson A, Stone J, Hibberd C, Murray G, Duncan R, Coleman R, et al. Disability, distress and unemployment in neurology outpatients with symptoms "unexplained by organic disease.". J Neurol Neurosurg Psychiatry. 2011;82(7):810–3.
41. Stone J, Sharpe M, Binzer M. Motor conversion symptoms and pseudoseizures: a comparison of clinical characteristics. Psychosomatics. 2004;45(6):492–9.
42. Libbon R, Baker S, Watson M, Natvig C, Strom L, Mikulich S. Sex effects on coping, dissociation, and PTSD in patients with non-epileptic seizures. Curr Psychiatry Rep. 2020;22(12):69.
43. Lanzillotti AI, Sarudiansky M, Scévola L, Oddo S, Korman GP, D'Alessio L. Sexual abuse, post-traumatic stress disorder and psychopathological characteristics in women with functional/dissociative seizures. Actas Esp Psiquiatr. 2024;52(5):616–24.
44. Kaplan MJ, Privitera MD, Meziane-Tani A. Characteristics of men with conversion disorder. Epilepsy Behav. 2021;114(Pt A):107556.
45. Reuber M, Elger CE. Psychogenic nonepileptic seizures: review and update. Epilepsy Behav. 2003;4(3):205–16.
46. Reuber M, Pukrop R, Bauer J, Helmstaedter C, Tessendorf N, Elger CE. Ann Neurol. 2003;53(3):305–11.

Part VI

Special Populations

Gender Interventions in Child and Adolescent Psychiatry

27

Álvaro Tamayo Saiz, Olga Anabitarte Bautista, and Beatriz Paya Gonzalez

27.1 Contextualizing: The Concepts of Sex and Gender

The first issue we need to resolve is defining the key terms regarding the topic we are discussing. When we talk about "gender interventions," we are appealing directly to the concept of gender, a problematic construct that has been around for centuries. The first distinction to make is between gender and sex, which takes us fully into feminist theory—a relevant ethical and philosophical current since the Enlightenment. When we talk about "sex," we are referring to the sexual dimorphism of the human species, with two sexes, male and female, that have different sexual characteristics which are essential for human reproduction. Gender, on the other hand, is a controversial concept. It refers to the social definition of the sexes and how society generates ideologies, norms, and stereotypes about sex [2, 3]. While sex belongs to biology, gender falls within the remit of philosophy, psychology, sociology, and politics, and has been a topic of conflict for centuries. Women have always been discriminated against on the basis of sex: they have been

Á. T. Saiz
Psychiatry Service. Child and Adolescent Psychiatry Section, Marqués de Valdecilla University Hospital, Santander, Spain
e-mail: alvaro.tamayo@scsalud.es

O. A. Bautista
Psychiatry and Mental Health Service, Fundacion Jimenez Diaz (CS Pontones). Quirón Salud, Madrid, Spain

B. P. Gonzalez (✉)
Psychiatry Service. Child and Adolescent Psychiatry Section, Marqués de Valdecilla University Hospital, Santander, Spain

Research Group on mental illnesses. IDIVAL, Santander, Spain
e-mail: mbeatriz.paya@scsalud.es

M. López-Atanes, M. Sáenz-Herrero (eds.), *Applying the Gender Perspective in Psychiatry and Psychotherapy*, https://doi.org/10.1007/978-3-032-17883-1_27

mistreated, denigrated, and ignored [2]. Since at least the seventeenth century, there has been a social and political movement to emancipate women.

Feminism aims to abolish gender by ending the ideologies, norms, and stereotypes that determine people's lives based on their sex. It seeks to end "patriarchy," the domination of women by men, and achieve equal rights and opportunities. Amelia Valcárcel defined feminism as "the set of theories, agenda and political practices that has guided and guides the defence of equality and citizenship for women, as well as the systematic abrogation of male privilege in society" [4].

While this may seem irrelevant to psychiatry, it's important to understand that "gender interventions" and "gender perspective" are at the crossroads where clinical practice, investigation, and political action intersect. By advocating for a gender perspective in mental health interventions, we acknowledge and address existing inequalities in how professionals approach our interventions with minors and families. The point is to ensure that gender-based disparities that occur in the broader social context are not replicated in our clinical practice.

27.2 Gender Differences in Epidemiology

Adolescence is the period of the lifespan when most of the major mental disorders begin, such as alcohol and other drug misuse and emotional, behavioral, psychotic, and eating disorders [1]. Epidemiological studies carried out in Spain, according to Polo Usaola [5, p. 104], indicate that women are diagnosed with depression, anxiety, and somatizations and consume anxiolytics and antidepressants around two to three times more often than men. For their part, men are diagnosed with addiction and substance use disorders five times more frequently than women in some age groups [5]. According to the Annual Report of the National Health System, published on August 5, 2024, anxiety disorders, which affect 10% of the population—making them the most prevalent disorders in the general population—affect twice as many women as men (14% vs 7%). The National Health Survey in Spain (ENSE) confirms that "the social gradient and the gender gap are present in all mental health indicators in adults" [6]. Regarding the child and adolescent population, the ENSE reflects that the prevalence of childhood mental health disorders is higher in males, except for depression/anxiety. The greatest gender difference was reported in behavioral disorders (including hyperactivity), 2.8% in boys and 0.7% in girls. The ENSE data also indicate that both chronic anxiety and depression occur in women aged 15 years or older twice as frequently as in men [6].

27.3 Clinical Implications

The first thing that needs to be considered when discussing the study of the relationships between gender and mental health is the existence of a basic limitation in much of the scientific research in this area. As Rippon [7] points out, there is a sexist bias in much of the research on the subject, to the extent that it would fall, when accounting for the supposed male/female differences, into an essentialism that is sometimes biological, sometimes psychological. In this sense, sometimes the research will deal with the "biological bases," the "neurological substrate," the "hormonal component" of previously observed male/female differences. On other occasions, it will be a question of searching for the "psychological bases," the "neuropsychological substrate" or the "neurocognitive component" of the aforementioned male/female differences. The problem is that both models ignore part—at best—or directly all—at worst—of the cultural, historical, and sociological variables that would be intervening in the formation of our "biology" and our "psyche," this error also being observed in mental health research. More specifically, the context that this research ignores is that of patriarchy, that of men's definition of what a man and a woman should be, and of the rules of hierarchy and domination over women that men also define. That is to say, this research paradigm attempts to abstract our brains, our psyches, and the psychological suffering from the sexist context in which they develop, resorting to an essentialism that attempts to reify our nervous system and our complex psyche as self-generated entities, acquiring a quasi-mystical quality, and outside of any influence from the culture in which they have grown up. This failure of this scientific tradition is particularly questionable at a time when research increasingly supports the hypothesis of the bidirectionality of the relationships between our nervous system and our psyche—healthy or ill—and the elational, cultural, social, etc., context in which they grow, not to mention the advances in epigenetics [8].

Research suggests that there are gender-related processes that influence the development of mental health problems. Gender intensification theory postulates that socialization pressures in early adolescence lead to the adoption of traditional gender roles, particularly in middle adolescence [9]. This could be understood as pressure on adolescents to assume traditional gender roles, which may determine their propensity to develop mental health problems.

Young people experience mental health problems and greater emotional distress during their transition to adolescence, with significant differences between boys and girls [10]: female adolescents report a higher level of distress than males. These results point to the role of gender as a factor in explaining differences in subjective well-being between boys and girls in adolescence. In childhood, no such differences are observed [11], suggesting that the gender gap in subjective well-being begins with puberty and the development of secondary sexual characteristics.

From the clinical point of view, girls show more internalizing symptoms than boys, in whom a more externalizing type of symptoms predominates [12–14]. These differences in the way men and women develop a mental disorder may explain the findings related to indicators of frequency of use of mental health services [15], age of referral [16], and willingness to use mental health services [17]. Boys have been found to be referred at an earlier age and are less willing to use mental health services than girls [18].

To understand gender differences in psychological suffering, we need to consider predisposing factors for mental disorders, which can also be mediated by gender. Research shows that more women than men experience multiple trauma (41% vs

27%), and that having experienced multiple traumas can lead to mental illness, especially in women [19]. From the perspective of therapy, we therefore want to highlight the need to improve the early detection and intervention of situations of abuse and mistreatment, especially in the female population, which challenges all health service workers in general, and in particular, professionals from mental health and primary care teams.

Premature pubertal development in girls has been linked to gender differences in depression [20, 21]. Studies indicate that girls with earlier sexual maturation show higher depressive symptoms than those with similar development to their female peers [22]. Given the sexist nature of society, it is relevant to consider that the development of secondary sexual attributes at puberty may be a determining milestone for girls. This stage may mark the beginning of a more sexualized perception [34, p. 202], contributing to emotional distress and the development of depressive symptoms.

Peer relationships are also a risk factor for sex differences in mental disorders. During adolescence, peer relationships influence adolescents' attitudes, activities, and emotional well-being [23]. Girls show greater sensitivity to other children's distress, greater empathy, and greater fear of rejection [24], which could influence the higher prevalence of internalizing symptoms in girls [20]. A study by Purdie and Downey [24] investigated the variable "rejection sensitivity" in adolescent females in the context of romantic relationships. The authors hypothesize that rejection-sensitive adolescents will display hypervigilant behaviors and maladaptive reactions to rejection. Thus, women with these characteristics, in order to preserve their romantic relationship, may adopt behaviors that increase their risk of victimization or other negative effects. In this study, rejection sensitivity predicted greater insecurity about the romantic relationship, a willingness to engage in inappropriate behaviors aimed at maintaining the relationship, greater physical aggression, and greater hostility in romantic conflict. Another interesting aspect of this study is that it postulates that sensitivity to rejection would have its origin in previous experiences of rejection and abuse, thus emphasizing the importance of the relational and traumatic life experiences in the configuration of a psychological variable such as "sensitivity to rejection," a variable that, on the other hand, has been associated with the presence of psychopathology, for example anxiety, depression and externalizing problems [25]. Again, we want to appeal to all professionals who work with children and adolescents so that, in a more or less informal way, they can work with boys and girls on issues of sexual and couples education.

In line with the above, according to a 2010 study [26], rejection sensitivity influences social and emotional development during adolescence and predicts the development of depressive and anxiety symptoms. At 16 and 17 years of age, fear of rejection affects men and women equally, but men show greater expectations of rejection. This is explained by "gender socialization" since boys have more difficulty than girls in moving toward establishing more emotionally complex relationships. Men are less capable of forming intimate relationships and are more sensitive to signs of rejection that affect their social status [26]. Furthermore, they would be more sensitive to rejection cues that would affect their social status, which could be interpreted from the theory of motivational systems [27]: boys would be more likely than girls, under certain circumstances, to enter into a hierarchical mode in the context of their interpersonal relationships.

Research suggests that sex differences in stress management and coping may also play a role in psychopathology. A New Zealand study showed that teenage girls face more stress and psychological disturbances than boys, while boys use less healthy coping strategies than girls (avoidance vs social support) [28]. This raises the question: can girls use healthier coping strategies to deal with stress, yet experience more psychological problems? We want to emphasize that these differences in stress coping strategies between men and women are the result of different learning within traditional gender roles. Related to the above, research highlights that women tend to use more prosocial coping strategies than men [29]. That is, the support strategies based on seeking social support observed in girls and adolescents are maintained into adulthood. This is consistent with what is observed in daily clinical practice in children's mental health services: mothers are the ones who most accompany their children, are most aware of their suffering, and are most often involved in the therapeutic process. This could also determine issues such as the willingness to attend mental health services for treatment, awareness of the illness, and adherence to treatments, which become points of interest for future research in this field.

27.4 Interventions with a Gender Perspective

Gender aspects in mental health care for children and adolescents are crucial for effective programs. As Pederson and colleagues [3] point out, health promotion activities with a gender perspective seek to improve health at the same time that counteract gender stereotypes.

Gender-focused intervention programs for children and adolescents emerged in the mid-1990s due to an increase in substance abuse problems among women and perceived ineffectiveness of existing treatment programs [30, 31]. These programs emphasized a family intervention to improve relationships and the family climate. Family relationships were identified as a specific risk factor for female substance abuse. Also, the first gender-specific interventions for aggressive behavior were developed [31], focusing on the different expression of aggression in girls and boys (relational vs physical aggression).

Despite initial advances in interventions incorporating a gender perspective, there is little literature on the subject, and publications on gender issues in the field of child and adolescent mental health interventions are still rare.

A recent systematic review on this topic includes 43 articles [10]. Most interventions were in North America and Europe, primarily in school or community settings, and mostly aimed at preventing addictive disorders or eating disorders. This review's findings on gender-sensitive interventions for mental disorders are presented below.

Three studies on mood disorders [32–34] aimed to address depression and suicide in young sexual and gender minorities. Conducted in community, family, and individual contexts, the studies' specific objectives were to meet the mental health needs of sexual or gender minority youth with depressive symptoms and/or suicidal tendencies. Programs addressed issues like invalidation and bullying, using gender-specific role models (e.g., from the same sexual or gender minority group).

Five studies on interventions for trauma and stress-related disorders have been identified [35–39]. These focused mainly on traumatized or sexually abused girls, with most interventions being community-based. As with other programs, the interventions address gender-specific mental health needs in this group, acknowledging the higher risk of sexual abuse in girls living in residential facilities. Many interventions also address risk factors (e.g., guilt and shame) and strengths (e.g., individual skills) in these youths. The Project Kealahou [38], implemented in the Hawaiian population, provides trauma-responsive care for girls. These include prosocial activities and peer girls' groups. Treatment, delivered mainly by female staff, is designed to be a safe, supportive space for this vulnerable group.

Interventions focusing on eating disorders mainly targeted female populations in school settings, with some addressing mixed groups [40–42]. Universal interventions focus on sociocultural aspects influencing body image, particularly feminine beauty ideals and myths, recognized as risk factors for developing eating disorders. Most universal interventions aim to promote body acceptance. One example is "Happy Being Me," a gender-specific program addressing both feminine and masculine beauty ideals, promoting body acceptance [40]. Prevention programs also highlight feminine beauty ideals and sociocultural pressures as gender-specific risk factors. One such program is "PriMa," which addresses risk and protective factors for anorexia nervosa in girls, including feminine beauty ideals, media literacy, and body image [43].

Most gender-focused interventions for behavioral disorders target women, with the majority being conducted in residential [44] or community settings [45]. Many studies evaluate gender-adapted programs developed due to a lack of interventions for female aggression [46]. These interventions address the different forms of aggressive behavior in women and men. Relational aggression is more prevalent among women, which reflects the traditional gender model. These treatments address risk factors, including previous experiences of violence and coping strategies. Elements also covered include relational aspects of aggression, gender-specific conflicts and problems, and aspects of gender role socialization. Furthermore, interventions promote empowerment and a positive self-image [10].

Studies of gender interventions for substance abuse in women have been conducted in various settings. Most are preventive interventions and address gender-specific factors such as stress, mood, and self-efficacy. Some also strengthen the mother-daughter bond and self-image [47–49]. There exist some gender-adapted dialectical behavioral therapy programs [50].

Most effective programs demonstrate effectiveness at the end of treatment and in subsequent follow-ups. Gender-specific concepts play a role in preventive interventions, though not in treatment programs. Although some treatment programs have been described according to the aforementioned premises, gender-specific approaches have not yet developed in the field of treating children and adolescents with mental health problems. Most studies evaluate interventions exclusively for girls, which should not be surprising given the gender gap in diagnoses and intervention design. Women have been neglected in substance abuse interventions, which has resulted in the development of specific treatments for them. Few studies have focused exclusively on boys with eating disorders, despite the fact that they are also an at-risk population.

Gender specificity in the studies is implemented differently depending on the problem and population. For example, addressing family support and minority stressors appears to be an important aspect of treating mood disorders in sexual and gender minority youth, whereas interventions for eating disorders focus primarily on beauty ideals and body acceptance for girls.

27.5 Recommendations and Future Directions

The harm caused to women by the sexist sociocultural context of Western societies has been discussed, with its traditional feminine identity focusing on emotions, relationships, and caring for others [5]. Numerous "gender mandates" exist including caring for children, partners, parents, and friends; maintaining an attractive appearance; being in a relationship and being a mother; taking on domestic chores and work; and accepting sexualization and the demand to satisfy others, which creates additional adolescent conflict, discomfort, and dissonance, and so all variables should be taken into consideration for prevention. Gender roles also affect asking for help. Mothers more often than fathers notice their children's distress and want to go with them to appointments. Also, they tend to feel more responsible for their children's suffering than males. There are also gender mandates for the construction of a traditional masculine identity, one of them being the denial or avoidance of discomfort, or at least of its expression. From this perspective, we see how men can often avoid asking for help or ask for it when the discomfort has already overwhelmed all coping strategies and the psychopathology has worsened, which could hinder the success of the interventions. Thus, it would be essential, both for mental health prevention and therapy, to focus on externalizing symptoms or substance use as potential maskers of affective symptoms.

Throughout the chapter, we have critically reflected on the sexist bias presented by classical neuroscience research, according to which the differences observed between men and women at the psychological and neurobiological level would be explained according to an acontextual essentialist metaphysics, and we have argued that in order to understand the differences that can be observed between men and women we must take into account the broader sociocultural context, which is still an environment riddled with sexist ideology.

Now, moving into the field of child and adolescent mental health professionals, we propose two approaches to clinical work with a gender perspective in mental health: one focused on diagnosis and the other on intervention, and finally, a note on prevention. First, we consider that it is vitally important to detect and compensate for the gender stereotypes that influence diagnosis. From this perspective, it is essential to consider how traditional gender stereotypes "prescribe" the expression of discomfort and to ask ourselves whether our patient could be being influenced by this view. Thus, as previously expressed, and in accordance with epidemiological data, we know that boys are more likely to present externalizing disorders and girls are more likely to present internalizing disorders. In this sense, we must question whether many of the conduct disorders, alterations in the level of activity such as hyperactivity or certain aggressive behaviors that children present could not in fact be speaking of the fact that the youth in question is in a situation of risk, neglect, or abuse, and that the symptoms expressed, in this case, should be understood as an emotional manifestation [51], as we have already mentioned. We must also question the role that body image and aesthetic pressure play on girls and adolescents, to the extent that this is a key social factor in understanding eating disorders. This topic is a classic topic widely studied in other texts [52]. With respect to neurodevelopmental disorders, for example, Baron-Cohen and colleagues point out the bias toward men observed in the diagnosis of several neurodevelopmental disorders, specifically autism spectrum disorders, Tourette syndrome, attention deficit hyperactivity disorder, specific language impairment, dyslexia, and learning disabilities [53]. Facing these disorders, we must pay attention during diagnoses, so we don't miss these kinds of symptoms in females.

Continuing with the lines of action we propose for child and adolescent mental health with a gender perspective, focusing now on interventions, we recommend taking into consideration and intervening on the psychological harm that can be caused by socialization in traditional gender roles. Thus, the first step toward correcting these attitudes is simply to become aware of the sexist context in which we are immersed and which is present in the therapeutic relationship. The next level involves compensating for traditional gender roles and attitudes within the scope of our therapeutic work. We understand that the core, fundamental change on which the rest of the interventions are built has to do with resisting traditional gender mandates in the field of therapy, both those that impact women and those that influence men. Specifically, and as a general principle, we understand that in the scope of our office, we must resist the vision of women as chronic, hyper-indulgent caregivers, whose identity is defined primarily by their role as partner and mother, relegated to the domestic sphere, and who would be the sole person responsible for child-rearing. Likewise, we believe we must appeal to men's responsibility in child-rearing, equate the importance of fatherhood with that of motherhood, and work openly in therapy to promote the equitable distribution of childcare between fathers and mothers, identifying men as capable of also taking on the emotional care of children. Furthermore, we must also include a gender perspective in individual therapy with children. We must explain to girls and adolescents what traditional gender roles are and help them understand that there are many ways to be a woman and that all are valid. We also believe it's important to work with boys to balance certain harmful attitudes inherent in their sexist upbringing: knowing that boys express their discomfort more through their behavior, we must help them put their emotions into words. And, just as with girls, we must help them understand that there are many ways to be a boy, and that all of them are appropriate. Also, we believe it's vitally important to address the issue of romantic relationships with adolescents, as this is sadly one of the contexts where the power relations typical of traditional masculinities and femininities are most clearly expressed. In this sense, we believe that, in many cases, sex education should be part of the therapeutic process with adolescent boys and girls, while helping them understand that they should aspire to build a relationship of mutual care that goes beyond feelings of romantic love. We must feel fully authorized, when clinically relevant, to explore all of these aspects with families and adolescents, thus incorporating into the clinical setting macro variables of the social context that are undoubtedly impacting, through various avenues of action, the mental state of our patients.

Finally, in terms of prevention, we need to improve the early identification and intervention of abuse and mistreatment of women. This is a challenge for all health professionals, especially mental health and primary care professionals. Psychoeducational work with parents and families on traditional gender roles and the gender perspective is vital, as families are the main vehicle for transmitting these values. This work can be done within the context of the assistance of mental health professionals across the diagnostic and intervention process. Also, in units where possible—day hospitals or inpatient units, for example—more specific work on the topic can be done, through parent groups.

We believe that work with a gender perspective should not be the sole responsibility of mental health professionals. All institutions that work with youths—health, education, justice, social services—should incorporate the principles outlined in this chapter. In particular, we would like to focus on the importance of the education system, as it is another important setting for the socialization of gender roles. Therefore, in our opinion, it would be very relevant for educational centers to include emotional education work in both early and late adolescence, with the aim of addressing the socialization of traditional gender roles and other predisposing factors already discussed.

References

1. Organización Mundial de la Salud. La salud mental de los adolescentes [Internet]. 2024 [cited 2025 Mar 28]. Available from: https://www.who.int/es/news-room/fact-sheets/detail/adolescent-mental-health
2. Miyares A. Delirio y misoginia trans. DEl sujeto transgénero al transhumanismo. 2a. Los libros de la catarata. 2023;
3. Pederson A, Greaves L, Poole N. Gender-transformative health promotion for women: a framework for action. Health Promot Int. 2015;30(1):140–50.
4. Valcárcel A. La civilización feminista. La esfera de los libros; 2023.
5. Polo Usaola C. La perspectiva de género en terapia familiar sistémica. In: Manual de terapia sistémica: Principios y herramientas de intervención. Desclee de Brouwer; 2014. p. 99–103. (Biblioteca de psicología).
6. Ministerio de Sanidad. Encuesta Nacional de Salud ENSE. 2017.
7. Rippon G. El género y nuestros cerebros: La nueva neurociencia que rompe el mito del cerebro femenino. Galaxia Gutenberg; 2020.

8. McEwen BS, Nasca C, Gray JD. Stress effects on neuronal structure: hippocampus, amygdala, and prefrontal cortex. Neuropsychopharmacol Off Publ Am Coll Neuropsychopharmacol. 2016;41(1):3–23.
9. Klaczynski PA, Felmban WS, Kole J. Gender intensification and gender generalization biases in pre-adolescents, adolescents, and emerging adults. Br J Dev Psychol. 2020 Sep;38(3):415–33.
10. Herrmann L, Reiss F, Becker-Hebly I, Baldus C, Gilbert M, Stadler G, et al. Systematic review of gender-specific child and adolescent mental health care. Child Psychiatry Hum Dev. 2024;55(6):1487–501.
11. Esteban-Gonzalo S, Esteban-Gonzalo L, Cabanas-Sánchez V, Miret M, Veiga OL. The investigation of gender differences in subjective wellbeing in children and adolescents: the UP&DOWN study. Int J Environ Res Public Health. 2020;17(8):2732.
12. Nolen-Hoeksema S, Girgus JS. The emergence of gender differences in depression during adolescence. Psychol Bull. 1994;115(3):424–43.
13. Lewinsohn PM, Gotlib IH, Lewinsohn M, Seeley JR, Allen NB. Gender differences in anxiety disorders and anxiety symptoms in adolescents. J Abnorm Psychol. 1998;107(1):109–17.
14. Keyes KM, Platt JM. Annual research review: sex, gender, and internalizing conditions among adolescents in the 21st century – trends, causes, consequences. J Child Psychol Psychiatry. 2024;65(4):384–407.
15. Cuffe SP, Waller JL, Addy CL, McKeown RE, Jackson KL, Moloo J, et al. A longitudinal study of adolescent mental health service use. J Behav Health Serv Res. 2001 Feb;28(1):1–11.
16. Griffin JA, Cicchetti D, Leaf PJ. Characteristics of youths identified from a psychiatric case register as first-time users of services. Psychiatr Serv. 1993;44(1):62–5.
17. Chandra A, Minkovitz C. Stigma starts early: gender differences in teen willingness to use mental health services. J Adolesc Health. 2006;38(6):754.e1–8.
18. Yoon L, Keenan KE, Hipwell AE, Forbes EE, Guyer AE. Hooked on a thought: associations between rumination and neural responses to social rejection in adolescent girls. Dev Cogn Neurosci. 2023;64:101320.
19. Yapp E, Booth T, Davis K, Coleman J, Howard LM, Breen G, et al. Sex differences in experiences of multiple traumas and mental health problems in the UK Biobank cohort. Soc Psychiatry Psychiatr Epidemiol. 2023;58(12):1819–31.
20. Yoon Y, Eisenstadt M, Lereya ST, Deighton J. Gender difference in the change of adolescents' mental health and subjective wellbeing trajectories. Eur Child Adolesc Psychiatry. 2023;32(9):1569–78.
21. Lewis G, Ioannidis K, van Harmelen AL, Neufeld S, Stochl J, Lewis G, et al. The association between pubertal status and depressive symptoms and diagnoses in adolescent females: a population-based cohort study. PLoS One. 2018;13(6):e0198804.
22. Mendle J, Ryan RM, McKone KMP. Age at menarche, depression, and antisocial behavior in adulthood. Pediatrics. 2018;141(1):e20171703.
23. McDonald KL, Bowker JC, Rubin KH, Laursen B, Duchene MS. Interactions between rejection sensitivity and supportive relationships in the prediction of adolescents' internalizing difficulties. J Youth Adolesc. 2010;39(5):563–74.
24. Purdie V, Downey G. Rejection sensitivity and adolescent girls' vulnerability to relationship-centered difficulties. Child Maltreat. 2000;5(4):338–49.
25. LoParo D, Fonseca AC, Matos AP, Craighead WE. A developmental Cascade analysis of peer rejection, depression, anxiety, and externalizing problems from childhood through young adulthood. Res Child Adolesc Psychopathol. 2023;51(9):1303–14.
26. Marston EG, Hare A, Allen JP. Rejection sensitivity in late adolescence: social and emotional sequelae: rejection sensitivity in late adolescence. J Res Adolesc. 2010;20(4):959–82.
27. Liotti G, Intreccialagli B. Los sistemas comportamentales interpersonales en la relación terapéutica. Rev Psicoter. 1996;7(26–27):13–24.
28. Eschenbeck H, Kohlmann CW, Lohaus A. Gender differences in coping strategies in children and adolescents. J Individ Differ. 2007;28(1):18–26.
29. Hobfoll SE, Dunahoo CL, Ben-Porath Y, Monnier J. Gender and coping: the dual-axis model of coping. Am J Community Psychol. 1994;22(1):49–82.

30. Kumpfer KL, Smith P, Summerhays JF. A wakeup call to the prevention field: are prevention programs for substance use effective for girls? Subst Use Misuse. 2008;43(8–9):978–1001.
31. Friedrich A, Mendez L, Mihalas S. Gender as a factor in school-based mental health service delivery. Sch Psych Rev. 2010;39(1):122–36.
32. Diamond GM, Diamond GS, Levy S, Closs C, Ladipo T, Siqueland L. Attachment-based family therapy for suicidal lesbian, gay, and bisexual adolescents: a treatment development study and open trial with preliminary findings. Psychotherapy. 2012;49(1):62–71.
33. Lucassen M, Merry S, Hatcher S, Frampton C(. Rainbow SPARX: a novel approach to addressing depression in sexual minority youth. Cogn Behav Pract 2015;22(2):203–216.
34. Craig S, Austin A. The AFFIRM open pilot feasibility study: a brief affirmative cognitive behavioral coping skills group intervention for sexual and gender minority youth. Child Youth Serv Rev. 2016;64:136–44.
35. Arnold EM, Kirk RS, Roberts AC, Griffith DP, Meadows K, Julian J. Treatment of incarcerated, sexually-abused adolescent females: an outcome study. J Child Sex Abuse. 2003;12(1):123–39.
36. O'Callaghan P, McMullen J, Shannon C, Rafferty H, Black A. A randomized controlled trial of trauma-focused cognitive behavioral therapy for sexually exploited, war-affected Congolese girls. J Am Acad Child Adolesc Psychiatry. 2013;52(4):359–69.
37. Smith DK, Chamberlain P, Deblinger E. Adapting multidimensional treatment foster care for the treatment of co-occurring trauma and delinquency in adolescent girls. J Child Adolesc Trauma. 2012;5(3):224–38.
38. Suarez E, Jackson DS, Slavin LA, Michels MS, McGeehan KM. Project Kealahou: improving Hawai'i's system of care for at-risk girls and young women through gender-responsive, trauma-informed care. Hawaii J Med Public Health J Asia Pac Med Public Health. 2014;73(12):387–92.
39. Whaling KM, der Sarkissian A, Sharkey J, Akoni LC. Featured counter-trafficking program: resiliency interventions for sexual exploitation (RISE). Child Abuse Negl. 2020;100:104139.
40. Bird EL, Halliwell E, Diedrichs PC, Harcourt D. Happy being me in the UK: a controlled evaluation of a school-based body image intervention with pre-adolescent children. Body Image. 2013;10(3):326–34.
41. Weigel A, Gumz A, Uhlenbusch N, Wegscheider K, Romer G, Löwe B. Preventing eating disorders with an interactive gender-adapted intervention program in schools: study protocol of a randomized controlled trial. BMC Psychiatry. 2015;15(1):21.
42. Gumz A, Weigel A, Daubmann A, Wegscheider K, Romer G, Löwe B. Efficacy of a prevention program for eating disorders in schools: a cluster-randomized controlled trial. BMC Psychiatry. 2017;17(1):293.
43. Adametz L, Richter F, Strauss B, Walther M, Wick K, Berger U. Long-term effectiveness of a school-based primary prevention program for anorexia nervosa: a 7-to 8-year follow-up. Eat Behav. 2017;25:42–50.
44. Goldstein NES, Giallella CL, Haney-Caron E, Peterson L, Serico J, Kemp K, et al. Juvenile Justice Anger Management (JJAM) treatment for girls: results of a randomized controlled trial. Psychol Serv. 2018;15(4):386–97.
45. Pepler D, Walsh M, Yuile A, Levene K, Jiang D, Vaughan A, et al. Bridging the gender gap: interventions with aggressive girls and their parents. Prev Sci. 2010;11(3):229–38.
46. Cummings AL, Hoffman S, Leschied AW. A psychoeducational group for aggressive adolescent girls. J Spec Group Work. 2004;29(3):285–99.
47. Elliot DL, Goldberg L, Moe EL, DeFrancesco CA, Durham MB, Hix-Small H. Preventing substance use and disordered eating: initial outcomes of the ATHENA (Athletes Targeting Healthy Exercise and Nutrition Alternatives) program. Arch Pediatr Adolesc Med. 2004;158(11):1043.
48. Fang L, Schinke SP. Two-year outcomes of a randomized, family-based substance use prevention trial for Asian American adolescent girls. Psychol Addict Behav. 2013;27(3):788–98.
49. Goldberg L, MacKinnon DP, Elliot DL, Moe EL, Clarke G, Cheong J. The adolescents training and learning to avoid steroids program: preventing drug use and promoting health behaviors. Arch Pediatr Adolesc Med. 2000;154(4):332.

50. Heider J, Fleck A, Peteler C, Anker S, Lieb S, Behrens M, et al. Dialektisch-Behaviorale Therapie für männliche Jugendliche mit Symptomen einer Borderline-Persönlichkeitsstörung. Prax Kinderpsychol Kinderpsychiatr. 2017;66(2):104–20.
51. Al Odhayani A, Watson WJ, Watson L. Behavioural consequences of child abuse. Can Fam Physician Med Fam Can. 2013;59(8):831–6.
52. Aparicio-Martinez P, Perea-Moreno AJ, Martinez-Jimenez MP, Redel-Macías MD, Pagliari C, Vaquero-Abellan M. Social media, thin-ideal, body dissatisfaction and disordered eating attitudes: an exploratory analysis. Int J Environ Res Public Health. 2019;16(21):4177.
53. Baron-Cohen S, Lombardo MV, Auyeung B, Ashwin E, Chakrabarti B, Knickmeyer R. Why are autism spectrum conditions more prevalent in males? PLoS Biol. 2011;9(6):e1001081.

Transcultural Mental Health Care and Gender: Specific Challenges for Migrant and Refugee Women

28

Melav Bari

Women with a migration and refugee background belong to the most vulnerable groups in terms of psychological stress. They experience an exceptionally high burden of mental health disorders, with significantly elevated rates of depression, anxiety, and post-traumatic stress disorder (PTSD) compared to the general population. Multiple studies have confirmed that this population is disproportionately affected by psychological distress due to pre-migration trauma, gender-based violence, forced displacement, and post-migration stressors [4, 7].

Studies indicate that between 30% and 65% of refugee and migrant women suffer from PTSD, a stark contrast to the 1–3% prevalence in the general population [7]. Depression is also widespread, affecting 40–55% of refugee women, while the prevalence in the general population is estimated at only 7–10%. Similarly, 30–50% of refugee women experience anxiety disorders, including generalized anxiety disorder and panic disorder [4].

Research further indicates that women are disproportionately affected by these disorders compared to refugee and migrant men, primarily due to higher exposure to gender-based violence, sexual exploitation, and structural inequalities in host countries [7].

While these figures apply to refugee and migrant women in general, research highlights that perinatal women are particularly vulnerable. One study found that rates of perinatal depression and PTSD among migrant women were significantly higher than in non-migrant populations, illustrating the added burden during pregnancy and the postnatal period [30].

M. Bari (✉)
University Medical Center Hamburg-Eppendorf and Centra – Coordinating centre for traumatised refugees, Hamburg, Germany
e-mail: m.bari@uke.de

M. López-Atanes, M. Sáenz-Herrero (eds.), *Applying the Gender Perspective in Psychiatry and Psychotherapy*, https://doi.org/10.1007/978-3-032-17883-1_28

28.1 Transcultural Psychiatry and Psychotherapy

Transculturality describes the dynamic interactions between cultures, which are no longer perceived as closed, homogeneous units but rather as overlapping and interconnected systems. In the context of psychiatry and psychotherapy, this means that mental health, concepts of illness, and therapeutic approaches exist within an intercultural field of tension and are shaped by migration processes, hybrid cultures, and cultural plurality [17].

While intercultural psychiatry primarily focuses on acknowledging and accommodating cultural differences, transcultural psychiatry takes a more integrative approach, viewing culture as a fluid, interactive, and evolving system. It incorporates diverse cultural perspectives into diagnosis, treatment, and the therapeutic relationship, emphasizing the influence of global interconnectedness and migration on mental health care [24].

In the psychotherapeutic context, transculturality implies that patients may develop multiple, intersecting cultural identities that should be recognized and addressed in therapy. Mental health disorders are not only shaped by biological and individual factors but also by cultural background, migration experiences, and societal narratives [9]. A flexible, culturally adaptive approach is essential, as rigid cultural frameworks may fail to capture the complexities of identity and mental health in an increasingly interconnected world [1].

28.2 Migrant and Refugee Women

The experiences of migrant and refugee women are characterized by multiple trauma extending across various phases of their lives [4]. This phenomenon is a result of a range of interacting factors spanning the entire migration process: pre-migratory stressors in their countries of origin, traumatic experiences during displacement, and post-migratory challenges in host countries. These stressors often interact cumulatively, significantly impairing mental health [22].

28.2.1 Pre-Migratory Stressors

Before fleeing their countries, many women are already exposed to extreme forms of violence, oppression, and systemic discrimination. In conflict-affected regions, they frequently experience sexual violence, torture, forced displacement, domestic abuse, and forced marriages. Research indicates that up to 70% of refugee women from war zones have experienced sexual violence [2]. The psychological consequences of these traumatic events often include chronic stress, dissociation, and long-term emotional dysregulation, especially when there is no access to mental health support [23].

A particularly harmful pre-migratory experience is female genital mutilation (FGM). FGM, deeply rooted in cultural and social norms in several regions, causes lasting physical and psychological harm. Women who have undergone FGM are at a significantly higher risk for PTSD, depression, and anxiety disorders [16]. The psychological impact of FGM is often compounded by persistent pain, sexual dysfunction, and difficulties during childbirth, leading to chronic distress and re-traumatization, especially in medical and gynecological settings [13].

28.2.2 Traumatic Experiences During Displacement

The migration journey itself is marked by violence, exploitation, and inhumane conditions while fleeing their home countries, which intensify existing trauma. Women are especially vulnerable to human trafficking, sexual assault by smugglers or border officials, and abuse in transit camps. Estimates suggest that up to 50% of refugee women experience sexual violence during displacement [12].

In addition, many women are forced to leave behind their families, leading to profound grief, loss, and loneliness. Family separation often intensifies the emotional trauma, particularly for those who have lost partners or children due to war or violence [11].

The prolonged uncertainty in transit countries further exacerbates mental health problems. Many women spend months or even years in limbo, facing legal and social insecurity, poor living conditions, and limited access to healthcare. Such conditions contribute to a constant state of fear and helplessness, which can lead to persistent anxiety, hypervigilance, and emotional numbing—key symptoms of PTSD. Chronic exposure to stressors during migration can also affect emotional regulation and increase vulnerability to long-term psychiatric disorders [6].

28.2.3 Post-migratory Stressors in the Host Country

Upon arrival in the host country, refugee and migrant women often expect safety, support, and stability. However, post-migratory stressors frequently become a new source of psychological distress, making the recovery process difficult. One of the most significant challenges is the uncertainty of asylum procedures. Lengthy and complex asylum procedures leave many women in a state of chronic insecurity, preventing them from establishing a sense of normality and exacerbating symptoms of stress, anxiety, and depression.

Social isolation is another key factor. Language barriers, cultural differences, and a lack of social support networks often lead to marginalization and disconnection from society. Many struggle to access healthcare and mental health services due to structural barriers and a lack of culturally sensitive care [12]. Without adequate support, many women experience hopelessness and withdrawal.

Discrimination and racism also play a significant role in the deterioration of mental health. Refugee women often face structural inequalities in employment, healthcare, and social interactions. Experiences of exclusion can reinforce feelings of inferiority, helplessness, and chronic stress, increasing the risk of psychosomatic symptoms and psychiatric disorders [22].

Another concerning factor is the persistence of domestic violence after migration. Economic stress, cultural expectations regarding gender roles, and difficulties in adjusting to a new society can intensify intimate partner violence in migrant communities. Many women remain in abusive relationships due to financial dependence, legal uncertainties, or social stigma. The continued exposure to domestic violence further deteriorates mental health and often leads to chronic trauma, suicidal ideation, and substance abuse [8].

For survivors of FGM, post-migratory stressors can be severe. Many experience re-traumatization in medical settings, as gynecological exams, pregnancy, and childbirth may resurface memories of their initial trauma. Additionally, living in a country where FGM is outlawed and widely condemned can create internal conflicts, shame, and identity struggles for some women, particularly if they still have ties to communities that support the practice [27].

28.3 Challenges in Psychiatric and Psychotherapeutic Care

The stigmatization of mental illness is one of the most significant barriers preventing refugee women from accessing psychiatric and psychotherapeutic care. In many countries of origin, deeply rooted cultural beliefs associate mental disorders with negative stereotypes, shame, and social exclusion [7]. Women experiencing psychological distress often hide their symptoms to avoid social isolation or family conflict. Fear of being labeled as “mentally ill” can prevent them from seeking professional help, leading to delayed diagnoses and untreated psychiatric conditions.

28.3.1 Concealed Symptoms and Alternative Coping Strategies

Due to social and cultural stigma, many refugee women do not openly acknowledge or discuss their psychological symptoms. Instead of seeking psychiatric or psychotherapeutic care, they often turn to alternative healing methods, such as spiritual practices, religious rituals, or traditional healers [26]. As a result, mental health conditions often remain undiagnosed until they manifest as chronic psychosomatic symptoms or severe trauma-related disorders.

A systematic review found that in several migrant communities, mental disorders are not recognized as medical conditions but rather perceived as spiritual, moral, or social problems [10]. For instance, in some cultures, depression is not considered a psychiatric disorder but rather a loss of balance between body and soul or even punishment for past misdeeds. These beliefs affect both the perception of illness and the acceptance of treatment, as Western psychiatric and psychotherapeutic models are often seen as incompatible with these cultural explanations.

28.3.2 Fear of Social Exclusion and Negative Consequences

In addition to personal barriers, social stigma within migrant communities also discourages refugee women from seeking professional mental health care. Many women fear that a psychiatric diagnosis or attending therapy could compromise their social standing within their families and communities [7]. In traditional societies where a woman's social status can limit marriage opportunities, mental disorders may be seen as a disadvantage or weakness that reduces her value. One major reason is the fear that a mental health diagnosis could reduce their chances of getting married. Additionally, they worry about being labeled as "crazy" or "incapable" by others. Seeking help for mental illness may also be seen as conflicting with cultural expectations that emphasize resilience and inner strength [3].

This fear of social rejection often leads women to deny or suppress their symptoms, seeking medical care only when their psychiatric condition significantly affects their daily functioning. This poses a serious risk for chronic PTSD, major depression, and suicidal crises.

28.3.3 Lack of Trust in Psychiatric and Psychotherapeutic Services

Besides social stigma, many refugee and migrant women experience a general distrust of psychiatric and psychotherapeutic treatments, particularly when treatment models seem incompatible with cultural beliefs. Women with a history of forced migration may view Western psychiatric models as too individualistic or incompatible with their cultural values [15].

In some countries of origin, psychiatric institutions are associated with social control, coercion, or poor healthcare quality. Past experiences with authoritarian regimes that misused psychiatric diagnoses for political repression may further contribute to a lack of trust in mental health services [18].

Additionally, some women express hesitation about being prescribed psychotropic medication, fearing dependency or loss of control. Concerns about confidentiality also play a crucial role—especially in close-knit communities where trust in institutions may be low. Women often worry that sensitive information shared in therapy might not remain private. Finally, there is often significant uncertainty regarding the purpose and outcomes of psychotherapy, as well as a general lack of knowledge about therapeutic methods. These doubts can foster mistrust and prevent engagement with mental health services [19].

Moreover, language barriers often reinforce distrust in psychiatric care. If professional interpreters are not available and untrained family members act as translators, misunderstandings and cultural taboos can make open communication difficult [10].

28.4 Improving Psychiatric and Psychotherapeutic Care for Refugee and Migrant Women

28.4.1 Addressing Stigma and Cultural Interpretations of Illness

Stigmatization of mental illness is a key reason why many refugee women avoid psychiatric services. In several countries of origin, mental disorders are associated with weakness, spiritual failure, or moral transgression. A psychiatric diagnosis may compromise social standing or marriage prospects, especially in conservative communities. Therefore, psychoeducation tailored to cultural contexts is essential. These interventions must legitimize mental health care and actively challenge harmful illness attributions [21].

Moreover, cultural interpretations of psychological distress must be taken seriously. In many cultures, depression and anxiety are expressed somatically or interpreted through religious and spiritual frameworks. Rather than dismissing these perspectives, clinicians must engage with them and offer integrative approaches that combine scientifically grounded approaches with cultural relevance [14].

28.4.2 Language, Communication, and Trust

Communication challenges are a frequent source of misdiagnosis, therapeutic breakdown, and disengagement. Refugee women often face difficulties articulating symptoms due to limited language proficiency. When untrained family members are used as interpreters, confidentiality, autonomy, and therapeutic alliance are compromised [20].

To build trust and ensure accurate care, systems must offer professional, gender-matched, and trauma-informed interpreters trained specifically for mental health contexts [25].

28.4.3 Gender-Responsive Therapeutic Structures

The gender of therapists and the safety of the setting are critical factors in the treatment of women with trauma histories. Many survivors of sexual violence, domestic abuse, or trafficking are unwilling to participate in mixed-gender therapy or male-led sessions [28].

Research consistently shows that access to female therapists, women-only therapy groups, and trauma-informed protocols increases participation and improves outcomes [31]. Flexible service models such as mother-child programs, mobile clinics, and on-site counseling in shelters further reduce access barriers.

28.4.4 Community-Based and Culturally Adapted Approaches

Cultural competence goes beyond translation. Therapists must be trained in cultural humility, understand patients' value systems, and respect non-Western healing practices. Incorporating traditional belief systems or involving spiritual leaders, where appropriate, may enhance engagement.

Community-based peer support programs, such as those led by trained facilitators with shared backgrounds, foster trust and bridge cultural gaps. Programs like Mind-Spring (the Netherlands) and Project Refugio (Berlin, Germany) have demonstrated the effectiveness of such approaches in improving psychological resilience and service utilization [5, 29].

28.4.5 Interdisciplinary Best Practices

Comprehensive care for refugee women must include legal, social, medical, and psychological dimensions. Interdisciplinary centers integrate psychotherapy with legal aid, social services, and interpretation. Evaluations confirm that this model reduces treatment delays and builds trust [5].

Such collaborative structures allow professionals to coordinate care and address the multifaceted needs of women affected by displacement, trauma, and structural vulnerability.

28.4.6 Empowerment and Participatory Models

Lasting improvement in mental health care must involve the active participation of refugee women. Participatory research and co-creation models allow women to contribute to the design, delivery, and evaluation of services. Empowering women as peer supporters, cultural mediators, or health trainers builds trust and ensures that interventions reflect community realities [10, 19]. These roles also provide avenues for social inclusion, self-efficacy, and long-term empowerment.

28.5 Conclusion

Refugee and migrant women are among the most vulnerable groups in mental health care, yet their specific burdens often remain unrecognized in clinical practice. Their lives are shaped by the intersection of gender-based violence, forced displacement, cultural dislocation, and structural inequality. These women frequently endure multiple, overlapping traumas—both before, during, and after migration—while navigating unfamiliar and often inaccessible mental health systems. Despite their strength and resilience, they encounter profound barriers to care, including stigma, language obstacles, and culturally mismatched therapeutic approaches.

Addressing these challenges requires a fundamental rethinking of psychiatric and psychotherapeutic care—one that centers on culture, gender, and context. Cultural identity profoundly shapes how psychological distress is experienced, expressed, and understood. Concepts of illness, healing, and personal suffering are deeply embedded in cultural traditions, narratives, and spiritual frameworks. Transcultural sensitivity is therefore not an optional addition to care but a foundational principle. Respecting and engaging with diverse cultural perspectives enables clinicians to recognize alternative understandings of trauma, to avoid pathologizing culturally rooted coping strategies, and to establish trust with women whose worldviews may differ significantly from Western clinical norms.

Effective mental health support must be intersectional, trauma-informed, and structurally inclusive. This includes training clinicians in gender- and culturally responsive approaches, offering access to female therapists and professional interpreters, and building flexible therapeutic settings that feel emotionally safe and accessible. It also calls for community-based peer programs that reflect cultural realities, and for interdisciplinary models that integrate psychological, social, medical, and legal support. Crucially, refugee women themselves must be included in the design and evaluation of mental health services so that care is not only provided for them, but shaped with them.

By embedding these values—cultural humility, gender awareness, and participatory care—into mental health frameworks, systems can begin to close the gap between institutional offerings and lived experience. In doing so, we move closer to a model of care that fosters healing, empowerment, and social inclusion for one of the most underserved and yet remarkably resilient groups in psychiatric care.

References

1. Antić A. Transcultural psychiatry: cultural difference, universalism and social psychiatry in the age of decolonisation. Cult Med Psychiatry. 2021;45(3):359–84. https://doi.org/10.1007/s11013-021-09719-4.
2. Blackmore R, Boyle JA, Fazel M, Ranasinha S, Gray KM, Fitzgerald G, Misso M, Gibson-Helm M. The prevalence of mental illness in refugees and asylum seekers: a systematic review and meta-analysis. PLoS Med. 2020;17(9):e1003337. https://doi.org/10.1371/journal.pmed.1003337.
3. Boettcher VS, Nowak AC, Neuner F. Mental health service utilization and perceived barriers to treatment among adult refugees in Germany. Eur J Psychotraumatol. 2021;12(1):1910407. https://doi.org/10.1080/20008198.2021.1910407.
4. Bohland HK, Kimbel R, Kegel P, Dietz P, Koestner C, Letzel S, Kurmeyer C, Jesuthasan J, Schouler-Ocak M, Zier U. Depression and anxiety in female refugees from East Africa and the Middle East displaced to Germany: cross-sectional results of the female refugee study, taking sociodemographic and migration-related factors into account. Front Psychol. 2024;14:1303009. https://doi.org/10.3389/fpsyt.2023.1303009.
5. Bundesweite Arbeitsgemeinschaft der Psychosozialen Zentren für Flüchtlinge und Folteropfer (BAfF). Versorgungsbericht 2024: Psychosoziale Versorgung für Geflüchtete und Überlebende von Folter in Deutschland. Berlin; 2024.

6. Collins CH, Zimmerman C, Howard LM. Refugee, asylum seeker, immigrant women and postnatal depression: rates and risk factors. Arch Womens Ment Health. 2011;14(1):3–11. https://doi.org/10.1007/s00737-010-0198-7.
7. DeSa S, Gebremeskel AT, Omonaiye O, Yaya S. Barriers and facilitators to access mental health services among refugee women in high-income countries: a systematic review. Syst Rev. 2022;11(1):62. https://doi.org/10.1186/s13643-022-01936-1.
8. Fellmeth G, Fazel M, Plugge E. Migration and perinatal mental health in women from low- and middle-income countries: a systematic review and meta-analysis. BJOG Int J Obstet Gynaecol. 2017;124(5):742–52. https://doi.org/10.1111/1471-0528.14184.
9. Grau L, Carretier E, Moro M-R, Revah-Levy A, Sibeoni J, Lachal J. A qualitative exploration of what works for migrant adolescents in transcultural psychotherapy: perceptions of adolescents, their parents, and their therapists. BMC Psychiatry. 2020;20(1):564. https://doi.org/10.1186/s12888-020-02970-w.
10. Gruner D, Magwood O, Bair L, Duff L, Adel S, Pottie K. Understanding supporting and hindering factors in community-based psychotherapy for refugees: a realist-informed systematic review. Int J Environ Res Public Health. 2020;17(13):Article 13. https://doi.org/10.3390/ijerph17134618.
11. Hameed S, Sadiq A, Din AU. The increased vulnerability of refugee population to mental health disorders. Kans J Med. 2018;11(1):20–3.
12. Hollander A-C, Bruce D, Burström B, Ekblad S. Gender-related mental health differences between refugees and non-refugee immigrants—a cross-sectional register-based study. BMC Public Health. 2011;11(1):180. https://doi.org/10.1186/1471-2458-11-180.
13. Im H, Swan LET, Heaton L. Polyvictimization and mental health consequences of female genital mutilation/circumcision (FGM/C) among Somali refugees in Kenya. Women Health. 2020;60(6):636–51. https://doi.org/10.1080/03630242.2019.1689543.
14. Kirmayer LJ, Narasiah L, Munoz M, Rashid M, Ryder AG, Guzder J, Hassan G, Rousseau C, Pottie K. Common mental health problems in immigrants and refugees: general approach in primary care. CMAJ. 2011;183(12):E959–67. https://doi.org/10.1503/cmaj.090292.
15. Kiselev N, Morina N, Schick M, Watzke B, Schnyder U, Pfaltz MC. Barriers to access to outpatient mental health care for refugees and asylum seekers in Switzerland: the therapist's view. BMC Psychiatry. 2020;20(1):378. https://doi.org/10.1186/s12888-020-02783-x.
16. Knipscheer J, Vloeberghs E, van der Kwaak A, van den Muijsenbergh M. Mental health problems associated with female genital mutilation. BJPsych Bull. 2015;39(6):273–7. https://doi.org/10.1192/pb.bp.114.047944.
17. Mahon D. Transcultural considerations. In: Cooper DB, editor. Alcohol use: assessment, withdrawal management, treatment and therapy: ethical practice. Springer; 2023. p. S. 33–55. https://doi.org/10.1007/978-3-031-18381-2_3.
18. Nyikavaranda P, Pantelic M, Jones CJ, Paudyal P, Tunks A, Llewellyn CD. Barriers and facilitators to seeking and accessing mental health support in primary care and the community among female migrants in Europe: a "feminisms" systematic review. Int J Equity Health. 2023;22(1):196. https://doi.org/10.1186/s12939-023-01990-8.
19. O'mahony J, Donnelly T. Immigrant and refugee women's post-partum depression help-seeking experiences and access to care: a review and analysis of the literature. J Psychiatr Ment Health Nurs. 2010;17(10):917–28. https://doi.org/10.1111/j.1365-2850.2010.01625.x.
20. Orang TM, Missmahl I, Thoele A-M, Valensise L, Brenner A, Gardisi M, Peter H, Kluge U. New directions in the mental health care of migrants, including refugees—a randomized controlled trial investigating the efficacy of value-based counselling. Clin Psychol Psychother. 2022;29(4):1433–46. https://doi.org/10.1002/cpp.2728.
21. Palic S, Elklit A. Psychosocial treatment of posttraumatic stress disorder in adult refugees: a systematic review of prospective treatment outcome studies and a critique. J Affect Disord. 2011;131(1):8–23. https://doi.org/10.1016/j.jad.2010.07.005.
22. Patanè M, Ghane S, Karyotaki E, Cuijpers P, Schoonmade L, Tarsitani L, Sijbrandij M. Prevalence of mental disorders in refugees and asylum seekers: a systematic review and meta-analysis. Global Ment Health. 2022;9:250–63. https://doi.org/10.1017/gmh.2022.29.

23. Rees SJ, Fisher JR, Steel Z, Mohsin M, Nadar N, Moussa B, Hassoun F, Yousif M, Krishna Y, Khalil B, Mugo J, Tay AK, Klein L, Silove D. Prevalence and risk factors of major depressive disorder among women at public antenatal clinics from refugee, conflict-affected, and Australian-born backgrounds. JAMA Netw Open. 2019;2(5):e193442. https://doi.org/10.1001/jamanetworkopen.2019.3442.
24. Robinson DM, Otonichar J, Torbey S, Moreno M, Merkel RL. From transcultural psychiatry to global mental health: the development of a global mental health program at the Department of Psychiatry and Neurobehavioral Sciences at the University of Virginia. In: Okpaku SO, editor. Innovations in global mental health. Springer; 2021. p. S. 633–53. https://doi.org/10.1007/978-3-030-57296-9_70.
25. Sander R, Laugesen H, Skammeritz S, Mortensen EL, Carlsson J. Interpreter-mediated psychotherapy with trauma-affected refugees—a retrospective cohort study. Psychiatry Res. 2019;271:684–92. https://doi.org/10.1016/j.psychres.2018.12.058.
26. Satinsky E, Fuhr DC, Woodward A, Sondorp E, Roberts B. Mental health care utilisation and access among refugees and asylum seekers in Europe: a systematic review. Health Policy. 2019;123(9):851–63. https://doi.org/10.1016/j.healthpol.2019.02.007.
27. Schouler-Ocak M, Moreno Leguizamon C, Kenneth Moran J, Sharif-Ali K, Gole J. Listening to refugee and vulnerable migrant women of Somali origin about the bodily and psychosocial consequences of female genital mutilation in Germany. Int J Arts Humanit Soc Sci (IJAHSS). 2022;3(11):Article 11. https://doi.org/10.56734/ijahss.v3n11a3.
28. Slobodin O, de Jong JT. Mental health interventions for traumatized asylum seekers and refugees: what do we know about their efficacy? Int J Soc Psychiatry. 2015;61(1):17–26. https://doi.org/10.1177/0020764014535752.
29. Sonne C, Carlsson J, Bech P, Elklit A, Mortensen EL. Treatment of trauma-affected refugees with venlafaxine versus sertraline combined with psychotherapy—a randomised study. BMC Psychiatry. 2016;16(1):383. https://doi.org/10.1186/s12888-016-1081-5.
30. Stevenson K, Fellmeth G, Edwards S, Calvert C, Bennett P, Campbell OMR, Fuhr DC. The global burden of perinatal common mental health disorders and substance use among migrant women: a systematic review and meta-analysis. Lancet Public Health. 2023;8(3):e203–16. https://doi.org/10.1016/S2468-2667(22)00342-5.
31. Taknint JT, Thomas FC, Gellatly R, Ameresekere M. Responding to trauma: a critical review of mental health and psychosocial interventions for refugee women. Curr Psychiatry Rep. 2024;26(12):866–76. https://doi.org/10.1007/s11920-024-01568-3.

On Mental Health in the LGBTQ+ Community

29

Marcus Rautenberg

29.1 Introduction

According to representative surveys [1] among 18–74-year-olds in 30 countries, up to 18% of Generation Z respondents identify as part of the LGBTQ+ community. The figures vary significantly by generation (11% for Millennials, 6% for Generation X, and 5% for Baby Boomers). Across all generations and countries, about 9% of respondents identify with LGBTQ+ regarding sexual orientation, and around 3% in terms of gender identity.

Although studies show high acceptance of the LGBTQ+ community and specific rights such as marriage and adoption in many countries (around 70% in Germany), many LGBTQ+ individuals in these countries still face everyday discrimination [2]. For example, in Germany—a country generally considered "queer-friendly"—over 80% of young people report experiencing discrimination due to their sexual orientation or gender identity at least once [3, 4].

Studies indicate that LGBTQ+ individuals are subject to numerous stress factors, including concealing their sexual or gender identity, facing rejection in family or social environments, and even experiencing violence. International studies suggest these stress factors lead to increased psychological vulnerability [5–7], commonly known as "minority stress."

This consistently reported elevated psychological vulnerability is likely also due to the absence of protective factors that usually support psychological resilience. In the LGBTQ+ community, such typical supports—like social acceptance from family or peer groups, or resources from work and leisure—are often missing (for more on resilience, see Ref. [8]). Consequently, the described high vulnerability often

M. Rautenberg (✉)
University Outpatient Clinic of the RPTU, Landau, Germany
e-mail: mail@psybera.org

M. López-Atanes, M. Sáenz-Herrero (eds.), *Applying the Gender Perspective in Psychiatry and Psychotherapy*, https://doi.org/10.1007/978-3-032-17883-1_29

leads to a significantly higher prevalence of mental health issues, and some studies indicate an increase in somatic illnesses as well (for an international overview, see Ref. [9]).

29.2 Psychotherapeutic Implications

Although the legal situation for LGBTQ+ individuals has improved significantly in many countries, studies suggest that general health care, including mental health services, has not yet adapted sufficiently to reflect these positive changes and the specific needs of affected individuals (for Germany, see Ref. [10]). Pöge et al. (2020) [11] identify a "heteronormative orientation of society" as one reason, as well as insufficient expertise and sensitivity regarding LGBTQ+ health topics. The authors also suggest that "internalized negative attitudes toward one's own gender or sexual orientation" significantly impact mental health, stating, "Gender or sexual orientation itself does not directly cause higher rates of depression or suicidality. Rather, a lack of acceptance, discrimination, and experiences of violence are psychologically stressful and can lead to mental illness" (ibid., pp. 19 ff.).

It should be emphasized that the needs within the LGBTQ+ community vary widely and are far from homogeneous. While one group may focus on issues related to sexual orientation (homosexual, bisexual), others face conflicts related to gender identity (transgender, nonbinary) and thus encounter greater social challenges in a society still "trapped in a binary gender model" [12]. While all may share a need for support in self- and external acceptance of their identities, distinct from hetero- and binary gender norms, transgender and nonbinary individuals often face challenges only after encountering pathologization or barriers within the healthcare system during their transition process (for definitions, see the following overview).

29.2.1 Definition of Terms

Gender Incongruence Describes when a person feels that they do not belong to the gender assigned to them at birth or the one corresponding to their physical sex characteristics.

Gender Dysphoria Refers to the subjective distress experienced due to the lack of alignment between one's biological sex and gender identity. Symptoms can include avoidant behavior, depressive reactions, and other forms of psychological adaptation.

Transition Process Encompasses the entire process from initial awareness of gender incongruence to medical or other measures aimed at reducing gender incongruence. Medical measures primarily include hormone substitution or "gender-affirming" surgeries. In many countries, including Germany, transgender and non-binary individuals are still required to undergo psychotherapy to access transition measures, even in the absence of accompanying mental health issues or complaints.

In fact, the "Standards of Care for the Health of Transsexual, Transgender, and Gender-Nonconforming People" (SOC) by the World Professional Association for Transgender Health (WPATH) [13] provides clear guidelines for appropriate support of transgender and gender nonconforming people within health care. These standards aim for reliable health care with individualized and flexible treatment to reduce distress (for an overview of specific psychotherapeutic support for transgender and nonbinary individuals, see Rautenberg [14] and Fröhlich and Rautenberg [15]). The SOC outlines basic principles that could be adapted to general professional work with LGBTQ+ individuals. These principles, modified by the author, are as follows:

- Treat people with nonhetero-, nonbinary-gender normative identities respectfully (do not pathologize differences in gender identity or sexual orientation).
- Provide treatment options (or refer to knowledgeable colleagues) and acquire expertise on LGBTQ+ health needs.
- Simplify access to appropriate health care.
- Obtain informed consent before beginning treatment and clarify the specific treatment goals.
- Offer continuous support.
- Show readiness to support individuals within their families and social environments (schools, workplaces, and other institutions).

In Germany, the SOC recommendations have largely been incorporated into the "S3-Guideline for the Diagnosis, Counseling, and Treatment of Gender Incongruence, Gender Dysphoria, and Trans Health," developed under the leadership of the "German Society for Sexual Research" (DGfS) [16]. This guideline, created by professional societies, trade, and advocacy groups, includes treatment recommendations and focuses on diagnosis, treatment advice, and psychosocial issues. It also offers general recommendations for psychotherapeutic support that can be applied to all LGBTQ+ individuals (see the following overview).

29.2.2 Recommendations for Psychotherapeutic Support

- Promote self-acceptance, self-esteem, and self-confidence.
- Address feelings of shame, guilt, and internalized trans negativity.
- Support identity development.
- Reflect on and address possible experiences and conflicts.
- Assist with the coming-out process.
- Provide support in making treatment decisions and offering continued guidance.

29.3 Conclusion and Outlook

In countries where the legal situation for LGBTQ+ individuals has improved in recent years, young people are increasingly willing to identify as LGBTQ+, at least in anonymous, representative surveys. Considering an additional unreported number, the global LGBTQ+ population may be significantly larger than previously estimated (at least 20%).

It is alarming that, even in these countries with legal protections and social acceptance, many still report experiences of discrimination and fear coming out, especially to healthcare professionals.

It is imperative to increase sensitivity and incorporate LGBTQ+-specific needs into training for healthcare workers. This would help prevent further pathologization and recognize that many mental health issues are simply reactions to discrimination. For transgender and nonbinary individuals, it is especially important to improve access to supportive treatment.

As professional companions, we should critically reflect on our, perhaps unconscious, hetero- and binary-gender-normative influences and remember what Carl Rogers (1957) described as a necessary condition for psychotherapy: "unconditional positive regard" [19].

References

1. Ipsos | LGBT+ Pride Study 2023, 2024 Global Survey.
2. FRA. LGBTIQ Equality at a Crossroads. 2024. https://fra.europa.eu/sites/default/files/fra_uploads/fra-2024-lgbtiq-equality_en.pdf
3. Krell C, Oldemeier C. „Coming-out – und dann…?!" Coming-out-Verläufe und Diskriminierungserfahrungen von lesbischen, schwulen, bisexuellen, trans* und queeren Jugendlichen und jungen Erwachsenen in Deutschland. 2017.
4. Heiligers N, Frohn D, Timmermanns S, Merz S, Moschner T. „How are you?" Die Lebenssituation von LSBTIQA* Jugendlichen und jungen Erwachsenen in Bayern. Bayerischer Jugendring (Hrsg.). 2023.
5. Meyer IH. Prejudice, social stress, and mental health in lesbian, gay, and bisexual populations: conceptual issues and research evidence. Psychol Bull. 2003;129:674–97. https://doi.org/10.1037/0033-2909.129.5.674.
6. Dürrbaum T, Sattler FA. Minority stress and mental health in lesbian, gay male, and bisexual youths: a meta-analysis. J LGBT Youth. 2020;17:298–314. https://doi.org/10.1080/19361653.2019.1586615.
7. de Lange J, Baams L, van Bergen DD, Bos HMW, Bosker RJ. Minority stress and suicidal ideation and suicide attempts among LGBT adolescents and young adults: a meta-analysis. LGBT Health. 2022;9:222–37. https://doi.org/10.1089/lgbt.2021.0106.
8. Fröhlich-Gildhoff K, Rönnau-Böse M. Resilienz. 5th ed. Stuttgart: UTB; 2019.
9. Hwahng SJ, Kaufman MR, editors. Global LGBTQ Health. Global LGBTQ Health. https://doi.org/10.1007/978-3-031-36204-0_3.
10. Beigang S, Fetz K, Kalkum D, et al. Diskriminierungserfahrungen in Deutschland – Ergebnisse einer Repräsentativ- und einer Betroffenenbefragung. Baden-Baden: Antidiskriminierungsstelle des Bundes; 2017.

11. Pöge K, Dennert G, Koppe U, Güldenring A, Matthigack EB, Rommel A. Die gesundheitliche Lage von lesbischen, schwulen, bisexuellen sowie trans- und intergeschlechtlichen Menschen. J Health Monit. 2020;5(S1):1–30. https://doi.org/10.25646/6448.
12. Sigusch V. Sexuelle Störungen und ihre Behandlung. Göttingen: Vandenhoeck & Ruprecht; 1997.
13. Coleman E, Radix AE, Bouman WP, Brown GR, de Vries ALC, Deutsch MB, Ettner R, Fraser L, Goodman M, Green J, Hancock AB, Johnson TW, Karasic DH, Knudson GA, Leibowitz SF, Meyer-Bahlburg HFL, Monstrey SJ, Motmans J, Nahata L, Nieder TO, Reisner SL, Richards C, Schechter LS, Tangpricha V, Tishelman AC, Van Trotsenburg MAA, Winter S, Ducheny K, Adams NJ, Adrián TM, Allen LR, Azul D, Bagga H, Başar K, Bathory DS, Belinky JJ, Berg DR, Berli JU, Bluebond-Langner RO, Bouman M-B, Bowers ML, Brassard PJ, Byrne J, Capitán L, Cargill CJ, Carswell JM, Chang SC, Chelvakumar G, Corneil T, Dalke KB, De Cuypere G, de Vries E, Den Heijer M, Devor AH, Dhejne C, D'Marco A, Edmiston EK, Edwards-Leeper L, Ehrbar R, Ehrensaft D, Eisfeld J, Elaut E, Erickson-Schroth L, Feldman JL, Fisher AD, Garcia MM, Gijs L, Green SE, Hall BP, Hardy TLD, Irwig MS, Jacobs LA, Janssen AC, Johnson K, Klink DT, Kreukels BPC, Kuper LE, Kvach EJ, Malouf MA, Massey R, Mazur T, McLachlan C, Morrison SD, Mosser SW, Neira PM, Nygren U, Oates JM, Obedin-Maliver J, Pagkalos G, Patton J, Phanuphak N, Rachlin K, Reed T, Rider GN, Ristori J, Robbins-Cherry S, Roberts SA, Rodriguez-Wallberg KA, Rosenthal SM, Sabir K, Safer JD, Scheim AI, Seal LJ, Sehoole TJ, Spencer K, St C, Amand TD, Steensma JF, Strang GB, Taylor K, Tilleman GG, T'Sjoen LN, Vala NM, Van Mello JF, Veale JA, Vencill B, Vincent LM, Wesp MA, West, Arcelus J. Standards of care for the health of transgender and gender diverse people, Version 8. Int J Transgend Health. 2022;23(Sup 1):S1–S259. https://doi.org/10.1080/26895269.2022.2100644.
14. Rautenberg M. Transgender und non-binäre Menschen in der Psychotherapie: Diagnostik, Beratung und Begleitung. Göttingen: Hogrefe; 2022.
15. Fröhlich M, Rautenberg M. Psychotherapeutische Begleitung von Transgender und non-binären Menschen. Ein Manual für die Gruppentherapie. Göttingen: Hogrefe; 2025.
16. AWMF. Geschlechtsinkongruenz, Geschlechtsdysphorie und Trans-Gesundheit: S3-Leitlinie zur Diagnostik, Beratung und Behandlung. 2019.
17. https://dgvn.de/meldung/wie-steht-es-um-die-globale-psychische-gesundheit-ein-ueberblick#:~:text=Laut%20des%20Hohen%20Kommissariats%20der,waren%2C%20um%2025%20Prozent%20zu. Abgerufen am 30.10.2024.
18. Bellach BM, Knopf H, Thefeld W. Der Bundesgesundheitssurvey 1997/98. Gesundheitswesen. 1998;60(2):59–68.
19. Rogers CR. The necessary and sufficient conditions of therapeutic personality change. J Consult Psychol. 1957;21:95–103.

Sexual Violence and Mental Health

30

Sandra Muñoz Sánchez, Marina de la Hermosa Lorenci, and Cristina Polo Usaola

30.1 The Discovery of Sexuality as a Starting Point

30.1.1 Rape Culture and Sexual Consent

The conceptualization of sexual violence has been transformed throughout history due to the sociocultural changes in the domination systems over women [1]. Under the constructs of heteronormativity, feminine pleasure has traditionally been forbidden and scarcely recognized [2], with the consequence that women have behaving according to the physical, psychological, and mental needs of men [3]. Women's bodies and psychic have historically been subjects of fantasized or real violence, and the sexual act between a man and a woman has always been presented as consented due to rape culture.

It was only at the end of the nineteenth century that sexual violence began to be considered under different parameters [4]. Female writers and thinkers with different perspectives addressed this field, making it possible for sexual violence to start being perceived as an attack on the sexual identity of women [5]. Despite all of that, female sexuality today can still be configured as a power structure that produces violence, in which myths that have supported and justified sexual violence as natural and expected by default continue to be perpetuated [6].

In the most recent discourses about sexual violence, sexual consent has been the main reference used to differentiate what we can consider sexual violence. Consent is understood as an act that is free, voluntary, without coercion, deception, or fraud involved. In this act, the person expresses, verbally or not, the will to participate in that sexual activity, and it must be communicated in a way that is recognizable to others. Different thinkers have addressed the complexity of this concept [7, 8] and

S. M. Sánchez (✉) · M. de la Hermosa Lorenci · C. P. Usaola
Hortaleza Mental Health-Care Service, Hospital Ramón y Cajal, Madrid, Spain

M. López-Atanes, M. Sáenz-Herrero (eds.), *Applying the Gender Perspective in Psychiatry and Psychotherapy*, https://doi.org/10.1007/978-3-032-17883-1_30

pointed out the difficulties in establishing clear lines between the acts of consent, giving in, or desiring sexual relationships. That implies that not all the subjective experiences of sexual assault result in an understanding of explicit violence for the victim, and there can be situations in which the violence goes unnoticed or is not fully recognized.

Given the diversity of violence detected in the feminine sexual sphere, it becomes especially relevant to understand the structural character of this type of violence, so that we can analyze in a more integrative way the scope and repercussions of this sexual aggression in the psyche and identity of the victims.

30.2 First Sexual Relationships in Teenagers: A Focus on Sexual Violence

Teenage years are characterized by numerous and strong changes that individuals experience in their interpersonal relationships. At the beginning of the youth, the need to find one's own sense of self emerges, and the sexual and romantic relationships start to be defined for those interested in them. At the same time, with the group codes and values that appear, it becomes more difficult to differentiate and express the expectations, desires, and worries around sexuality. The impact of the gender stereotypes in this relationship dynamics, the idealization and lack of experience in romantic and sexual relationships, implies that female teenagers have a higher vulnerability to gender violence in romantic relationships and/or associated sexual violence.

In the last years, , an incongruence between formal discourse and real-life actions has been observed in teenage population [9]. On the one hand, female teenagers would express a discourse that is apparently more egalitarian around their sexual relationships. On the other hand, there would still be traditional ideas present around the different ways to conceive masculine and feminine sexual freedom. Social media wouldn't be of help to minimize this ambivalence, facilitating the female teenagers to find themselves sometimes in sexual dynamics that situate them in places of vulnerability or risk through new mechanisms, like revenge porn, sextortion, grooming, or more subtle control strategies [10].

In a similar way, the relationship that could exist between mainstream pornography and the learning of sexually violent conducts is present in the actual debate [11]. The use of this type of pornography, in the way that is conceived nowadays, can interfere with beliefs about sexual practices, normalizing acts that imply violence against women or non-desired submissive attitudes for them during sexual experiences. Therefore, normative references for sexual learning could impact the configuration of sexual identities, facilitating unequal sexual dynamics or asymmetric power relationships that promote the exposition of teenage girls to sexual violence.

30.3 Mental Health Consequences of Sexual Violence

In this part, we are going to address the most frequent impacts on the mental health of victims of sexual violence. We would like to specify that in this chapter, we understand victim as any cis or trans woman, with diverse coexistent identity components that modulate different subjective experiences of sexual violence.

The impact of sexual violence on the mental health of the victims has traditionally been invisibilized by different disciplines, but this dynamic has changed in the last decades, and there are several publications that address the consequences of sexual violence on the mental and physical health of women [12].

Even though there can be common characteristics in the victims of this type of violence, it is important to demystify and question the universality of these characteristics, because factors like age, frequency of aggressions, substance abuse, traumatic antecedents, or the reaction of the environment can have an important impact on the type of mental health consequences and their intensity. We also need to take into account that the consequences can appear not immediately after the aggression, making the difference between short- and long-term signs, although in many cases they can overlap.

30.4 Short-Term and Medium/Long-Term Consequences

One of the clinical diagnoses more frequently used in short-term cases of sexual violence is acute stress disorder [13], which can regularly appear with feelings of fear, shame, anger, or guilt. Attending to the guilt feeling, there are two types that have been differentiated: behavioral guilt and character guilt. The first one appears when the person thinks that the violent act was triggered by their own behavior, the second one is more related to self-esteem and identity, and the person feels guilty because of their own way of being. In the case of the victims of sexual violence, the behavioral guilt is more frequent. However, if the violence appears in a reiterated way, the characterial guilt would be more present.

On the other hand, the immobilization or paralysis reactions are the most frequently ignored in nonclinical contexts. This lack of knowledge has contributed to the lack of credibility and/or blaming of the victims, because this type of reaction was not understood in a situation of sexual aggression. Even though this mechanism has been explained through the theory named the Polyvagal theory by Porges [14], which gets activated in situations of threat that exceed the vital resources of the person, as it happens with rape victims.

In this context, it would be interesting to take into account the concept of epistemic injustice [15], including both testimonial injustice and hermeneutical one. The first one occurs when the knowledge of a person is ignored, or their credibility diminishes because the person belongs to a specific social group, and the second one is described when there are no concepts created that a person can use to identify or put in words their lived experiences. Given that, for years, there did not exist in the social imaginary or in the professional discourse descriptions of the trauma produced by sexual violence, the oppression situation of the victim would have been increased, with the inability to enunciate their experience, provoking a particular effect on the feminine identity and subjectivity [16].

In relation to the midterm and long-term psychological consequences, the most frequent diagnosis for women who have suffered a sexual assault is post-traumatic stress disorder [13]. Although this diagnosis appears to include the effects of the war on soldiers, in the 1970s, it was made visible that the most frequent post-traumatic disorders were not the ones that appeared after a warlike conflict, but the ones suffered by women in all stages of their lives when they experienced gender-related violence [17]. This clinical picture can include dissociative symptoms, affecting memory, identity, or perception.

Besides post-traumatic stress disorder, a higher risk for depression, suicidal attempts, use of substances, anxiety and panic attacks, eating disorders, obsessive compulsive disorder, and bipolar disorder has been described in victims of sexual violence [18]. Taking into account that one of the factors that impacts the most on the severity of the symptoms after the traumatic experience is the reaction that the woman finds in her environment; reactions like being ignored, lack of recognition of her experience, or blame, can make the clinical picture worse and make the recovery more difficult [19].

30.5 Complex Post-Traumatic Stress Disorder and Effects on Social Identity

The concept of complex post-traumatic stress disorder (complex PTSD) was created by Judith Herman in 1992. This concept was developed to hold the psychological consequences experienced by people who suffer from repeated and prolonged interpersonal traumatic experiences, whose symptoms were not represented enough in the diagnosis of post-traumatic stress disorder. Among the consequences listed in this diagnosis, we can include prolonged sexual and psychological abuses, neglect and child abuse, and sexual exploitation. This diagnosis includes alterations in emotional and impulse regulation, attention, consciousness, perception of themselves, perception of the aggressor, in relationships with other people, and in their own system of beliefs in life.

On the other hand, a cultural dimension of trauma has been described too [20]. In sexual aggression, despite what happens to any other victims, the debate is frequently focused on the credibility of the facts, whether there is a manipulation for concrete purposes by the victim, or if there has been consent. These manifestations not only put in question the credibility of the victims, but also the credibility of the professionals who intervene in post-traumatic situations. These difficulties demand that we be aware of the traumatic reality, and there is a need for social movements that give voice to the situations and make their roots visible, without pretending that the survivor victims have to adjust to any given stereotype.

30.6 Specific Forms of Sexual Violence

30.6.1 Particularities of Sexual Violence Within Heterosexual Partnerships

Sexual violence in heterosexual relationships is often invisibilized, and it is frequently not noticed, both in personal and professional contexts. The fact that the perpetrator is the romantic partner contributes to questioning the aggressions, and this type of violence can be more traumatic than when it is perpetrated by unknown men [21]. There is a confusion added in this situation that is not present in other types of abuse, and it can happen for the victim that she thinks that there is an individual sexual issue, instead of identifying themselves as a true victim.

The fact that this violence happens in a context of an interpersonal relationship that is assumed to be a space of love and protection provokes a breach of trust, adding psychological consequences characteristic of this type of violence. More severity in depression has been described, and also a more acute negative self-image, more suicidal ideation, or an increase in the number of suicidal attempts, in comparison to groups of women who have not experienced sexual violence or have not been in a romantic relationship [12, 22]. At the same time, in this context, the vulnerability of women with severe mental health suffering can be increased [23], and other simultaneous forms of violence can happen in the relationship.

30.7 Child Sexual Violence and Its Consequences

Childhood is understood as the period of the vital cycle in which the physical, psychological, and emotional development of a person happens. It is an especially sensitive and vulnerable stage, where every type of sexual contact between a child and an adult is considered abusive by itself, because of the obvious power difference that exists between them [24]. The responsibility of this abusive act would belong exclusively to the adult, because we understand that children are not able to consent to sexual contact because they don't have enough power to refuse, and they are not conscious of the implications of what they would be consenting to [25]. In the cases of intrafamilial violence, added to the traumatic experience itself, the child can also experience the breaking of the bond with the aggressor, and a possible rupture of trust in the family structure as a safe place [24].

The consequences on the mental health of the victims can be diverse, from a severe psychological impact to the absence of negative effects [26, 27]. In a generalized way, victims are going to experience the physical and psychological trauma of this experience through prolonged periods of apprehension, guilt, or fear of losing the attachment to this significant person, in a life stage in which there are no symbolic resources to explain what is happening around them.

Besides, child sexual violence consequences can appear psychologically already in the adult stage [27]. If the victim had an experience of negation and dissociation in childhood, the psychological impact will be more severe [26]. These women would present anxiety, inappropriate sexual worries or behaviors, anger, shame, or guilt throughout their lives [27]. They could have difficulties in their future romantic relationships, in their sexual relationships, or in motherhood [28], and also an increased risk of depression, suicidal attempts, borderline personality disorder, somatization disorders, substance abuse, or eating disorders [29].

In conclusion, it is important to note that child victims of sexual abuse have a higher risk of revictimization as adults, that is, they may have a higher risk of experiencing both sexual and physical violence [30, 31]. Revictimization in women has been connected to the difficulty in acquiring proper defense mechanisms under the post-traumatic consequences of child abuse [5], which is the reason why women with previous experiences of sexual abuse in childhood would have a higher possibility to present depression, post-traumatic stress disorder, substance abuse, or suicidal attempts after suffering a new sexual aggression as adults [18].

30.8 Sexual Violence in Women in Situations of Vulnerability: Severe Mental Illness

Most of the national and international bibliography that we reviewed remarks a higher frequency of all types of gender violence against women with mental health disorders diagnosed. The relationship between these two circumstances is bidirectional; thereby, there has been observed that suffering different types of violence during life, including sexual abuse in childhood, can have a psychological impact connected to the diagnosis of mental health disorders. At the same time, having mental health issues implies an element of vulnerability to be a victim of sexual aggression as an adult, both perpetrated by known people and by romantic and/or sexual partners.

Despite the higher vulnerability that affects these women, both the bibliography and the experience of the authors show that the professionals working in health, law, social services, and other areas give less credibility to women when they have been diagnosed with a severe mental health disorder. This contributes to revictimization and creates a tendency in them to not verbalize these experiences, due to the fear of not being believed.

This lack of credibility is partially connected with the fact that the professionals can attribute their narratives of their abuse experiences to the psychopathology they have been diagnosed with. Their lack of self-esteem, the discourse that can be disorganized, and the difficulties in some cognitive functions can have as a consequence that these narratives that have less appearance of coherence, and present memory gaps. When the perpetrators are their partners, or other apparently caring figures (health professionals included, in some cases), the difficulties for credibility increase. These women can also suffer isolation and a lack of access to information and resources. On the other hand, some professionals who work with these women are afraid that if they make visible violent situations, it can have a negative impact on their mental suffering, a fear that lacks scientific support.

30.9 Other Psychosocial Factors that Enhance Sexual Violence

In these places where the prevalence of sexual violence is higher, there are also higher rates of other types of violence [32]. Therefore, it would be important to reflect on the psychosocial factors that can enhance or mitigate this type of violence, because depending on the environment, the social structure, or identity variables, sexual violence could be enhanced, avoided, and/or prevented.

We think that, in order to do that analysis, we need to take into account the concept of intersectionality, a theoretical approach that remarks that gender, race, class, age, or sexual orientation (within other social categories) are factors that relate to each other in order to enhance the places of privilege and oppression depending on the context.

The female racialized thinkers put into relevance the sexism, classism, and racism that would have been promoted through history in thinking lines that were far from the recognition of the social reality of black women, invisibilizing the needs and fights of poor and racially oppressed women [33]. From the hegemonic white context, the masculine norm would have taken over the female racialized body to appropriate the erotization of their black bodies and turn them into their own object of desire.

On the other hand, gender and class would also be complementary dimensions in the general process of social stratification. In general lines, in mid-high socioeconomic sectors, women can have more resources and tools that allow them to partly minimize gender asymmetries [34].

Following this reflection line, sexual violence would not occupy the same place or would have the same consequences depending on the place that the victim occupies. Higher-class, white women, with economic and/or intellectual resources, could count on more physical tools that can imply a more integral recuperation of trauma.

However, in our social frame, if the violence is directed at a woman in social exclusion risk, racialized, who comes from a culture that is unknown or non-understandable to us, or has some type of disability, her vulnerability would be increased, and the recognition of the sexual violence situation that she went through can be distorted.

That is why we think that in the evaluation of sexual violence, it is necessary to incorporate an intersectional perspective, to give proper value to possible silenced discrimination factors.

Most of the investigations, theory, and training around sexual violence are focused on cis-heterosexual abled women, despite the fact that it is described as a higher risk of sexual violence against women with both physical and intellectual disability [35], and the risk is also higher for trans women, especially racialized trans women [36]. In the case of lesbian women, corrective sexual violence, as a way to punish and "cure" homosexuality, also has a higher impact on black lesbian women [37]. Lesbians are also more exposed to sexual violence in contexts of armed conflict than heterosexual women [38], in which sexual violence is frequently used as a war weapon against all women, as a type of violence that is perpetrated systematically, publicly, on a mass scale, with strategically focused intentions [39].

Despite all these realities, most mental health professionals are not trained to work with the intersection of identity, sexual orientation, race, physical and intellectual disability, and sexual violence, and this has an impact on the access of these women to mental health services and their possibilities of recovery.

30.10 Notes on Professional Intervention

It is needed to dismantle the stereotypes associated with sexual violence victims, enlarging the reference frame and making other perspectives possible. In the case of women, victims can offer resistance, or not, can have different behavioral responses to the traumatic experience, or can have psychological sequels diverse in terms of intensity and temporality. Also, demystifying other social constructs, sexual assaults are not perpetrated more commonly by strangers in an alley, but by men that the victim knows, family or friends, and it doesn't always happen at night, but can happen anywhere, anytime. Understanding one only way of reaction for the victims could imply excluding other women acting in a different way, so it is necessary to note that the responses and consequences of sexual violence are as diverse as the women who suffer it.

As a general indication for the intervention with sexual violence victims, we want to point out the importance of listening to the victim's needs, and not ours, attending to her desire to report to the authorities or not, or how and when to receive health care. We also need to consider that the characteristics of the narrative can be very different, including narratives that show struggles to explain what happened, and others full of doubts, disorganized and organized, contradictory or coherent, with gaps or detailed. Emotionally, the responses can happen in a wide range, with victims overwhelmed by emotion and lacking it [40].

Fear, shame and/or guilt are usually direct feelings associated with sexual violence, that a lot of times are not expressed spontaneously. We will usually find predominantly numbness, freezing, or anxiety, and also feelings of hopelessness, anger, or rage. Detecting alert, hypervigilance, and difficulties in making decisions is also common, and in some cases it is not possible in the first evaluations to obtain all the information necessary for the person who is attending to the victim.

It would be needed to highlight that long-term consequences of sexual aggression can also appear in the physical and behavioral spheres, with changes in desire, and also possible consequences in the gynecological and reproductive health areas, symptoms that frequently go unnoticed or are not taken into account.

The ignorance about the variability of consequences and behaviors that women who suffer sexual violence can present can aggravate the neglect in intervention spaces or the doubts around the narrative when there are emotional responses that are not interpreted as valid. The numerous specialists that the victim might have to go through in her process (health, social, legal, etc.), suppose a successive re-experimentation of the traumatic event, being the questioning and disbelief when the victim doesn't adjust to the established canon, one of the most frequent institutional violences.

Impact of sexual violence on professionals who intervene with victims of sexual abuse. The care of the professional.

Working with sexual violence victims has numerous impacts on the mental health of professionals. The frequent exposure to violence narratives, the identification of risk and revictimization situations, the difficulties to intervene, etc., frequently produce feelings of frustration, impotence, and wear that can end up in a burnout syndrome, vicarious traumatization, and the activation of present or past violence experiences [41].

In order to avoid these effects, to improve attention to the victims and take care of the social, legal, and health professionals, it is necessary to develop strategies that can help us improve the professional practice and mitigate the pain.

Neutrality toward trauma, especially when it is caused by another human being, is impossible. As professionals, we are going to navigate a group of reactions that range from over-implication to rejection of the victim. We would analyze here some factors that can impact the professional's reactions:

- Myths and beliefs around women and sexuality
- A lot of professionals believe that they are not able to guide and treat these situations, and that they don't have enough time to do it.
- A lot of professionals feel frustrated because they understand that the success of any intervention is to get the victim to report the aggression, and, in case the aggressor is their partner, to break up with him.
- Countertransference aspects.

30.11 Concluding Remarks

Should the frame of not prioritizing all parts involved in pleasure in sexual relationships still be normalized? The higher visibilization of sexual violence lately has given more relevance to the sufferings of women in sexual and romantic relationships, and we are experiencing a transit period that allows us to expose dynamics far from mutual respect that have been silenced until now.

However, facts like dressing in a certain way, drug use, playing with seduction and erotism, or having identity components of social oppression, are understood by some men as an excuse to keep exposing women to non-desired situations and/or to perpetrate sexual violence. Taking into account that the presentation of bodies and sexual conduct can create a variety of responses in others, this would never be a reason to attribute the right to invade the sexuality of a woman, molest them, or place a man in a power position that attacks the sexual integrity of victims.

Before finishing, we would like to point out that this chapter doesn't pretend to be an instructor for an adequate way of intervention in every context. We are aware of the complexity of this phenomenon and the multiple edges that this presents, and that is the reason why we understand that addressing it from an integrative perspective can facilitate a better intervention in any discipline. Thereby, reflecting on the roots and motivations of sexual violence allows us to understand in a wider way the diverse psychological consequences that it can provoke in the victims. Getting closer to this knowledge and the awareness of its complexity can facilitate for all the professionals involved in the recovery process to evaluate them, understand them, and avoid the revictimization, as harmful in some occasions as the sexual violence itself.

References

1. Vigarello G, Vigarello G. Historia de la violación: siglos XVI – XX. Madrid: Ed. Cátedra [u.a.]; 1999. 394 p. (Colección feminismos).
2. Benjamin J, Benjamin J. Los lazos de amor: psicoanálisis, feminismo y el problema de la dominación. 1st ed. Buenos Aires: Paidós; 1996. p. 354. (Psicología profunda)
3. Millett K. Sexual politics. Repr. London: Rupert Hart-Davis; 1971.
4. Pateman C. The sexual contract. Nachdr. Stanford: Stanford University Press; 2009. p. 264.
5. Herman JL. Trauma and recovery: the aftermath of violence – from domestic abuse to political terror. 20th ed. New York: BasicBooks; 2003. p. 290.
6. Mackinnon C. FEMINISMO INMODIFICADO I DISCURSOS SOBRE LA VIDA Y EL DERECHO [Internet]. 2024 [citado 29 de octubre de 2024]. Disponible en: https://traficantes.net/libros/feminismo-inmodificado
7. Serra C. El sentido de consentir. Editorial Anagrama; 2024.
8. Leguil C. Ceder No Es Consentir: Un Abordaje Clínico y Político Del Consentimiento. 1st ed. Barcelona: Ned Ediciones; 2023. p. 1.
9. Martínez I, Amigot PA, Bayot A, Bonilla A, Castillo MGL. Imaginario cultural, construcción de identidades de género y violencia: formación para la igualdad en la adolescencia; 2018.
10. Rey A. Acoso y abuso sexual en las redes sociales. Instituto asturiano de la mujer del principado de Asturias; 2017.
11. Hughes DM, Stoner JR, editores. The social costs of pornography: a collection of papers. Princeton: Witherspoon Institute; 2010. p. 259.
12. San Vicente A, M MSN, Polo C. Violencia sexual: efectos sobre la identidad y la salud mental de las mujeres. In: Sáenz Herrrero M, editor. Psicopatología en mujeres Incorporando la perspectiva de género en la psicopatología descriptiva. Springer; 2019.
13. Diagnostic and statistical manual of mental disorders. DSM-5. 5th ed. Bangkok: IGroup Press; 2013. p. 947.
14. Porges SW, Buczynski, Ruth. Psicoterapia Bilbao. 2012. La Teoría Polivagal para El Tratamiento del Trauma [Internet]. Disponible en: https://psicoterapiabilbao.es/wp-content/uploads/2015/11/la_teoria_polivagal_1_.pdf
15. Fricker M. Epistemic injustice: power and the ethics of knowing. Oxford/New York: Oxford University Press; 2007. p. 18.
16. Carmona Osorio M. Paradigmas en estallido: epistemologías para una ¿post?psiquiatría. Rev Asoc Esp Neuropsiquiatría. diciembre de. 2017;37(132):509–28.
17. Paricio R, Franquelo A, Usaola C, Vega C. Las huellas de la violencia: una aproximación al trastorno por estrés postraumático complejo. 20 de mayo de. 2019;20:45–56.
18. Cruz Fortún MÁ de la. Factores predictivos del impacto psicopatológico en víctimas de agresión sexual. 5 de mayo de 2014 [citado 29 de octubre de 2024]; Disponible en: https://hdl.handle.net/20.500.14352/38347
19. Sarasua B, Zubizarreta I, de Corral P, Echeburúa E. Factores de Vulnerabilidad y de Protección del Impacto Emocional en Mujeres Adultas Víctimas de Agresiones Sexuales. Ter Psicológica. diciembre de. 2012;30(3):7–18.
20. Serrano C. La costilla rota de Adán: costes humanos de la violencia de género. Primera edición. Barcelona: B; 2022. 326 p. (Sinequanon).

21. Velázquez S. Violencias cotidianas, violencia de género: escuchar, comprender, ayudar. Reimpr. Buenos Aires: Paidós; 2004. p. 334. (Psicologia, psiquiatria, psicoterapia)
22. Martínez Sanz A. Estudio de la violencia sexual sobre las mujeres en la relación de pareja, y las repercusiones de la violencia en pareja sobre la sexualidad de las mujeres. Estudio realizado en servicios públicos de la Comunidad Valenciana. 2016 [citado 29 de octubre de 2024]; Disponible en: http://rua.ua.es/dspace/handle/10045/64881
23. Polo C, M L, Fernández P, Muñoz S, San Vicente A. Visibilización de la Violencia de Género en consultas sanitarias. Un proyecto de Atención Primaria y Salud Mental. Buenas Prácticas en el Sistema Sanitario de Salud. 2015.
24. Barudy Labrin J. El dolor invisible en la infancia: una lectura ecosistémica del maltrato infantil [Internet]. 1998 [citado 29 de octubre de 2024]. Disponible en: https://dialnet.unirioja.es/servlet/libro?codigo=135940
25. Finkelhor D. Sexually victimized children. In: Violence against women: classic papers, vol. 2005. Auckland: Pearson Education New Zealand; 1979. p. 42–56.
26. Cole PM, Putnam FW. Effect of incest on self and social functioning: a developmental psychopathology perspective. J Consult Clin Psychol. abril de. 1992;60(2):174–84.
27. Murray LK, Nguyen A, Cohen JA. Child sexual abuse. Child Adolesc Psychiatr Clin N Am. abril de. 2014;23(2):321–37.
28. López S, Faro C, Lopetegui L, Pujol Ribera E, Monteagudo M, Cobo Gómez JV, et al. Impacto del abuso sexual durante la infancia-adolescencia en las relaciones sexuales y afectivas de mujeres adultas. Gac Sanit Órgano Of Soc Esp Salud Pública Adm Sanit. 2017;31(3):210–9.
29. Satyanarayana VA, Chandra PS, Vaddiparti K. Mental health consequences of violence against women and girls. Curr Opin Psychiatry. septiembre de. 2015;28(5):350–6.
30. Polo Usaola C, López Gironés M, Escudero Nafs A, Olivares Zarco D, Rodríguez Vega B, Fernández LA. Abuso sexual infantil: coexistencia con otros tipos de maltrato en edad infantil y adulta. Arch Psiquiatr. 2006:133–44.
31. Werner KB, McCutcheon VV, Challa M, Agrawal A, Lynskey MT, Conroy E, et al. The association between childhood maltreatment, psychopathology, and adult sexual victimization in men and women: results from three independent samples. Psychol Med. febrero de. 2016;46(3):563–73.
32. Mondéjar LL. La Opinión de Murcia. 2018 [citado 29 de octubre de 2024]. ¿Qué quieren las mujeres? O por qué a Lilith no le gustaba la postura del misionero. Disponible en: https://www.laopiniondemurcia.es/opinion/2018/03/07/quieren-mujeres-o-lilith-le-31750435.html
33. Davis AY. Women, race and class. London: Women's Press; 1994. p. 271.
34. Ariza M, de Oliveira O. Inequidades de género y clase. Nueva Soc. 1999;164:70–81.
35. Iglesias M. La violencia sexual en las mujeres con discapacidad [Internet]. AIES. [citado 29 de octubre de 2024]. Disponible en: https://iniciativasyestudiossociales.org/violencia-sexual-mujeres-discapacidad/
36. Ussher JM, Hawkey A, Perz J, Liamputtong P, Sekar J, Marjadi B, et al. Crossing boundaries and fetishization: experiences of sexual violence for trans women of color. J Interpers Violence. 1 de marzo de. 2022;37(5–6):NP3552-84.
37. Doan-Minh S. Corrective rape: an extreme manifestation of discrimination and the state's complicity in sexual violence. Hastings Womens Law J. 2019;30:167.
38. HaleyNelson C. Sexualized violence against lesbians. Peace Rev. 1 de abril de. 2005;17(2–3):163–80.
39. Meger S. Sexual violence as a weapon of war. En: Meger S, editor. Rape Loot Pillage: The Political Economy of Sexual Violence in Armed Conflict [Internet]. Oxford University Press; 2016 [citado 29 de octubre de 2024]. p. 0. Disponible en: https://doi.org/10.1093/acprof:oso/9780190277666.003.0006
40. Consejería de Sanidad de la Comunidad de Madrid. Protocolo de asistencia sanitaria urgente y coordinada a mujeres víctimas de violencia sexual en la Comunidad de Madrid (Código VISEM). 2023.
41. Ojeda T. El autocuidado de los profesionales de la salud que atienden a víctimas de violencia sexual. Rev Peru Ginecol Obstet. 2006;52(1):21–7.

Gender Issues in Perinatal Mental Health 31

Mihika Shidore, Rabab Lotiya, and Prabha S. Chandra

31.1 Introduction

Ms. S is a 38-year-old banker who was raised by her single mother following the early death of her father. Her mother had a history of severe anxiety and practiced an authoritarian parenting style, as her grandmother had, and frequently emphasized rigid moral values and would often discriminate between her brother and her. During childhood, she endured sexual abuse by a close relative, an experience she has not fully processed. Her married life is fraught with constant discord and instances of violence from her husband. S is currently pregnant, in the third trimester, and has developed significant anxiety. Her anxiety is particularly focused on fears related to giving birth to a girl child, a concern influenced by familial and cultural expectations. She has also started reliving her past early childhood traumatic experiences and fears that she will not handle childbirth well.

31.2 Echoes of the Past: The Hidden Burden of Childhood Trauma in the Perinatal Period

31.2.1 What Is Trauma?

Trauma encompasses a wide variety of events, experiences, and affects involving betrayal or fear that can impact individuals in different ways. When trauma is cumulative, developmental, and interwoven into attachment and relationships, it constitutes *complex trauma* that can change one's perception of the self and the world.

M. Shidore · R. Lotiya · P. S. Chandra (✉)
National Institute of Mental Health ad Neurosciences, Bangalore, India
e-mail: chandra@nimhans.ac.in

M. López-Atanes, M. Sáenz-Herrero (eds.), *Applying the Gender Perspective in Psychiatry and Psychotherapy*, https://doi.org/10.1007/978-3-032-17883-1_31

When experienced in childhood, trauma changes the trajectory of life [42]. Adverse childhood experiences (ACEs) are traumatic events that happen during childhood, such as emotional or physical abuse, neglect, or living in a dysfunctional household. These experiences can negatively impact a child's development and overall health by disrupting the normal functioning of the nervous, endocrine, and immune systems due to prolonged stress. ACEs may include abuse (physical, emotional, sexual), neglect (physical and emotional), and household dysfunction, including factors such as domestic violence, the loss of a parent, parental separation, substance abuse within the home, having an incarcerated family member, or the presence of mental illness in the household. Additionally, exposure to violence can involve community violence, bullying, or experiences of collective violence [8].

31.2.2 How Does Trauma Affect the Brain?

The association between childhood ACEs and perinatal mental health disorders has multiple biological explanations. Studies have indicated that childhood maltreatment leads to morphological alterations in the brain [95]. Childhood exposure to any traumatic event can lead to activation of the hypothalamic-pituitary axis, causing increased corticosteroid production that may lead to an impact on cognitive and physical functions [21]. Young children are particularly susceptible to excessive exposure to corticosteroids caused by frequent stressful events, making them more likely to develop stress-related disorders later in life [15]. During pregnancy, the placenta releases corticotropin-releasing hormone, which triggers the pituitary gland to stimulate the adrenal glands, resulting in the production of corticosteroids. Research has shown that individuals with a history of adverse childhood experiences (ACEs) tend to exhibit increased HPA axis activity and elevated cortisol levels while pregnant [79]. Additionally, the adverse childhood experiences (ACEs) and co-occurring maternal mental health conditions can negatively affect a mother's resilience and ability to cope with the inherent stressors of pregnancy, childbirth, and the transition to parenthood. The presence of a mentally ill person in a family can increase the genetic risk of developing mental illness in an individual, and emotional neglect operates through low perceived support and poor resilience to stress, and contributes to the development of perinatal depression (PND).

31.2.3 Can Childhood Trauma Shroud the Experience of Motherhood?

ACEs are linked to a multitude of psychiatric conditions in adulthood in women, especially in the perinatal period. They can be associated with *perinatal depression (PND)* through psychobiological pathways [18] as well as an increased association to psychiatric disorders in general, which leads to an increased predisposition to the development of PND [15]. A nationwide study on Icelandic women done in 2023 suggested that cumulative ACEs bear a *dose–response relationship* with the occurrence of PND. This association was most significant in women presenting with persistent (antenatal and postnatal depression) and was strongly seen with emotional neglect, having someone mentally ill at home, and a history of emotional abuse, in addition to other events like domestic violence and bullying in childhood. This study also showed that ACEs can lead to PND in women with or without psychiatric comorbidities, underscoring that ACEs can be an independent risk factor [8].

The impact of childhood ACEs extends beyond perinatal depression. The strength of the associations indicates that ACEs are more strongly linked to symptoms of *postpartum post-traumatic stress disorder (PTSD)*, which aligns with existing evidence that *trauma begets trauma.*

Perinatal trauma refers to any extremely distressing or frightening experience reported by a woman that has the potential to cause psychological harm. To qualify, the event must be associated with conception, pregnancy, childbirth, or occur within the first year after giving birth. People with ACEs may experience various peripartum medical events as traumatic and have higher rates of development of PTSD following unexpected birth outcomes. A study found that the most commonly endorsed perinatal traumatic event was the fear that their unborn child was in danger or going to die. Women with multiple ACEs present more with pregnancy-related problems, have more frequent/unplanned medical visits, and are more anxious [60]. ACEs, especially child maltreatment and a higher number of events is strongly associated with the development of anxiety and PTSD in both pregnancy and the postpartum period, as well as increased rates of suicide. ACEs also led to increased substance use and perinatal deaths associated with overdose. Interestingly, for individuals in the perinatal period—when distressing, intrusive thoughts or images about potential harm to one's baby are fairly common—a mother's history of adverse childhood experiences (ACEs), particularly those involving a lack of safety or protection, may play a significant role in shaping the nature or intensity of postpartum obsessive–compulsive symptoms.

31.2.4 Does Trauma Flow Through Generations?

In a systematic review done in 2015, childhood maltreatment emerged as a major risk factor for perinatal depression as well as post-traumatic stress disorder, although this association can be moderated by early protective relationships [18]. The cycle of maltreatment hypothesis suggests that a parent's own history of being maltreated can raise the likelihood that their children will also experience maltreatment [98]. In addition to the direct transmission of ACEs, recent studies have found that a parent's history of adverse childhood experiences is also linked to health issues in their children, emphasizing the intergenerational transmission of trauma [65]. The time spanning from pregnancy through the first three years after birth—commonly known as "the first 1000 days"—is a vital period for brain development and represents a phase of increased vulnerability to adversity in children [46]. Poor maternal mental health during this period may trigger frequent and prolonged toxic stress responses in children, propagating the intergenerational cycle of health issues in families [10].

The results of a recent cohort study (GMATCH cohort) done in 2025 indicated that the effects of adverse childhood experiences (ACEs) on health can extend from pregnancy through the postpartum years, emphasizing the importance of sustained mental health support for mothers, not just during pregnancy but also afterward, especially for those who have experienced ACEs in the past. The impact of mothers' ACEs not just affects early life experiences in offspring but can persist into adulthood. In addition to biological links, poor parenting practices and disadvantaged caregiving may lead to maladaptive stress responses and foster attachment issues in children. Additionally, sex differences in how the HPA axis is shaped during early life, particularly in females during early childhood, play a role in increased sensitivity and vulnerability to the effects of adverse childhood experiences (ACEs). The study also showed that the intergenerational transmission of the impact of ACEs was more pronounced in those belonging to the lower socioeconomic class, rural background, and having lower educational levels [101].

Early sexual abuse can be an important risk factor for the development of perinatal mental health disorders. A cross-sectional study involving 500 women identified a strong link between experiences of physical and sexual abuse and the development of postpartum mental health disorders. A history of sexual abuse may affect a procedure as basic as prenatal examinations for fear of intimate contact and may impact care during pregnancy. Certain experiences of pregnancy and postpartum, like childbirth and breastfeeding, may exacerbate the trauma of sexual abuse. Maternal child sexual abuse (CSA) increases the chances of negative birth perceptions and increased fear of delivery.

31.2.5 Beyond the Emotional Impact

ACEs not only lead to adverse mental health outcomes, but are also responsible for adverse pregnancy outcomes, early cessation of breastfeeding due to painful breastfeeding experience [9], and disrupted mother-infant bonding with higher chances of emotional and physical difficulties in the infant [75]. Child sexual abuse (CSA) in the mother has been found to be an independent risk factor for complicated delivery, higher chances of caesarean section, and giving birth to babies with low birth weight, as well as higher chances of preterm birth [9]. The history of maternal CSA also affects the mother-infant bonding and decreases parenting efficacy and morale. CSA victims may have reduced empathetic awareness, harsher punishment attitudes, and may victimize their children. This is usually mediated by depression or substance use [9].

31.2.6 The Role of Violence

Apart from ACEs, one of the factors that can significantly contribute to negative perinatal mental and physical outcomes is intimate partner violence. *Perinatal intimate partner violence (IPV)* refers to experiences of abuse—whether physical, emotional, sexual, or psychological—that occur within the time frame starting *one year before pregnancy*, continuing *throughout the pregnancy*, and extending *up to one year after childbirth* [78]. IPV can be unilateral or bilateral, involving victimization and perpetration by both partners. Violence can be physical or psychological that involves threats of harm to the body that may or may not be enacted. A study done on the impact of IPV in adolescent pregnant women showed that bilateral IPV in pregnancy had worse mental health outcomes in the form of high prevalence of anxiety and depression [97].

Perinatal IPV is more common among women who are younger, unmarried, have lower socioeconomic status, unstable housing, Medicaid coverage, or less education. Rates are slightly higher before pregnancy (4.7%) than during pregnancy (3.7%) [34].

IPV often involves repeated abuse by a partner on whom the victim may depend for emotional, financial, or practical support, making it especially distressing. The fear of future harm and the invasive, ongoing nature of IPV significantly increase the risk of developing mental health symptoms. About 40% of low-income pregnant women who suffered IPV met the criteria of PTSD [47], which can last months into the postpartum period [13]. In Silverman et al. [82], the records between 2003 and 2007, it was found that 54.3% of mothers who ended their lives with suicide had experienced IPV [73]. Prolonged stress and fear associated with IPV can lead to increased drug use. Although most women try to abstain from it during pregnancy, some end up using it as a coping mechanism, as it may mitigate the distress associated with IPV [49].

In addition to adverse mental health outcomes, IPV is related to multiple obstetric complications. Stress from IPV can cause dysregulation of the HPA axis and various autoimmune and inflammatory responses [24]. The chronic stress from IPV can negatively affect obstetric health. Women exposed to perinatal IPV are at higher risk for complications such as high blood pressure, bleeding, infections, and preterm birth. Both prepregnancy and during pregnancy, IPV is linked to poor health outcomes, but certain risks—like vaginal bleeding, severe nausea, and kidney infections—may be more pronounced when abuse occurs in the year before pregnancy. Women exposed to IPV are five times more likely to experience placental abruption, a serious complication linked to fetal growth restriction, preterm birth, and stillbirth [57]. Miscarriages, preterm birth, and diminished intrauterine growth can occur in women experiencing IPV. Psychological IPV impacts infant birth weight more than physical IPV [103]. The effects of IPV can persist long term in children of parents born to victims of IPV in the form of development of internalizing and externalizing disorders [12], neurodevelopmental delays, and disorders of executive functioning [1]. Perinatal IPV may also lead to an adverse impact on mother-baby bonding and attachment. It reduces the maternal responsiveness and increases negative cognitions about parenting and self-efficacy, leading to hostile and neglectful caregiving [40]. Thus, perinatal IPV casts a long shadow, endangering both mother and child with lasting wounds that begin before birth.

Another stressor predisposing to perinatal mental health illness is a history of infertility. It is defined as failure to achieve a clinical pregnancy within 12 months of regular unprotected sexual intercourse. Although artificial reproductive techniques are an effective solution to this predicament, the experience of infertility and its treatment may be extremely stressful. Its diminishing effect on the couple's marital satisfaction [94], self-esteem, and quality of life may last long into pregnancy and postpartum and can increase the risk of developing perinatal depression [77]. The question is whether infertility treatments also play a role in the development of perinatal depression. A meta-analysis conducted in 2019 shows that women receiving infertility treatments are not at a greater risk of developing perinatal depression than the controls [16].

This discussion highlights how perinatal trauma, influenced by adverse childhood experiences and maternal mental health challenges, can deeply affect a woman's resilience and coping during pregnancy and postpartum. The case vignette exemplifies these concepts, illustrating how a distressing event related to childbirth triggered psychological distress compounded by prior trauma and existing mental health conditions. By understanding these interrelated factors, we can better appreciate the complexities faced by the woman in the vignette and the importance of targeted support during the perinatal period.

Ms. A is a 29-year-old first-time mother who delivered a healthy baby girl two weeks ago following a prolonged and painful labor that ended in a forceps-assisted vaginal delivery. During delivery, she experienced significant perineal trauma and blood loss, resulting in an extended hospital stay. Since returning home, Ms. A reports feeling overwhelmed and exhausted. Although her baby is thriving, Anjali avoids physical closeness; she hesitates to hold her baby and often leaves her in the crib, responding to her cries only after prolonged periods. When she does pick the baby up, she appears tense and avoids eye contact. Feeding is mechanical and hurried. She expresses frustration, saying, "I don't feel anything for her. I'm just going through the motions." She has also begun to express guilt and shame, fearing she is a "bad mother," and frequently asks her mother-in-law to take over caregiving duties so she can spend time alone in her room.

31.3 The Early Connection: Determinants of Maternal–Infant Relationship

Maternal–infant bonding is the development of a reciprocal emotional relationship between a mother and her infant, primarily initiated and driven by the mother. It refers to the strong feelings of affection, protectiveness, and connection that a mother develops toward her baby, typically beginning in the early postpartum period [7, 19, 85]. This distinct role is influenced by biological factors such as the physical connection established during pregnancy, the hormonal and emotional responses associated with breastfeeding, and the caregiving responsibilities that mothers often assume. While other caregivers—such as fathers or extended family members—can contribute to the attachment process, the mother's role is particularly vital during the early months of the infant's life. Forming a secure attachment in the postpartum period is crucial, as it significantly influences a child's long-term mental health and well-being. Securely attached children tend to have better emotional regulation, social skills, and stress resilience [48, 93, 102].

31.3.1 Neurobiological Foundations

Oxytocin plays a key role in maternal care by activating neural networks involved in bonding and infant recognition. High oxytocin receptor density in the medial preoptic area, ventral tegmental area, and nucleus accumbens (NA) supports caregiving behavior. fMRI studies show oxytocin-linked brain activation when mothers view their own infants. During pregnancy, plasma oxytocin levels correlate with maternal bonding, attachment, and concern for infant well-being. Oxytocin also predicts the quality of caregiving behaviors in both mothers and fathers [27, 29, 92]. The pattern of dopamine release correlates closely with maternal behavior. The ventral tegmental area (VTA) and substantia nigra (SN) are key sources of dopamine that facilitate caregiving. Selective destruction of monoaminergic neurons in these regions impairs maternal behavior. Similarly, transgenic mice lacking the dopamine transporter also show disrupted maternal responses [14]. Maternal attachment is underpinned by distinct neural systems mediating reward and stress, which together shape caregiving behavior. Key limbic structures—the nucleus accumbens (NAcc) and amygdala—play central roles in assigning emotional valence to infant cues and have been shown to be critical in maternal bonding across mammalian species. The NAcc, a core component of the mesolimbic dopaminergic reward pathway, provides motivational reinforcement for maternal behaviors. In contrast, the amygdala, a central hub for emotional and threat processing, contributes to the stress-related aspects of maternal care. It is involved in maternal vigilance and social affiliation, with lesions resulting in reduced maternal responsiveness. These subcortical structures interact with cortical regions, such as the medial preoptic area (MPOA)—which integrates infant sensory cues to promote caregiving, as well as the anterior cingulate cortex (ACC) and dorsomedial prefrontal cortex (dmPFC), both implicated in empathy and theory of mind. These higher-order cortical systems may enhance the mother's ability to interpret and respond appropriately to her infant's needs. Together, this integrated network of reward, stress, and social cognition systems provides the neural scaffolding for maternal motivation, attachment, and sensitive caregiving [11, 56, 92].

31.3.2 Psychological and Emotional factors

Mother–infant bonding is an emotional and psychological process that begins in pregnancy and evolves through infancy. Key psychological factors influencing this bond include maternal mental health, attachment style, reflective functioning, and responsiveness to infant cues.

31.3.2.1 Attachment Representations

A mother's internal working models of attachment—shaped by her own early caregiving experiences—also play a critical role. Mothers with secure attachment styles are more likely to interpret their infant's cues accurately and respond sensitively [70, 104]. In contrast, mothers with unresolved trauma or insecure attachment histories may experience difficulties forming an emotional connection with their baby or may exhibit inconsistent caregiving patterns. These internal models act as templates for caregiving behavior and emotional responses [59].

31.3.2.2 Reflective Functioning and Mentalization

Reflective functioning, or the ability to understand the infant as a separate individual with independent mental states, is essential for maternal sensitivity and bonding [83]. High reflective functioning allows mothers to interpret crying or fussiness not as personal rejection, but as communication of need. This capacity helps buffer the impact of infant distress and promotes emotional regulation in both mother and child [58]. Deficits in mentalization are often observed in mothers with borderline personality traits or those with histories of trauma and neglect, which may result in inconsistent or intrusive responses to infant cues [26, 90].

31.3.2.3 Maternal Sensitivity and Responsiveness

Maternal sensitivity, the ability to perceive, interpret, and respond appropriately to infant signals, is a key predictor of secure attachment and healthy bonding. Sensitive mothers foster a sense of trust and safety, which is foundational for the infant's emotional development [2]. Conversely, intrusiveness or inconsistency in caregiving can undermine the infant's confidence in the caregiver and lead to attachment difficulties.

31.3.2.4 Maternal Mental Health

Maternal mental health is a critical psychological factor influencing maternal–infant bonding. Postpartum depression (PPD), anxiety, and post-traumatic stress disorder (PTSD) can impair emotional availability and responsiveness, which are essential for secure attachment. PPD is particularly associated with bonding difficulties, including emotional withdrawal, reduced maternal sensitivity, and negative perceptions of the infant [23, 50]. A 2020 systematic review found that early-onset depression (within six months postpartum), its severity, and diagnosis through structured instruments were more strongly linked to impaired bonding [84]. Findings on maternal anxiety are mixed; some studies report reduced sensitivity [68], while others describe more intrusive, critical, or less warm behaviors [44, 71, 99]. Additionally, maternal and neonatal complications during childbirth—such as poor pain control or unplanned/emergency caesarean sections—have been associated with postpartum PTSD, which carries an elevated risk of bonding disorders [52]. Sleep disturbances in the postpartum period can reduce maternal emotional sensitivity and availability. Poor sleep often worsens mood and heightens anxiety, creating a cycle that negatively impacts bonding. Prolonged sleep disruption may also lead to fatigue, emotional instability, and irritability, further hindering secure attachment with the infant [55].

31.3.3 The Role of Neonatal and Obstetric Factors

Obstetric Complications The mode and experience of childbirth significantly shape initial maternal–infant interaction. Traumatic birth experiences, including emergency caesarean sections, excessive pain, or feelings of loss of control, can negatively affect early bonding. Women who perceive their childbirth as traumatic are more likely to experience acute stress symptoms, which can interfere with their emotional availability and responsiveness to the infant. Evidence on factors such as unplanned pregnancy, unplanned caesarean delivery, delivery examinations, higher birth order, mode of delivery, the absence of breastfeeding, and infant gender remains inconsistent, with some studies linking these variables to poorer maternal–infant bonding. These discrepancies may reflect underlying sociocultural variations across study populations [17, 36, 55, 62].

Infant health is a significant determinant of maternal bonding. Preterm birth, low birth weight, or neonatal complications can disrupt the natural bonding process. These infants may be separated from their mothers due to medical needs, limiting physical contact and impairing maternal responsiveness during the critical early period [54]. Mothers of preterm or medically fragile infants often experience heightened anxiety, feelings of helplessness, or difficulty relating to the child, which can delay or weaken the emotional connection [74].

Difficult infant temperament has been linked to negative maternal responses, reduced sensitivity, parenting stress, and mutual rejection, though its direct role in maternal–infant bonding is less studied. High infant negative emotionality and low positive emotionality were associated with poorer bonding, independent of maternal depression and anxiety, highlighting the need to consider both maternal and infant factors together [69, 100]. While maternal–infant bonding is associated with infant temperament, the relationship is complex and likely bidirectional, shaped by reciprocal dysfunctional interactions between mother and infant [35].

31.4 Sociocultural Factors

Cultural beliefs, family support, and social context significantly influence maternal–infant bonding. Supportive partners and stable home environments enhance bonding, while stressors like intimate partner violence, low social support, and poverty can impair maternal emotional availability. Though poverty and adverse conditions may not directly affect bonding, they are closely linked to maternal depression, which can indirectly disrupt it. In patriarchal societies with strong son preference, having a female infant has been associated with postpartum depression and impaired bonding [25, 53]. A cross-sectional study in southern India found poor maternal–infant bonding significantly associated with joint or extended family living, possibly due to reduced direct interaction and increased maternal workload limiting time and emotional availability for bonding [96]. Exposure to intimate partner violence (IPV) can have profound effects on parent–infant relationships. In households where IPV occurs, the ability of parents to form secure, responsive bonds with their infants may be compromised. Emotional availability is often diminished following conflict; parents may become less attuned to their infant's needs and less responsive in caregiving interactions. This emotional withdrawal can hinder the development of early attachment [6, 51].

In conclusion, maternal–infant bonding is shaped by a dynamic and multifactorial process influenced by the mother's internal state, the surrounding environment, and the early caregiving context. Disruptions in this delicate process can arise from both emotional and situational challenges, often interacting in complex ways. Recognizing the nuanced pathways through which bonding can be impaired is essential for early identification and intervention. By fostering supportive environments, addressing maternal well-being, and promoting sensitive caregiving, it is possible to strengthen the foundations of a secure mother–infant relationship and support long-term developmental outcomes.

Ms. P, a 30-year-old primigravida, underwent an emergency caesarean section after a prolonged, painful labor that deviated significantly from her birth plan. She felt ignored by staff, uninformed about procedures, and powerless throughout the process. In the weeks following delivery, she experienced intrusive flashbacks of the birth, emotional numbness, and avoided discussing the experience. She became increasingly withdrawn, tearful, and struggled to bond with her baby. A postpartum assessment revealed she met criteria for post-traumatic stress disorder (PTSD) related to childbirth. With trauma-focused therapy and support, Ms. P gradually processed the experience and reconnected with her infant.

31.5 The Impact of Childbirth Experience on Perinatal Mental Health

Childbirth is a transformative event in a woman's life, encompassing physical, emotional, and psychological dimensions. While the medical aspects of childbirth often receive the most attention, the subjective experience of childbirth, how a woman perceives and emotionally processes the event, is usually overlooked and can have profound implications for her mental health during the perinatal period.

The childbirth experience is shaped not only by medical outcomes but also by personal, cultural, relational, and systemic factors. Two women with similar clinical events may report vastly different emotional responses, underscoring the importance of subjective perception [38]. A positive pregnancy experience encompasses multiple dimensions: maintaining physical and sociocultural normality, ensuring a healthy pregnancy for both mother and baby (including prevention and management of risks, illness, and mortality), supporting an effective transition to positive labor and birth, and facilitating the achievement of positive motherhood, which includes the development of maternal self-esteem, competence, and autonomy [22].

A systematic review found that the prevalence of negative childbirth experiences ranged from 6.8% to 44%, influenced by multiple factors. Individual contributors include age, parity, childbirth fear, low self-efficacy, lack of control, unmet expectations, and poor preparation. Interpersonal factors such as insufficient partner or caregiver support also play a role. Additionally, unexpected medical interventions—like prolonged labor, induction, instrumental delivery, emergency caesarean, and adverse neonatal outcomes such as low Apgar scores or NICU admission—are linked to more negative perceptions of childbirth [39].

A negative subjective experience of childbirth has been shown to significantly contribute to the development of maternal depression and anxiety in the postpartum period [20, 64] Post-traumatic stress symptoms were assessed using the impact of event scale (IES), objective birth experiences were recorded through birth journals, and subjective birth experiences were evaluated using three structured questions. Subjective birth experience showed the strongest association with post-traumatic stress symptoms and mediated the effects of both predisposing factors and objective events, highlighting its key role in postpartum psychological outcomes [30]. Childbirth-related PTSD was found to negatively impact marital relationships, with many women reporting sexual dissatisfaction due to fear of another traumatic birth [4]. A systematic review examined 12 studies, out of which five articles found a positive association between women's negative childbirth experience and their unwillingness to have more children; three studies found a positive association between women's negative childbirth experience and their willingness to postpone their next pregnancy; and six studies showed a positive association between women's negative childbirth experience and their request for a C-section in their subsequent pregnancies [81]. A negative childbirth experience is associated with a reduced willingness to conceive again and a preference to avoid vaginal birth in subsequent pregnancies [32].

Women retain a vivid and lasting memory of their childbirth experience, even years after delivery, particularly when assessed using validated tools. This underscores the critical impact of childbirth on long-term outcomes, including mental health, sexual satisfaction, exclusive breastfeeding, and preferences for future birth modes. Given these far-reaching effects, it is essential for healthcare professionals to recognize and support women who report negative birth experiences, especially during the postpartum period, to promote psychological well-being and improve maternal and child health trajectories.

31.6 Cultural Factors Impacting Perinatal Mental Health

31.6.1 Gender Discrimination and Patriarchy

Discrimination of societal roles and expectations based on gender can impact a woman's well-being in many ways, especially in sensitive phases like pregnancy, postpartum, and perimenopausal periods. This is compounded by the pressure to give birth to a male child in many cultures, further affecting mental health during this period of time.

Gender discrimination can appear in numerous forms, including biased interpersonal interactions, discriminatory institutional practices, and systemic barriers that limit access to education, career advancement, financial resources, and political participation. It also includes unequal treatment within families, workplaces, and institutional settings, as well as more subtle forms such as microaggressions, objectification, the use of sexist language, and underlying assumptions that women are intellectually or physically inferior. Crucially, similar to other types of discrimination, perceived gender discrimination can be a significant source of psychological stress. It is often considered more harmful than other stressors due to its uncontrollable nature and its connection to deeply held and immutable aspects of one's identity [86].

A study conducted in the Czech Republic among child-bearing women showed that gender discrimination is associated with depressive symptoms due to the stress from perceived discrimination as well as financial and social disadvantage caused by discrimination [86]. Another study conducted by the same research group followed up the children of this cohort to look for the impact of maternal gender discrimination on children. The children born to these women had more emotional problems between 7 and 15 years of age as compared to the control group. First, children and boys displayed greater problems than children of married mothers. This intergenerational transmission can occur through the presence of maternal depression and financial disadvantage, highlighting the fact that gender discrimination is not just a woman's problem, but rather a societal menace [87].

It's crucial to understand how patriarchy and expected gender roles affect help-seeking in women with perinatal depression, in addition to contributing to it. A recent systematic review highlighted the impact of sociocultural beliefs on help-seeking in Indian women with perinatal depression. It's a common cultural belief that pregnancy is a potential cure for existing depression and resolution of spousal conflict, minimizing the need for medical consultation. Additionally, the stigma and shame associated with suffering from depression in a period of life that should be ideally considered "happy" and the need to be a "good mother" despite perceived suffering, negatively affect disclosure in women [45]. Women are typically expected to serve as the primary caregivers for their infants, even when they are struggling with functional impairments due to perinatal depression (PND). In addition to childcare, they are also expected to meet the growing demands of their families and society—taking on roles such as a dutiful daughter-in-law, a cheerful new mother, and a supportive wife—while also managing domestic responsibilities. These long-standing cultural norms are deeply rooted in patriarchal ideologies that remain prevalent in Indian society. As a result, many women in the perinatal period internalize these expectations and, rather than showing themselves compassion, tend to be self-critical when they feel they are falling short [61, 80].

An important cause of anxiety during pregnancy is the pressure of birthing a male child, especially in cultures where the birth of a female child is perceived as an economic and social liability due to prevailing social evils like the dowry system. In addition to societal pressure, many women also display this gender preference due to beliefs like bearing a male child only can propagate the family, sense of social and financial security provided by sons, and the need for a son to perform final rites. One of the strongest factors causing postpartum depression in Indian women was the sadness about the baby's gender. This is also mediated through the increased risk of violence perpetrated on women bearing girl infants. In a study conducted among pregnant women in the urban population of an Indian state, 47.9% of the women reported any gender preference, and 27.5% of the women had a male gender preference. Higher rates of stress and anxiety were found among women, spouses, or families with male gender preference as compared to those with female or no gender preference [91].

31.6.2 Adolescence and Motherhood

Adolescent pregnancy and motherhood are significant public health concerns. Even though the postpartum phase can be challenging for mothers of all ages, adolescent motherhood is fraught with unique stressors. Factors like low age, early dropout from school, low access to healthcare, less support networks, being abandoned by the child's father, and societal stigma can lead to worries about the future of the unsupported baby and immense anxiety during pregnancy [72]. Other risk factors may include high levels of perceived stress, a previous history of depression, and experiences of sexual or physical abuse, how the adolescent views her pregnancy, criticism from family members, low self-confidence and self-worth, substance use, parental stress, exposure to community violence, anxiety, and being of African-American background [76]. A study conducted in Kenya revealed that one-fourth of adolescent mothers in study population experienced depressive symptoms. Having parents who supported their education and a female friend to confide in emerged as protective factors [31]. Understanding the risk factors and protective factors may help in a more sensitive approach toward the identification and treatment of perinatal mental health disorders in adolescent girls.

31.6.3 Displacement, Migration, and Social Discrimination

Perinatal mental health is shaped not only by biological and psychological factors but also by culture. Cultural beliefs influence how women perceive pregnancy, childbirth, and motherhood, shaping emotional responses and coping strategies. Rituals, family roles, and expectations can provide support or create pressure, impacting mental well-being. In some cultures, distress is expressed through physical symptoms or spiritual beliefs, which may obscure underlying psychiatric conditions. Stigma and gender norms often affect help-seeking behavior. Understanding these cultural dynamics is crucial for accurate assessment and effective care.

The term *migrant* encompasses a heterogeneous population ranging from refugees and asylum seekers to economic migrants, each with diverse legal statuses and reasons for migration. Perinatal mental health in migrant women is shaped by displacement, trauma, and marginalization, requiring culturally and contextually sensitive care that acknowledges the complexities of their migration experience [3, 41].

Emerging evidence indicates that the prevalence of mental disorders among migrants and refugees is significantly higher than that of host populations, with considerable variability in different migrant subgroups. A systematic review reported that one in four migrant women during pregnancy or the postpartum period experience perinatal depression, one in five experience perinatal anxiety, and one in 11 are affected by perinatal post-traumatic stress disorder (PTSD) [88]. Migrant women are disproportionately affected by socioeconomic disadvantage, with the majority originating from low- and middle-income countries [3, 66]. Risk factors frequently associated with poor perinatal mental health outcomes in migrant women include language barriers, inadequate social support, minority ethnic status, and heightened vulnerability to interpersonal violence [28, 63, 89].

In addition to structural barriers, cultural norms around emotional expression may impede detection and treatment. In contrast to Western clinical frameworks that emphasize affective symptoms such as sadness and guilt, many non-Western cultures, including Hispanic, Asian, and African populations, commonly express emotional distress through somatic complaints. These may include fatigue, pain, generalized body discomfort, or gynecological symptoms such as vaginal discharge, especially among South Asian women. Somatization serves as a culturally acceptable means of articulating distress in contexts where direct disclosure of emotional suffering may be stigmatized or discouraged [5, 37, 67].

Pregnancy-related discrimination, such as unequal treatment in the workplace, denial of maternity rights, or social exclusion, has been identified as a significant psychosocial stressor during the perinatal period. Such discrimination can contribute to feelings of worthlessness, chronic stress, and reduced self-efficacy, all of which are established risk factors for perinatal depression and anxiety. Emerging evidence suggests that women who experience pregnancy discrimination are at greater risk for adverse mental health outcomes, including depressive symptoms, heightened anxiety, and lower perceived social support. Despite its relevance, pregnancy discrimination remains an under-recognized determinant in perinatal mental health research, warranting further investigation and targeted policy interventions [33, 43].

In conclusion, discrimination emerges as a critical yet under-recognized determinant of perinatal mental health. Addressing these systemic inequities through inclusive policies, culturally sensitive care, and targeted psychosocial interventions is essential for improving perinatal mental health outcomes among affected populations.

References

1. Aarnoudse-Moens CSH, Weisglas-Kuperus N, Van Goudoever JB, Oosterlaan J. Meta-analysis of neurobehavioral outcomes in very preterm and/or very low birth weight children. Pediatrics. 2009;124(2):717–28. https://doi.org/10.1542/PEDS.2008-2816.
2. Ainsworth MDS, Blehar MC, Waters E, Wall S. Patterns of attachment: a psychological study of the strange situation; 1978.
3. Anderson FM, Hatch SL, Comacchio C, Howard LM. Prevalence and risk of mental disorders in the perinatal period among migrant women: a systematic review and meta-analysis. Arch Women's Mental Health. 2017;20(3):449–62. https://doi.org/10.1007/S00737-017-0723-Z/FIGURES/1.

4. Ayers S, Eagle A, Waring H. The effects of childbirth-related post-traumatic stress disorder on women and their relationships: a qualitative study. Psychol Health Med. 2006;11(4):389–98. https://doi.org/10.1080/13548500600708409.
5. Bashiri N, Spielvogel AM. Postpartum depression: a cross-cultural perspective. Primary Care Update OB/GYNS. 1999;6(3):82–7. https://doi.org/10.1016/S1068-607X(99)00003-7.
6. Boeckel MG, Wagner A, Grassi-Oliveira R. The effects of intimate partner violence exposure on the maternal bond and PTSD symptoms of children. J Interpers Violence. 2017;32(7):1127–42. https://doi.org/10.1177/0886260515587667;JOURNAL:JOURNAL:JIVA;REQUESTEDJOURNAL:JOURNAL:JIVA;PAGE:STRING:ARTICLE/CHAPTER.
7. Bowlby J. The making and breaking of affectional bonds. I. Aetiology and psychopathology in the light of attachment theory. An expanded version of the Fiftieth Maudsley Lecture, delivered before the Royal College of Psychiatrists, 19 November 1976. Br J Psychiatry. 1977;130(3):201–10. https://doi.org/10.1192/BJP.130.3.201.
8. Bränn E, Vaina A, Daníelsdóttir HB, Thordardottir EB, Yang Q, Jakobsdóttir J, Aspelund T, Hauksdóttir A, Valdimarsdóttir UA, Lu D. Association between adverse childhood experiences and perinatal depressive symptoms: a cross-sectional analysis of 16,831 women in Iceland. Arch Women's Mental Health. 2023;26(6):839–49. https://doi.org/10.1007/S00737-023-01369-2.
9. Brunton R. Childhood abuse and perinatal outcomes for mother and child: a systematic review of the literature. PLoS One. 2024;19(5):e0302354. https://doi.org/10.1371/JOURNAL.PONE.0302354.
10. Bucci M, Marques SS, Oh D, Harris NB. Toxic stress in children and adolescents. Adv Pediatr. 2016;63(1):403–28. https://doi.org/10.1016/j.yapd.2016.04.002.
11. Cardinal RN, Parkinson JA, Hall J, Everitt BJ. Emotion and motivation: the role of the amygdala, ventral striatum, and prefrontal cortex. Neurosci Biobehav Rev. 2002;26(3):321–52. https://doi.org/10.1016/S0149-7634(02)00007-6.
12. Carlson BE. Children exposed to intimate partner violence: research findings and implications for intervention. Trauma Violence Abuse. 2000;1(4):321–42. https://doi.org/10.1177/1524838000001004002;SUBPAGE:STRING:ABSTRACT;WEBSITE:WEBSITE:SAGE;WGROUP:STRING:PUBLICATION.
13. Cerulli C, Talbot NL, Tang W, Chaudron LH. Co-occurring intimate partner violence and mental health diagnoses in perinatal women. J Women Health. 2011;20(12):1797–803. https://doi.org/10.1089/JWH.2010.2201.
14. Champagne FA, Chretien P, Stevenson CW, Zhang TY, Gratton A, Meaney MJ. Variations in nucleus Accumbens dopamine associated with individual differences in maternal behavior in the rat. J Neurosci. 2004;24(17):4113–23. https://doi.org/10.1523/JNEUROSCI.5322-03.2004.
15. Chapman DP, Whitfield CL, Felitti VJ, Dube SR, Edwards VJ, Anda RF. Adverse childhood experiences and the risk of depressive disorders in adulthood. J Affect Disord. 2004;82(2):217–25. https://doi.org/10.1016/J.JAD.2003.12.013.
16. Chen S, Wang T, Zhang S, Zhao L, Chen L. Association between infertility treatment and perinatal depressive symptoms: a meta-analysis of observational studies. J Psychosom Res. 2019;120:110–7. https://doi.org/10.1016/J.JPSYCHORES.2019.03.016.
17. Chen R, Zhan FY, Lutkiewicz K, Hailemeskel HS, Shimels Hailemeskel H, Kebede AB, Fetene MT, Dagnaw FT. Mother-infant bonding and its associated factors among mothers in the postpartum period, Northwest Ethiopia, 2021. Front Psychiatry. 2022;13:893505. https://doi.org/10.3389/FPSYT.2022.893505.
18. Choi KW, Sikkema KJ. Childhood maltreatment and perinatal mood and anxiety disorders: a systematic review. Trauma Violence Abuse. 2016;17(5):427–53. https://doi.org/10.1177/1524838015584369.
19. Condon JT, Corkindale CJ. The assessment of parent-to-infant attachment: development of a self-report questionnaire instrument. J Reprod Infant Psychol. 1998;16(1):57–76. https://doi.org/10.1080/02646839808404558;JOURNAL:JOURNAL:CJRI20;PAGE:STRING:ARTICLE/CHAPTER.

20. Coo S, García MI, Mira A. Examining the association between subjective childbirth experience and maternal mental health at six months postpartum. J Reprod Infant Psychol. 2023;41(3):275–88. https://doi.org/10.1080/02646838.2021.1990233.
21. De Kloet ER, Oitzl MS, Joëls M. Stress and cognition: are corticosteroids good or bad guys? Trends Neurosci. 1999;22(10):422–6. https://doi.org/10.1016/S0166-2236(99)01438-1.
22. Downe S, Finlayson K, Tunçalp, Metin Gülmezoglu A. What matters to women: a systematic scoping review to identify the processes and outcomes of antenatal care provision that are important to healthy pregnant women. BJOG Int J Obstetr Gynaecol. 2016;123(4):529–39. https://doi.org/10.1111/1471-0528.13819;SUBPAGE:STRING:FULL.
23. Doyle FL, Dickson SJ, Eapen V, Frick PJ, Kimonis ER, Hawes DJ, Moul C, Richmond JL, Mehta D, Dadds MR. Towards preventative psychiatry: concurrent and longitudinal predictors of postnatal maternal-infant bonding. Child Psychiatry Hum Dev. 2023;54(6):1723–36. https://doi.org/10.1007/S10578-022-01365-0/TABLES/6.
24. Dutton MA, Green BL, Kaltman SI, Roesch DM, Zeffiro TA, Krause ED. Intimate partner violence, PTSD, and adverse health outcomes. J Interpers Violence. 2006;21(7):955–68. https://doi.org/10.1177/0886260506289178.
25. Edhborg M, Nasreen HE, Kabir ZN. Impact of postpartum depressive and anxiety symptoms on mothers' emotional tie to their infants 2–3 months postpartum: a population-based study from rural Bangladesh. Arch Women Mental Health. 2011;14(4):307–16. https://doi.org/10.1007/S00737-011-0221-7/TABLES/4.
26. Ensink K, Berthelot N, Bernazzani O, Normandin L, Fonagy P. Another step closer to measuring the ghosts in the nursery: preliminary validation of the trauma reflective functioning scale. Front Psychol. 2014;5(DEC):115791. https://doi.org/10.3389/FPSYG.2014.01471/BIBTEX.
27. Febo M, Numan M, Ferris CF. Functional magnetic resonance imaging shows oxytocin activates brain regions associated with mother–pup bonding during suckling. J Neurosci. 2005;25(50):11637–44. https://doi.org/10.1523/JNEUROSCI.3604-05.2005.
28. Fellmeth G, Plugge E, Paw KM, Charunwatthana P, Nosten F, McGready R. Pregnant migrant and refugee women's perceptions of mental illness on the Thai-Myanmar border: a qualitative study. BMC Pregnancy Childbirth. 2015;15(1):1–11. https://doi.org/10.1186/S12884-015-0517-0/FIGURES/1.
29. Francis DD, Champagne FC, Meaney MJ. Variations in maternal behaviour are associated with differences in oxytocin receptor levels in the rat. J Neuroendocrinol. 2000;12(12):1145–8. https://doi.org/10.1046/J.1365-2826.2000.00599.X.
30. Garthus-Niegel S, Von Soest T, Vollrath ME, Eberhard-Gran M. The impact of subjective birth experiences on post-traumatic stress symptoms: a longitudinal study. Arch Women Mental Health. 2013;16(1):1–10. https://doi.org/10.1007/S00737-012-0301-3.
31. Gebrekristos LT, Ajayi AI, Groves AK, Kabiru CW. Examining the associations between social support and postpartum depression symptoms among adolescent mothers in Nairobi, Kenya. Reprod Health. 2025;22(1):11. https://doi.org/10.1186/S12978-025-01943-0.
32. Ghanbari-Homayi S, Mohammad-Alizadeh-Charandabi S, Meedya S, Jafarabadi MA, Mohammadi E, Mirghafourvand M. The impact of first childbirth experience on women's attitude towards having another child and subsequent vaginal birth. Curr Women Health Rev. 2020;17(3):244–50. https://doi.org/10.2174/1573404816999200930161803/CITE/REFWORKS.
33. Hackney KJ, Daniels SR, Paustian-Underdahl SC, Perrewé PL, Mandeville A, Eaton AA. Examining the effects of perceived pregnancy discrimination on mother and baby health. J Appl Psychol. 2021;106(5):774–83. https://doi.org/10.1037/APL0000788.
34. Hahn CK, Gilmore AK, Aguayo RO, Rheingold AA. Perinatal intimate partner violence HHS public access. Obstet Gynecol Clin N Am. 2018;45(3):535–47. https://doi.org/10.1016/j.ogc.2018.04.008.
35. Hairston IS, Solnik-Menilo T, Deviri D, Handelzalts JE. Maternal depressed mood moderates the impact of infant sleep on mother–infant bonding. Arch Women Mental Health. 2016;19(6):1029–39. https://doi.org/10.1007/S00737-016-0652-2/FIGURES/1.

36. Hairston IS, Handelzalts JE, Lehman-Inbar T, Kovo M. Mother-infant bonding is not associated with feeding type: a community study sample. BMC Pregnancy Childbirth. 2019;19(1):125. https://doi.org/10.1186/S12884-019-2264-0.
37. Halbreich U, Alarcon RD, Calil H, Douki S, Gaszner P, Jadresic E, Jasovic-Gasic M, Kadri N, Kerr-Correa F, Patel V, Sarache X, Trivedi JK. Culturally-sensitive complaints of depressions and anxieties in women. J Affect Disord. 2007;102(1–3):159–76. https://doi.org/10.1016/J.JAD.2006.09.033.
38. Hodnett ED. Pain and women's satisfaction with the experience of childbirth: a systematic review. Am J Obstet Gynecol. 2002;186(5):S160–72. https://doi.org/10.1016/S0002-9378(02)70189-0.
39. Hosseini Tabaghdehi M, Kolahdozan S, Keramat A, Shahhossein Z, Moosazadeh M, Motaghi Z. Prevalence and factors affecting the negative childbirth experiences: a systematic review. J Matern Fetal Neonatal Med. 2020;33(22):3849–56. https://doi.org/10.1080/14767058.2019.1583740;REQUESTEDJOURNAL:JOURNAL:IJMF20;WGROUP:STRING:PUBLICATION.
40. Huth-Bocks AC, Krause K, Ahlfs-Dunn S, Gallagher E, Scott S. Relational trauma and posttraumatic stress symptoms among pregnant women. Psychodyn Psychiatry. 2013;41(2):277–302. https://doi.org/10.1521/PDPS.2013.41.2.277.
41. Iliadou M, Papadakaki M, Sioti E, Giaxi P, Leontitsi E, Petelos E, Van den Muijsenbergh M, Tziaferi S, Mastroyiannakis A, Vivilaki VG. Addressing mental health issues among migrant and refugee pregnant women: a call for action. Eur J Midwifery. 2019;3(May):9. https://doi.org/10.18332/EJM/108626.
42. Isobel S, Goodyear M, Foster K. Psychological trauma in the context of familial relationships: a concept analysis. Trauma Violence Abuse. 2019;20(4):549–59. https://doi.org/10.1177/1524838017726424.
43. Kachi Y, Fujiwara T, Inoue A, Baba S, Eguchi H, Ohta H, Tsutsumi A. The effects of pregnancy discrimination on postpartum depressive symptoms: a follow-up study. BMC Pregnancy Childbirth. 2022;22(1):1–8. https://doi.org/10.1186/S12884-022-05148-2/TABLES/3.
44. Kaitz M, Maytal HR, Devor N, Bergman L, Mankuta D. Maternal anxiety, mother–infant interactions, and infants' response to challenge. Infant Behav Dev. 2010;33(2):136–48. https://doi.org/10.1016/J.INFBEH.2009.12.003.
45. Kalra H, Tran T, Romero L, Sagar R, Fisher J. National policies and programs for perinatal mental health in India: a systematic review. Asian J Psychiatr. 2024;91:103836. https://doi.org/10.1016/J.AJP.2023.103836.
46. Kang NR, Kwack YS, Song JK, Kim MD, Park JH, Kim BN, Moon DS. The impact of maternal adverse childhood experiences on offspring's internalizing and externalizing problems. Psychiatry Investig. 2021;18(11):1050–7. https://doi.org/10.30773/PI.2021.0343.
47. Kastello JC, Jacobsen KH, Gaffney KF, Kodadek MP, Bullock LC, Sharps PW. Posttraumatic stress disorder among low-income women exposed to perinatal intimate partner violence: posttraumatic stress disorder among women exposed to partner violence. Arch Women Mental Health. 2016;19(3):521–8. https://doi.org/10.1007/S00737-015-0594-0.
48. Khan F, Fraley RC, Young JF, Hankin BL. Developmental trajectories of attachment and depressive symptoms in children and adolescents. Attach Hum Dev. 2020;22(4):392–408. https://doi.org/10.1080/14616734.2019.1624790.
49. Khantzian EJ. The self-medication hypothesis of substance use disorders: a reconsideration and recent applications. Harvard Rev Psychiatry. 1997;4(5):231–44. https://doi.org/10.3109/10673229709030550.
50. Kidd KN, Prasad D, Cunningham JEA, de Azevedo Cardoso T, Frey BN. The relationship between parental bonding and mood, anxiety and related disorders in adulthood: a systematic review and meta-analysis. J Affect Disord. 2022;307:221–36. https://doi.org/10.1016/J.JAD.2022.03.069.
51. Kitzmann KM. Effects of marital conflict on subsequent triadic family interactions and parenting. Dev Psychol. 2000;36(1):3–13. https://doi.org/10.1037/0012-1649.36.1.3.

52. Kjerulff KH, Attanasio LB, Sznajder KK, Brubaker LH. A prospective cohort study of post-traumatic stress disorder and maternal-infant bonding after first childbirth. J Psychosom Res. 2021;144:110424. https://doi.org/10.1016/J.JPSYCHORES.2021.110424.
53. Klainin P, Arthur DG. Postpartum depression in Asian cultures: a literature review. Int J Nurs Stud. 2009;46(10):1355–73. https://doi.org/10.1016/J.IJNURSTU.2009.02.012.
54. Korja R, Latva R, Lehtonen L. The effects of preterm birth on mother-infant interaction and attachment during the infant's first two years. Acta Obstet Gynecol Scand. 2012;91(2):164–73. https://doi.org/10.1111/J.1600-0412.2011.01304.X.
55. La Rosa VL, Alparone D, Commodari E. Psychological and social factors influencing mother–child bonding in the first year after birth: a model for promoting infant and maternal well-being. Front Psychol. 2025;16:1588433. https://doi.org/10.3389/FPSYG.2025.1588433/BIBTEX.
56. Leckman JF, Herman AE. Maternal behavior and developmental psychopathology. Biol Psychiatry. 2002;51(1):27–43. https://doi.org/10.1016/S0006-3223(01)01277-X.
57. Leone JM, Lane SD, Koumans EH, Demott K, Wojtowycz MA, Jensen J, Aubry RH. Effects of intimate partner violence on pregnancy trauma and placental abruption. J Women Health. 2010;19(8):1501–9. https://doi.org/10.1089/JWH.2009.1716.
58. Luyten P, Nijssens L, Fonagy P, Mayes LC. Parental reflective functioning: theory, research, and clinical applications. Psychoanal Study Child. 2017;70(1):174–99. https://doi.org/10.1080/00797308.2016.1277901;WGROUP:STRING:PUBLICATION.
59. Lyons-Ruth K, Bronfman E, Parsons E. Atypical attachment in infancy and early childhood among children at developmental risk. IV. Maternal frightened, frightening, or atypical behavior and disorganized infant attachment patterns. Monogr Soc Res Child Dev. 1999;64(3):67–96. https://doi.org/10.1111/1540-5834.00034;PAGE:STRING:ARTICLE/CHAPTER.
60. Mackle T, Colodro-Conde L, de Dassel T, Braun A, Pope A, Bennett E, Kothari A, Bruxner G, Medland SE, Patterson S. "Echoes of a dark past" is a history of maternal childhood maltreatment a perinatal risk factor for pregnancy and postpartum trauma experiences? A longitudinal study. BMC Pregnancy Childbirth. 2023;23(1):397. https://doi.org/10.1186/S12884-023-05714-2.
61. Malhotra S, Shah R. Women and mental health in India: an overview. Indian J Psychiatry. 2015;57(Suppl 2):205–11. https://doi.org/10.4103/0019-5545.161479.
62. Mazúchová L, Kelčíková S, Porubská A, Malinovská N, Grendár M. Mother-infant bonding in the postpartum period and its predictors. Cent Eur J Nurs Midw. 2020;11(3):121–9. https://doi.org/10.15452/CEJNM.2020.11.0022.
63. Miszkurka M, Zunzunegui MV, Goulet L. Immigrant status, antenatal depressive symptoms, and frequency and source of violence: what's the relationship? Arch Women's Mental Health. 2012;15(5):387–96. https://doi.org/10.1007/S00737-012-0298-7/FIGURES/2.
64. Moniri M, Mirghafourvand M, Meedya S, Ghanbari-Homaie S. Can pregnancy experience predict birth experience, postpartum depression and anxiety? A Prospective Descriptive Study Nursing Open. 2024;11(12):e70116. https://doi.org/10.1002/NOP2.70116.
65. Moog NK, Cummings PD, Jackson KL, Aschner JL, Barrett ES, Bastain TM, Blackwell CK, Bosquet Enlow M, Breton CV, Bush NR, Deoni SCL, Duarte CS, Ferrara A, Grant TL, Hipwell AE, Jones K, Leve LD, Lovinsky-Desir S, Miller RK, Buss C. Intergenerational transmission of the effects of maternal exposure to childhood maltreatment in the USA: a retrospective cohort study. Lancet Public Health. 2023;8(3):e226–37. https://doi.org/10.1016/S2468-2667(23)00025-7.
66. National Collaborating Centre for Women's and Children's Health. National Collaborating Centre for Women's and Children's Health (UK). In: Pregnancy and complex social factors: a model for service provision for pregnant women with complex social factors. RCOG Press; 2010. https://www.ncbi.nlm.nih.gov/books/NBK62607/.
67. Neale A, Wand A. Issues in the evaluation and treatment of anxiety and depression in migrant women in the perinatal period. Australas Psychiatry. 2013;21(4):379–82. https://doi.org/10.1177/1039856213486215;PAGEGROUP:STRING:PUBLICATION.

68. Nicol-Harper R, Harvey AG, Stein A. Interactions between mothers and infants: impact of maternal anxiety. Infant Behav Dev. 2007;30(1):161–7. https://doi.org/10.1016/J.INFBEH.2006.08.005.
69. Nolvi S, Karlsson L, Bridgett DJ, Pajulo M, Tolvanen M, Karlsson H. Maternal postnatal psychiatric symptoms and infant temperament affect early mother-infant bonding. Infant Behav Dev. 2016;43:13–23. https://doi.org/10.1016/J.INFBEH.2016.03.003.
70. Nordahl D, Rognmo K, Bohne A, Landsem IP, Moe V, Wang CEA, Høifødt RS. Adult attachment style and maternal-infant bonding: the indirect path of parenting stress. BMC Psychol. 2020;8(1):1–11. https://doi.org/10.1186/S40359-020-00424-2/FIGURES/1.
71. O'Dea GA, Youssef GJ, Hagg LJ, Francis LM, Spry EA, Rossen L, Smith I, Teague SJ, Mansour K, Booth A, Davies S, Hutchinson D, Macdonald JA. Associations between maternal psychological distress and mother-infant bonding: a systematic review and meta-analysis. Arch Women's Mental Health. 2023;26(4):441–52. https://doi.org/10.1007/S00737-023-01332-1.
72. Osok J, Kigamwa P, Huang KY, Grote N, Kumar M. Adversities and mental health needs of pregnant adolescents in Kenya: identifying interpersonal, practical, and cultural barriers to care. BMC Womens Health. 2018;18(1):96. https://doi.org/10.1186/S12905-018-0581-5.
73. Palladino CL, Singh V, Campbell J, Flynn H, Gold KJ. Homicide and suicide during the perinatal period: findings from the national violent death reporting system. Obstet Gynecol. 2011;118(5):1056–63. https://doi.org/10.1097/AOG.0B013E31823294DA.
74. Pierrehumbert B, Nicole A, Muller-Nix C, Forcada-Guex M, Ansermet F. Parental post-traumatic reactions after premature birth: implications for sleeping and eating problems in the infant. Arch Dis Child Fetal Neonatal Ed. 2003;88(5) https://doi.org/10.1136/FN.88.5.F400.
75. Rariden C, SmithBattle L, Yoo JH, Cibulka N, Loman D. Screening for adverse childhood experiences: literature review and practice implications. J Nurs Pract. 2021;17(1):98–104. https://doi.org/10.1016/j.nurpra.2020.08.002.
76. Recto P, Champion JD. Psychosocial risk factors for perinatal depression among female adolescents: a systematic review. Issues Mental Health Nurs. 2017;38(8):633–42. https://doi.org/10.1080/01612840.2017.1330908.
77. Ross LE, McQueen K, Vigod S, Dennis CL. Risk for postpartum depression associated with assisted reproductive technologies and multiple births: a systematic review. Hum Reprod Update. 2011;17(1):96–106. https://doi.org/10.1093/HUMUPD/DMQ025.
78. Saltzman LE, Johnson CH, Gilbert BC, Goodwin MM. Physical abuse around the time of pregnancy: an examination of prevalence and risk factors in 16 states. Matern Child Health J. 2003;7(1):31–43. https://doi.org/10.1023/A:1022589501039.
79. Schreier HMC, Enlow MB, Ritz T, Gennings C, Wright RJ. Childhood abuse is associated with increased hair cortisol levels among urban pregnant women. J Epidemiol Community Health. 2015;69(12):1169–74. https://doi.org/10.1136/JECH-2015-205541.
80. Sharma I, Pathak A. Women mental health in India. Indian J Psychiatry. 2015;57(Suppl 2):201–4. https://doi.org/10.4103/0019-5545.161478.
81. Shorey S, Yang YY, Ang E. The impact of negative childbirth experience on future reproductive decisions: a quantitative systematic review. J Adv Nurs. 2018;74(6):1236–44. https://doi.org/10.1111/JAN.13534.
82. Silverman JG, Decker MR, Reed E, Raj A. Intimate partner violence victimization prior to and during pregnancy among women residing in 26 U.S. states: associations with maternal and neonatal health. Am J Obstet Gynecol. 2006;195(1):140–8. https://doi.org/10.1016/j.ajog.2005.12.052.
83. Slade A, Sadler L, De Dios-Kenn C, Webb D, Currier-Ezepchick J, Mayes L. Minding the baby: a reflective parenting program. Psychoanal Study Child. 2005;60(1):74–100. https://doi.org/10.1080/00797308.2005.11800747.
84. Śliwerski A, Kossakowska K, Jarecka K, Świtalska J, Bielawska-Batorowicz E. The effect of maternal depression on infant attachment: a systematic review. Int J Environ Res Public Health. 2020;17(8):2675. https://doi.org/10.3390/IJERPH17082675.

85. Spinner MR. Maternal-infant bonding. Can Family Phys Medecin de Famille Canadien. 1978;24:1151–3.
86. Stepanikova I, Acharya S, Abdalla S, Baker E, Klanova J, Darmstadt GL. Gender discrimination and depressive symptoms among child-bearing women: ELSPAC-CZ cohort study. EClinicalMedicine. 2020;20 https://doi.org/10.1016/j.eclinm.2020.100297.
87. Stepanikova I, Acharya S, Colón-López A, Abdalla S, Klanova J, Darmstadt GL. Maternal gender discrimination and child emotional and behavioural problems: a population-based, longitudinal cohort study in the Czech Republic. EClinicalMedicine. 2022;53:101627. https://doi.org/10.1016/J.ECLINM.2022.101627.
88. Stevenson K, Fellmeth G, Edwards S, Calvert C, Bennett P, Campbell OMR, Fuhr DC. The global burden of perinatal common mental health disorders and substance use among migrant women: a systematic review and meta-analysis. Lancet Public Health. 2023;8(3):e203–16. https://doi.org/10.1016/S2468-2667(22)00342-5.
89. Stewart DE, Gagnon AJ, Merry LA, Dennis CL. Risk factors and health profiles of recent migrant women who experienced violence associated with pregnancy. J Women Health. 2012;21(10):1100–6. https://doi.org/10.1089/JWH.2011.3415;JOURNAL:JOURNAL:JWH;PAGE:STRING:ARTICLE/CHAPTER.
90. Suchman NE, DeCoste C, Leigh D, Borelli J. Reflective functioning in mothers with drug use disorders: implications for dyadic interactions with infants and toddlers. Attach Hum Dev. 2010;12(6):567–85. https://doi.org/10.1080/14616734.2010.501988.
91. Supraja TA, Varghese M, Desai G, Chandra PS. The relationship of gender preference to anxiety, stress and family violence among pregnant women in urban India. Int J Cult Ment Health. 2016;9(4):356–63. https://doi.org/10.1080/17542863.2016.1205114.
92. Swain JE, Lorberbaum JP, Kose S, Strathearn L. Brain basis of early parent–infant interactions: psychology, physiology, and in vivo functional neuroimaging studies. J Child Psychol Psychiatry. 2007;48(3–4):262–87. https://doi.org/10.1111/J.1469-7610.2007.01731.X.
93. Tang Y, Li S, Ma L, Zheng Y, Li Y. The effects of mother-father relationships on children's social-emotional competence: the chain mediating model of parental emotional expression and parent-child attachment. Child Youth Serv Rev. 2023;155:107227. https://doi.org/10.1016/J.CHILDYOUTH.2023.107227.
94. Tao P, Coates R, Maycock B. Investigating marital relationship in infertility: a systematic review of quantitative studies. J Reprod Infertil. 2012;13(2):71–80. https://www.scopus.com/record/display.uri?eid=2-s2.0-84861122745&origin=inward
95. Teicher MH, Samson JA, Anderson CM, Ohashi K. The effects of childhood maltreatment on brain structure, function and connectivity. Nat Rev Neurosci. 2016;17(10):652–66. https://doi.org/10.1038/NRN.2016.111.
96. Thamby A, Bajaj A, Manoj L, Sunil Kumar G, Gokul G, Thennarasu K, Jaisoorya T. Impaired mother-infant bonding: a community study from India. J Reprod Infant Psychol. 2024;42(3):528–39. https://doi.org/10.1080/02646838.2022.2125938;JOURNAL:JOURNAL:CJRI20;PAGE:STRING:ARTICLE/CHAPTER.
97. Thomas JL, Lewis JB, Martinez I, Cunningham SD, Siddique M, Tobin JN, Ickovics JR. Associations between intimate partner violence profiles and mental health among low-income, urban pregnant adolescents. BMC Pregnancy Childbirth. 2019;19(1):1–8. https://doi.org/10.1186/S12884-019-2256-0/TABLES/2.
98. Thornberry TP, Knight KE, Lovegrove PJ. Does maltreatment beget maltreatment? A systematic review of the intergenerational literature. Trauma Violence Abuse. 2012;13(3):135–52. https://doi.org/10.1177/1524838012447697.
99. Tietz A, Zietlow AL, Reck C. Maternal bonding in mothers with postpartum anxiety disorder: the crucial role of subclinical depressive symptoms and maternal avoidance behaviour. Arch Women's Mental Health. 2014;17(5):433–42. https://doi.org/10.1007/S00737-014-0423-X/TABLES/4.
100. van den Bloom DC, Hoeksma JB. The effect of infant irritability on mother-infant interaction: a growth-curve analysis. Dev Psychol. 1994;30(4):581–90. https://psycnet.apa.org/buy/1994-37174-001

101. Wang H, Zhang Y, Ding W, Dai J, Zhu X, Xu X. Intergenerational association of adverse childhood experiences and perinatal mental health in adult female offspring: evidence from the longitudinal grandmothers, mothers, and their Children's health study in China. Lancet Reg Health Western Pac. 2025;59:101579. https://doi.org/10.1016/J.LANWPC.2025.101579.
102. Waters SF, Virmani EA, Thompson RA, Meyer S, Raikes HA, Jochem R. Emotion regulation and attachment: unpacking two constructs and their association. J Psychopathol Behav Assess. 2010;32(1):37–47. https://doi.org/10.1007/S10862-009-9163-Z/FIGURES/1.
103. Yost NP, Bloom SL, McIntire DD, Leveno KJ. A prospective observational study of domestic violence during pregnancy. Obstet Gynecol. 2005;106(1):61–5. https://doi.org/10.1097/01.AOG.0000164468.06070.2A.
104. Zdolska-Wawrzkiewicz A, Chrzan-Dętkoś M, Bidzan M. Maternal attachment style during pregnancy and becoming a mother in Poland. J Reprod Infant Psychol. 2018;36(1):4–14. https://doi.org/10.1080/02646838.2017.1395400.

Abortion and Mental Health

32

Marta B. Rondón

32.1 Introduction

About 34,000 women die every year due to the complications of unsafe abortion. Every year, between 2010 and 2014, there were about 55 million abortions, of which around 55%, that is 25 million, were unsafe. These are major contributors to maternal mortality and put women at risk of legal prosecution, stigmatization, and extreme morbidity.

According to the World Health Organization, abortion is the loss of the fetus before it is viable, and unsafe abortion is "a procedure for termination of a pregnancy done by an individual who does not have the necessary training or in an environment not conforming to minimal medical standards [1]." Around 97% of these occur in developing nations, located in Asia, Africa, or Latin America [2]. Recently, a distinction between "less unsafe" and "unsafe" was introduced to make way for a correct appraisal of medical abortion and manual vacuum aspiration as the less unsafe alternatives [3].

Pregnancy and postpartum have been recognized as periods when the well-being of the woman is challenged by several physical, social, and psychological demands. Even as maternity and motherhood have been romanticized in most cultures, it is currently understood that pregnancy does not protect from mental illnesses and that special attention must be paid to the woman's health, both physical and mental, during the perinatal period to ensure favorable outcomes for mother and child.

Recent data on the association of suicide and social determinants of health has identified being perinatal as one of the factors linked to high suicidality [4].

M. B. Rondón (✉)
Universidad San Martin de Porres, Facultad de Medicina Humana, Instituto de Investigación, Lima, Peru

M. López-Atanes, M. Sáenz-Herrero (eds.), *Applying the Gender Perspective in Psychiatry and Psychotherapy*, https://doi.org/10.1007/978-3-032-17883-1_32

Furthermore, intimate partner violence (IPV) has been identified as one of the strongest risk factors for suicidal ideation [4].

IPV, more prevalent in less affluent and industrialized countries, is linked to unwanted pregnancy, which in turn triggers anxiety, hostility, and depression. Vulnerable, victimized women find themselves trapped in desperate situations, unable to leave their aggressors. Involuntary motherhood may represent a very heavy physical and mental burden, and it may put a woman in dire danger of violence, poverty, or illness. It is one of the most powerful drivers of gender inequality.

The Beijing Platform for Action recognized that equal access to the highest attainable level of health is a strategic need for women to attain equality. This level of health can only be achieved if there is information and services for women to "have the capability to reproduce and the freedom to decide if, when, and how often to do so [5]."

Induced abortion to attain free, safe, and voluntary maternity is, of course, not desired by anybody. It is a difficult decision for any woman, and it shows how injustice, violence, and stereotypical roles harm women. It is the end result of social failures in education, health, and cultural and family pressures [6].

32.2 Maternal Mental Health and Pregnancy Intendedness

Unwanted pregnancy is the root cause of abortion [7]. In turn, several researchers on perinatal depression have found a link between unwanted pregnancy and depression during pregnancy and postpartum. Consequently, the prevention of unwanted pregnancy ought to lower the high prevalence of mood disorders during the peripartum period, which are pervasive mood disorders that affects both the mother and the child.

Perinatal depression, affecting between 15% and 44% of pregnant women in low- and middle-income countries, is a serious illness with clear neurobiological, psychological, and social determinants that causes disability and is comorbid with other physical and mental ailments that can end in suicide. It significantly interferes with the functioning of the affected person and diminishes his/her chances of achieving personal, academic, and work realization [8].

Depression poses other health risks for pregnant women too: it has been shown that depressed women have a higher chance of obstetric complications, such as emergency C-sections, instrumental deliveries, more epidural anesthetics, more admissions to intensive care units, and a higher rate of premature and small-for-gestational-age deliveries [9].

Suicide is not frequent during pregnancy; but, in some countries, it is the leading cause of maternal mortality, especially in younger women when they carry unwanted pregnancies in severely restrictive contexts, where no other way out seems possible [10–12].

Unwanted pregnancy has been recognized as one of the risk factors for perinatal, particularly postnatal depression. Fisher [13], in a review of 34 papers from 17 low- and middle-income countries reporting on depression in women who had given birth, found that the prevalence of postpartum depression was 19.8% (CI 95% 19.5–20.0) and identified the following risk factors:

Socioeconomic disadvantage OR range 2.1–13.2
Unwanted pregnancy OR range 1.6–8.8
Being younger OR 2.5–5.4
Being unmarried OR range 3.4–5. 8
Lacking intimate partner empathy and support OR range 2.0–9.4
Having hostile in-laws OR range 2.1–4.4
Experiencing intimate partner violence OR range 2.11–6.75
Having insufficient emotional and practical support OR range 2.8–6.1
In some settings: giving birth to a female OR range 1.8–2.6
Having a history of mental health problems OR range 5.1–5.6

Secondary analysis of the data from the Pregnancy Infection and Nutrition study (PIN3) has shown that pregnancy intention does indeed have an impact on postpartum mental health. Out of 680 women enrolled, 433 (64%) reported an intended pregnancy, 207 (30%) reported a mistimed pregnancy (they did want a child but not at that point in time), and 40 (6%) had an unwanted pregnancy. Although overall only 7.3% of the sample was depressed at 6 months postpartum and 6% was depressed at 12 months, the women who had reported an unwanted pregnancy had three times the rate of depression (15%) compared to those who had a desired pregnancy (5%) 3 months postpartum. At 12 months, the gap was much wider, with 20% of women with unwanted children depressed vs 3% of women who had wanted to be pregnant and 11% of those who reported mistimed pregnancies [14]. This study, done in a setting where abortion is legal, supports very clearly the plausibility of a link between unintended pregnancy and postpartum depression, especially in underprivileged populations. Women chose to keep the baby, and yet their mental health was harmed by the experience.

In a large study (982 women who started prenatal care before week 16), researchers found that women who reported unplanned pregnancies tended to have lower levels of brain-derived neurotrophic factor (BDNF). Women with the lower levels of BDNF in turn, were found to have 1.61 times higher odds of antepartum depression (OR = 1.61; 95% CI: 1.13–2.30) after adjusting for potential confounders such as maternal age, early maternal BMI, and parity [15]. This illustrates that probably the added stress of facing an unwanted pregnancy induces changes in the brain that are associated with an increased chance of suffering from depression.

Alterations in the metabolism of cortisol, assessed via hair cortisol concentration, may also be linked to unwanted or mistimed pregnancy. Unplanned pregnancy is so stressful that it causes prenatal depression in many cases [16]. The hypothalamus is stimulated under stress and secretes the corticotropin-releasing hormone (CRH), which triggers the secretion of the adrenocorticotropic hormone (ACTH) into the bloodstream, targeting the adrenal cortex. Cortisol is secreted there—and subsequently acts on maternal and fetal target tissues. There is evidence that elevated hair cortisol concentrations in the first trimester may be associated with preterm birth. The first trimester is when women discover themselves to be pregnant and are expected to deal with various emotions that depend on the woman's social and psychological context. This is the time to face partner abandonment, changes in plans and goals, and family rejection for those who are confronted with an unplanned pregnancy.

In settings where abortion is illegal, the untoward consequences of unwanted pregnancy may be worse. A lengthy follow-up study of women who were denied abortion in Czechoslovakia and their progeny shows that the mental health of the mother is affected for at least 7 years, and the physical and mental health of the children is permanently harmed [17].

Lara et al found that an unplanned pregnancy increased the odds of postpartum depression and postpartum depressive symptoms 2.71 times at 6 weeks postpartum and 2.81 times at 6 months postpartum. However, an unwanted pregnancy raised the odds by 3.87 times at 6 weeks postpartum and 2.71 times at 6 months postpartum [18]. The authors also note that circumstances such as pregnancy intention, low educational attainment, low income, and being unemployed are crucial factors in developing countries, but not in developed countries. Of particular importance is the observation that the burden (both financial and psychological) of an unwanted pregnancy may be higher for disadvantaged women, whose coping mechanisms are already overburdened.

32.3 Progress in Recent Years

In the past 30 years, more than 60 countries have liberalized their abortion laws. We can now state that the majority of women (60%) of the world live in places where legal abortion is available. In all, 34% of women live in countries where abortion is available on request. Twelve percent of women reside in countries where abortion is available to protect their health. This includes, in some cases, mental health, and there are special provisions for rape and some fetal malformations. There are 44 countries (where 20% of the world's women live) that only allow abortion to save the woman's life. Six percent live in countries where abortion is totally prohibited. Unfortunately, the regions of the world where abortion is restricted are regions with lower incomes and lower levels of overall development [19] (Fig. 32.1).

A seminal article by Sedgh et al. analyzes the trends in abortion in the different regions to dispel the myth that liberalization of abortion regulation causes an increase in the number of abortions. The rate of abortions has declined from 40 per 1000 women in 1990–94 to 35 in 2010–2014. The decline in the developed world has been 19 points; in the developing countries, the decline has been only 2%. Furthermore, Latin America and the Caribbean, a region with restrictive laws (except for Uruguay, Colombia, Mexico, and Argentina), shows an increase in the rate of abortions.

In the regions of the world where abortion is allowed only to save the woman's life or to protect her health, there is a higher chance that a woman in need of an abortion will resort to an unsafe procedure. Even if her health is at stake, there are

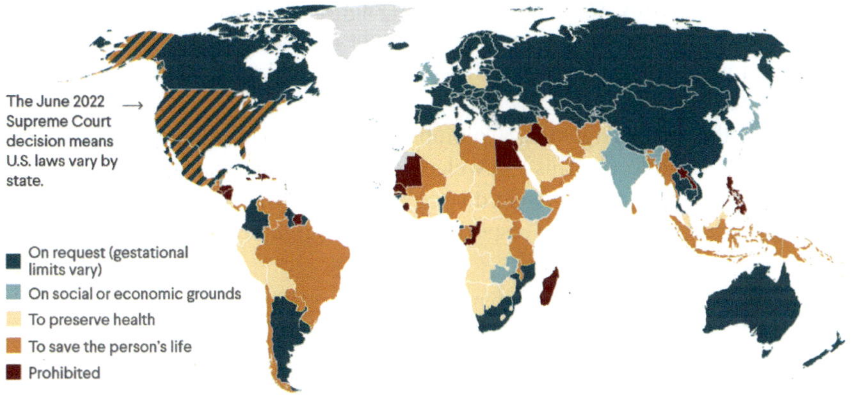

Fig. 32.1 Abortion laws around the world. FUENTE: CENTER FOR REPRODUCTIVE RIGHTS. Notes: Abortion laws vary by state in the United States and Mexico. Some countries that permit abortion to save the person's life, to preserve health, or on social or economic grounds also permit it in cases of rape, incest, or fetal impairment

issues that will prevent the woman from obtaining a safe termination in a health center; for instance, abortion services may be unavailable or difficult to access, there may be lack of awareness of what the law permits, both in the health providers and in the people; women may be prevented from seeking care due to cultural and religious ideas or fear of ill-treatment or legal reprisals, unwillingness from practitioners to implement abortion laws and recognize that women have a right; abortion services may be of low quality or too costly, or the attitudes of medical staff may discourage the women or conscientious objectors, not well regulated by local law, may deny women the treatment [20].

That a country has a legal provision to allow termination of pregnancy to protect a woman's health speaks of the preoccupation with the health—and dignity—of the woman, it emphasizes that a given society values the well-being of the woman. Abortion is a legal right and, in cases where the health of the woman is at stake, it is a human right.

In the Americas, the map of abortion has changed drastically. The overturn of Roe v Wade in the United States has introduced a powerful backward force, and women, as well as sexual and reproductive health professionals, now need to put up a fight to protect the right of women to self-determination. Recent literature has highlighted the increase in suicide risk in the United States due to provider-targeted abortion restrictions [21], which is to say that the denial of abortion causes anxiety and heightened stress in women. This additional load may give rise to severe psychopathology in vulnerable individuals, ending up in suicide.

Two other countries in Latin America (Nicaragua and El Salvador) and one in Europe (Poland) have hardened their restrictions. In El Salvador, 181 women who suffered obstetric emergencies resulting in miscarriage were jailed between 2000 and 2019 [22]. The International Human Rights Court finally issued a sentence on the lengthy "Caso Beatriz v. El Salvador," stating that the denial of a timely abortion to a woman suffering from lupus and carrying an anencephalic fetus constitute obstetric violence. As such, it violated her right to health and subjected Beatriz to unjustified anguish. It is expected that El Salvador will take steps to comply with this sentence [23].

On the other hand, Argentina, Colombia, and Mexico have made abortion available up to the 12th week. This is a welcome change in the area of the world where social and economic development do not go in hand with maternal mortality, intimate partner violence, and the respect for women's rights.

32.4 Abortion When Health Is at Risk

Health is defined as a state of complete physical, psychological, and social well-being, and not merely as the absence of disease.

Pregnancy may represent a risk to the mother's health as a consequence of physiological vulnerability, such as complications inherent to pregnancy itself, for instance, hyperemesis gravidarum or eclampsia; or it may interfere with the treatment of other potentially life-threatening conditions, such as cancer. A third case occurs when pregnancy coexists with other illnesses that may be aggravated by gestation.

Under these considerations, the possibility that a pregnancy may trigger or increase a woman's risk of depression or of not being able to receive adequate treatment for any other mental condition should immediately prompt the discussion of whether she wants to use her right to therapeutic abortion.

In this case, it is important to recognize that depression is a serious illness that causes disability, difficulties in interpersonal interactions, social and work dysfunction, leads to stigma and discrimination, and may end up in suicide.

However, mental health is much more than the absence of depression. It includes a positive state of well-being that allows the individual to have a clear vision of a meaningful present and a significant future; with mental health comes the promise of self-realization.

For adolescents who become pregnant, the fact that pregnancy will imperil their chances of graduating from secondary school or attending tertiary education, and that the processes of developing an identity of their own, forming relationships, and becoming financially independent will be irreversibly stopped, should prompt consideration of therapeutic abortion: the reason being the protection of mental health.

32.5 The Impact of Abortion on the Mental Health of the Woman

Research on the mental health consequences of abortion has been difficult to interpret because of methodological flaws. Steinberg has proposed that the ideal case/control study would include women who desired abortions and got them, and a control group of women who wanted an abortion but were denied. This method is followed in the cohort study led by Antonia Biggs, the TurnAway study, which demonstrated that women who had been denied abortions had worse mental health than those who got the procedure. Being denied an abortion was associated with a greater risk of adverse psychological outcomes in the first week after an abortion [24].

Furthermore, the 956 women enrolled were followed for 5 years, and depression was similar between the two groups at the end of the period. However, women who were denied the abortion had experienced increased poverty [24] and a higher risk of violence from the man involved in the pregnancy [25].

In Uruguay, women who had access to legal abortions reported satisfaction with the availability and quality of the services, although there was a high level of internalized and suffered stigma [26].

Mexico City public hospitals have provided legal abortions since 2012, allowing for interesting research on the emotional consequences in a very Catholic and conservative setting. Florez-Celis, Cordero-Oropeza, and Ramos-Lira [27] have found that stigma is highly prevalent among women who have abortions. In a cross-sectional study, they found that 15.8% of women presented with depressive symptoms 2 weeks after an abortion, and this was associated with stigma, previous experience of violence, and previous childless pregnancies [28].

In sum, newer research supports that abortion does not damage mental health; stigma seems to play a big role in unfavorable short-term emotional responses, and, in the long term, social health seems to be better in women who get abortions in comparison with those who do not.

32.6 Final Remark

The relationship between abortion and mental health is a complex one. On one hand, the notion that abortion may cause lasting depression, anxiety, or an ailment similar to posttraumatic stress is being dispelled by good-quality research. The role of stigma as a factor in the dynamics of depressive symptoms needs to be studied further.

On the other hand, a large proportion of women in the world have access to abortion to protect their health (physical and mental) only. The inclusion of a mental health component in access to abortion needs rejection of our traditional dualist conceptions of health as well as an emphasis on health being a state of well-being, not only the absence of disease.

It is timely to point out that "therapeutic" is a misnomer. Termination of pregnancy does not cure a mental illness, and this is not what is intended by allowing abortion "to protect the health of the woman." Rather, what is intended is that a woman is not subjected to undue suffering caused by an unwanted pregnancy, compounded by a personal history of previous depressive illness, childhood adversity, familial history of depression, obstetric complications, social and economic deprivation, interpersonal violence, or comorbid physical illness. These circumstances challenge the capacity of a person to cope with stress to the point where severe illness may follow. The rationale for allowing abortion in these cases is to protect the woman from depression and its complications, and to protect her right to the highest attainable level of health.

References

1. Ganatra B, Tunçalp Ö, Johnston HB, Johnson BR, Gülmezoglu A, Temmerman M. From concept to measurement: operationalizing WHO's definition of unsafe abortion. Bull World Health Organ. 2014;92:155.
2. WHO Worldwide, an estimated 25 million unsafe abortions occur each year. Press release; http://www.who.int/news-room/detail/28-09-2017-worldwide-an-estimated-25-million-unsafe-abortions-occur-each-year
3. Ganatra B, Gerdts C, Rossier C, Johnson BR Jr, Tunçalp Ö, Assifi A, Sedgh G, Singh S, Bankole A, Popinchalk A, Bearak J, Kang Z, Alkema L. Global, regional, and subregional classification of abortions by safety, 2010–14: estimates from a Bayesian hierarchical model. Lancet. 2017;390(10110):2372–81. https://doi.org/10.1016/S0140-6736(17)31794-4. Epub 2017 Sept 27
4. Na PJ, Shin J, Kwak HR, et al. Social determinants of health and suicide-related outcomes: a review of meta-analyses. JAMA Psychiatry. 2025;82(4):337–46. https://doi.org/10.1001/jamapsychiatry.2024.4241.
5. Fourth World Conference on Women, Beijing Declaration and Platform for Action, September 1995. Para 94, p. 95; http://www.un.org/womenwatch/daw/beijing/pdf/BDPfA%20E.pdf
6. Briozzo L. Aborto provocado: un problema humano. Perspectivas para su análisis – estrategias para su reducción. Rev Méd Urug [online]. 2003;19(3):188–200. Disponible en: http://www.scielo.edu.uy/scielo.php?script=sci_arttext&pid=S1688-03902003000300002&lng=es&nrm=iso. ISSN:1688-0390
7. Pinotti JA, Faundes A. Unwanted pregnancy: challenges for health policy. Int J Gynecol Obstet. 1989;3(Suppl 3):97–102.
8. Berndt ER, Koran LM, Finkelstein SN, Gelenberg AJ, Kornstein SG, Miller MI, Thase ME, Trapp GA, Keller MB. Lost human capital from earlyonset chronic depression. Am J Psychiatry. 2000;157(6):940–7.
9. Chung T, Lau T, Yip A, Chiu H, Lee D. Antepartum depressive symptomatology is associated with adverse obstetric and neonatal outcomes. Psychosom Med. 2001;63(5):830–4.
10. Department of Health. Report of the confidential enquiries into maternal deaths. London: Department of Health; 1999.
11. Brockington I. Suicide in women. Int Clin Psychopharmacol. 2001;16:S7–S19.
12. Frautschi S, Cerulli A, Maine D. Suicide during pregnancy and its neglect as a component of maternal mortality. Int J Gynaecol obstet. 1994;47:275–84.
13. Fisher J, Cabral de Mello M, Patel V, Rahman A, Tran T, Holton S, Holmes W. Prevalence and determinants of common perinatal mental disorders in women in low- and lower-middle-income countries: a systematic review. Bull World Health Organ. 2012;90(2):139G–49G. https://doi.org/10.2471/BLT.11.091850. Epub 2011 Nov 24
14. Mercier RJ, Garrett J, Thorp J, Siega-Riz AM. Pregnancy intention and postpartum depression: secondary data analysis from a prospective cohort. BJOG. 2013;120(9):1116–22.
15. Fung J, Gelaye B, Zhong QY, Rondon MB, Sanchez SE, Barrios YV, Hevner K, Qiu C, Williams MA. Association of decreased serum brain-derived neurotrophic factor (BDNF) concentrations in early pregnancy with antepartum depression. BMC Psychiatry. 2015;15:43. https://doi.org/10.1186/s12888-015-0428-7.

16. Faisal-Cury A, Menezes PR, Quayle J, Matijasevich A. Unplanned pregnancy and risk of maternal depression: secondary data analysis from a prospective pregnancy cohort. Psychol Health Med. 2017;22(1):65–74.
17. David H. Born unwanted, 35 years later: the Prague Study. Reprod Health Matt. 2006;14:181–90.
18. Lara MA, Navarrete L, Nieto L. Prenatal predictors of postpartum depression and postpartum depressive symptoms in Mexican mothers: a longitudinal study. Arch Womens Ment Health. 2016;19(5):825–34. https://doi.org/10.1007/s00737-016-0623-7.
19. Center for Reproductive Rights. A Global View of World's abortion laws. World Abortion Map. http://worldabortionlaws.com/about.html
20. World Health Organization. Unsafe abortion global and regional estimates of the incidence of unsafe abortion and associated mortality in 2008. p. 7.
21. Zandberg J, Waller R, Visoki E, Barzilay R. Association between state-level access to reproductive care and suicide rates among women of reproductive age in the United States. JAMA Psychiatry. 2023;80(2):127–34. https://doi.org/10.1001/jamapsychiatry.2022.4394. PMID: 36576746; PMCID: PMC9857811
22. Diario El País, 17 dic 2022; https://elpais.com/america-futura/2022-12-17/rosita-4934-noches-en-una-carcel-de-el-salvador-po. Accessed 12 Apr 2025.
23. Corte IDH. Caso Beatriz y otros Vs. El Salvador. Fondo, Reparaciones y Costas. Sentencia de 22 de noviembre de 2024. Serie C No. 549; https://jurisprudencia.corteidh.or.cr/es/vid/1061937459. Accessed 13 Apr 2022.
24. Biggs MA, Upadhyay UD, McCulloch CE, Foster DG. Women's mental health and well-being 5 years after receiving or being denied an abortion: a prospective, longitudinal cohort study. JAMA Psychiatry. 2017;74(2):169–78. https://doi.org/10.1001/jamapsychiatry.2016.3478. Erratum in: JAMA Psychiatry. 2017;74(3):303. doi:10.1001/jamapsychiatry.2016.4174. PMID: 27973641
25. Roberts SCM, Biggs MA, Chibber KS, Gould H, Rocca CH, Foster DG. Risk of violence from the man involved in the pregnancy after receiving or being denied an abortion. BMC Med. 2014;12:144.
26. Makleff S, Labandera A, Chiribao F, et al. Experiencia en la obtención de un aborto legal en Uruguay: conocimientos, actitudes y estigma entre las usuarias de aborto. BMC Women Health. 2019;19:155. https://doi.org/10.1186/s12905-019-0855-6.
27. Flores-Celis K, Cordero Oropeza M, Ramos-Lira LE. Psychosocial profiles of women who legally terminated a pregnancy in Mexico City. Salud Ment [online]. 2024;47(1):35–43. https://doi.org/10.17711/sm.0185-3325.2024.005. Disponible en: http://www.scielo.org.mx/scielo.php?script=sci_arttext&pid=S0185-33252024000100035&lng=es&nrm=iso. Epub 15-Abr-2024. ISSN 0185-3325
28. Ramos-Lira L, Karla FC, Moreno López M, Saltijeral M, Wagne F. Revista Latinoamericana de Psicología. 2023;55:64–72.

Prostitution and Mental Health

33

Marian Arias Roncero

33.1 Introduction

Askabide is a nonprofit, independent association that has been working since 1985 for the inclusion of people engaged in prostitution in the Basque Country, as well as women who are facing social exclusion.

To achieve this goal, our work is oriented to:

- Developing projects that attend to this collective, always starting from the concrete experience of direct dealings with these people, aiming to give a comprehensive response to all the needs they present.
- Developing projects of information, sensitization, and social denunciation of the situation in which this group finds itself.

In a continuous search for ways of approaching this reality, we work to find solutions to those aspects of marginalization and exclusion that are related to prostitution.

33.2 Situation of Prostitution in the Basque Country

Prostitution is a multifaceted issue that presents many faces and angles from which it can be approached in the social, legal, labor, health, immigration, and policies implemented by the different administrations. It is a complex reality, involving multiple agents and dynamics in continuous transformation.

M. A. Roncero (✉)
Responsible for Training and Sensitisation in Askabide, Basque Country, Spain
e-mail: marianarias@askabide.org

M. López-Atanes, M. Sáenz-Herrero (eds.), *Applying the Gender Perspective in Psychiatry and Psychotherapy*, https://doi.org/10.1007/978-3-032-17883-1_33

People engaged in prostitution (PEPs) constitute a group of people who are different in terms of sex, gender, sexual orientation and identity, nationality, age, or social and ecological characteristics that can determine a greater or lesser degree of social exclusion, as well as greater difficulty and inequality in accessing services and resources that guarantee their rights.

According to the study titled "Trafficking in Women and Girls for Sexual Exploitation", conducted by Carmen Meneses 2021, the fieldwork, developed in parallel and triangulated, allows us to estimate that in 2018, the number of women involved in prostitution in the Basque Country ranged between 1968 and 2308 women in Euskadi.

The working document prepared by the Department of Social Affairs of the Basque Government for the working group developed in 2012, titled Transition Model for the Incorporation into the Basque Social Services System of Interventions in the Field of Prostitution, outlines the main problems faced by this group:

- Irregular administrative situation is the main obstacle to social integration and access to resources.
- Widespread lack of knowledge of the existing socio-sanitary and socio-assistance resources of the public network.
- Limited access to decent housing and working conditions due, among other causes, to the high mobility in the exercise of prostitution.
- Incidence of depression and psychological disorders linked to stress, loneliness, fear, and social stigma, which prevent them from developing an autonomous and full life.
- Increased risk rates of HIV and other STI transmission and infection due to the increase in unsafe sexual practices, along with unwanted pregnancies among young women.
- Maintenance of situations of violence by partners and acceptance of risky practices by women, for fear of expulsion and to obtain income.
- Experience of situations of exploitation and violence linked to the existence of sexual exploitation and forced prostitution networks around macro-clubs, to which access is limited.

Although this study was carried out in 2012, the same problems of this group are still present today. Among the projects that we develop in Askabide, where we engage and work with these women, the field program called "Community intervention agents," which consists of establishing contact and intervening with the group of people engaged in prostitution (PEP) in Bizkaia, in the same places where they carry out their activities of prostitution (clubs, apartments, and streets) with intervention agents, who come from similar backgrounds as those they work with, play a key role in this effort.

The intervention agent is a woman with a background in prostitution whose profile is similar to that of the target group, and whose knowledge and life experience allow her to integrate easily into this context, understand the needs of those engaged in prostitution, and develop easily in this context, as well as identifying the needs of the group and determining the appropriate language to address them.

This methodology, based on the theory of peers, has proved very valid, since PEPs accept and receive information better when it is transmitted by a peer.

In 2024, thanks to this program, we have contacted 543 different people.

As for the profile of these people, 99% of these contacts have been with women (98% with cisgender women, 1% transgender women) and 1% with men.

It should also be noted that 98% of the contacts were with migrant women, 91% of whom were from Latin American countries.

Secondly, there is the "Welcome Center" program, which we define as a center for attention, information, and counseling in a specialized area such as prostitution and exclusion.

Our work at the reception center is to provide women in prostitution and/or in situations of exclusion with the necessary tools, through information, counseling, and support services in various areas, to respond to their needs and demands and promote real and full integration into our society.

In 2024, we have assisted 318 people in this program, of whom 94% were cis women, 4.5% transgender women, and 5% men.

In terms of age, 81% of the people we have assisted are between 30 and 64 years old, 15% are between 19 and 29 years old, and 4% are over 65 years old.

With regard to the level of education, 32% of the people assisted have no education and 34% have a high school diploma or basic education. About 12% have intermediate or higher studies and 13% have a high school diploma.

In terms of origin, 92% of the people served are migrants. About 37% come from Latin American countries, 26% from Maghreb countries, and 27% from other African countries, with only 7% representing the national women assisted.

Almost half of the people assisted (49%) are in a situation of administrative irregularity.

It should be noted that even though they are registered on the census, only 27% receive some kind of financial benefit, with almost 80% of the people assisted not receiving any type of benefit. In most cases, these people do not have a lease or sublease contract for the homes in which they live.

In summary, the main profile of the people we have assisted in the reception center has been female, migrant, without a social or family network, between 30 and 60 years old, and almost half of them in a situation of administrative irregularity; they are women who come from prostitution and face social exclusion, and none of them receive any form of financial support.

On the other hand, it is necessary to point out that the characteristics that define the phenomenon of prostitution in recent times are the heterogeneity of the group of people engaged in prostitution (PEP), the invisibility of the premises where prostitution is exercised and the high mobility of PEP from one premises to another.

The widespread use of the Internet as a means to offer and demand paid sexual services has contributed greatly to increasing the invisibility of the group and the places where the activity takes place. In addition to the discretion it offers, this form of contact has made it possible to diversify the environments in which prostitution can be practiced (apartments, residential premises, etc.), making access to PEPs and their clients increasingly difficult due to the impossibility of identifying them as such, beyond the places where prostitution is practiced.

These circumstances are added to the isolation resulting from the dynamics in which the activity is carried out (rotation system between premises, little social network beyond the premises, long working hours, etc.) and the lack of information that many of the PEPs have about their most basic rights (access to health, administrative and legal issues, knowledge of resources).

This adverse scenario is forcing PEPs to adapt to a new context where demand is compromised, increasing working hours, assuming greater risks, reducing negotiation time with clients, increasing their mobility from one location to another in search of more isolated and invisible spaces, in short, less accessible to outsiders.

As psychiatrist Marga Saenz-Herrero says, these women are the "Invisibles of the Invisibles."

33.3 Mental Health of Women in Prostitution

The World Health Organization (WHO) defines mental health as a state of well-being in which the individual is aware of his or her own capabilities, can manage the normal stresses of life, can work productively and fruitfully, and is able to contribute to his or her community.

Mental health includes our emotional, psychological, and social well-being. It refers to more than the absence of mental disorders; it is an integral part of health, so much so that there is no health without mental health and it is determined by multiple factors: socioeconomic, biological, and environmental.

Poor mental health is likewise associated with rapid social change, stressful working conditions, gender discrimination, social exclusion, unhealthy lifestyles, risks of violence, poor physical health, and human rights violations [14].

The context of prostitution, with which Askabide works, is a context of social exclusion conditioned, in general, by a situation of economic precariousness sometimes and especially social, which places them in a clear situation of vulnerability compared to other groups of people and more specifically women.

These women suffer multiple and intersecting forms of discrimination, including those related to their sex, age, social class, ability, race, ethnicity, sexual orientation, sexual identity, or migratory status.

It is obvious that engaging in prostitution entails a personal maladjustment, or at least some particular personal characteristics, in most of the people who participate in it.

The world of prostitution is a world apart from the so-called "normalized" one, with its own scale of values, forms of relationship, characteristics, interests, etc.

The following are some of the issues that seem to us to be decisive when dealing with the mental health problems of women in prostitution:

33.4 Stigma

Stigma is defined as "the mark or sign imposed by the other due to inadequate social behavior." The idea of stigmatization is close to the notion of deviance, which originates from a situation of control.

From this perception, the woman who engages in prostitution is seen as a person who assumes a deviant behavior and lives on the margins of society.

The stigma discriminates and excludes MEPs from the social environment, putting them at greater risk for their mental and physical stability. In addition, this branding makes society hold MEPs responsible for all the problems they suffer from, and in particular those related to the activity.

Women are relegated to a subcategory that increases their social isolation, increases the difficulty of adapting to new lifestyles, increases the difficulty of expanding and diversifying interpersonal relationships, and developing social and work skills.

The stigma that is socially identified as a consequence of the practice of prostitution becomes the protagonist of the problems of the PEPs, making the PEPs see themselves as incapable of improving their situation, hence the importance of the social stigma-look (bad women or worse than others for practising prostitution).

Another essential element is that the stigma causes them to feel that their credibility is continually questioned by authorities (police, social services, health personnel, etc.), and at the same time they are not considered valid interlocutors.

All this has an influence on their emotional relationships: partners, families, social environment, and in many cases, they are forced to lead a double life.

33.5 Migration

As we have already mentioned, most of the women currently engaged in prostitution in Bizkaia are foreigners, 95% of the women we attend to at Askabide.

They are far away from their country of origin, and they have to integrate and adapt to another culture. There is a great feeling of uprooting in them, because they come to an unknown place, where some of them do not understand the language, and where, in many cases, their life is reduced to work.

In addition to the problems related to the practice of prostitution, they must adapt to a new society, which generates additional psychosocial problems.

The situation of administrative irregularity, the fear of repatriation, the insecurity, the difficulty of access to resources and services, and the difficulties of finding alternative employment cause them a lot of stress and anxiety.

Because of their immigrant status, they suffer from discrimination and racism.

Women who have been settled here for some time suffer from depression due to loneliness and distance from their families of origin, especially their children.

33.6 Violence

The characteristics of people in prostitution, in relation to gender diversity, sexual orientation and identity, origin, culture, administrative, and legal status, or situations of social exclusion, are determining factors in their exposure to situations of violence.

These women also face situations of violence as a result of the insecurity and lack of protection in which prostitution is carried out.

Types of violence suffered by PEPs (Askabide table)

Direct physical violence	Beating, grabbing, suffocation; sexual assault and/or sexual abuse; robbery, holding against their will, murder
Direct verbal and/or psychological violence	Insults, threats, sexist humiliations; coercion through drug and alcohol consumption; harassment of clients; accusations of theft; deception or swindling about the type and price of the service
Structural violence	Lack of credibility, revictimization, social invalidation of their testimonies and voices, criminal impunity in the face of aggressions, sexist stereotype

The feeling of lack of protection and risk of future aggressions, distrust in the system, experiences of revictimization, misinformation, or the perception of MEPs of not having credibility for practicing prostitution, are some of the reasons that make it difficult to denounce situations of violence in the exercise of prostitution. Likewise, it is necessary to contemplate and consider the risk to which they are exposed by reporting, the lack of effective security measures in these environments (clubs, apartments, street), and the feeling of defenselessness and non-reparation of the damage in the case of activating the report.

Regarding experiences of violence and discrimination, we observed with great concern a normalization and acceptance of situations of violence as part of the fact of engaging in prostitution.

33.7 Studies on Prostitution and Mental Health

If we take a brief look at different studies on prostitution and mental health, we can first mention that, depending on the position on prostitution held by the person carrying out the study, the focus will be on the existence of mental health problems in these women for different reasons.

Those who support the legalization of prostitution see it as an opportunity to improve the mental health and general welfare of women in prostitution by offering a safer and more regulated environment, thus improving working conditions and, consequently, the mental health of sex workers. They argue that legalization can reduce the stigma associated with prostitution, which could lead to greater social acceptance and, consequently, better access to mental health services and psychological support.

In addition, they argue that by establishing a legal framework, protective measures can be implemented to help prevent violence and abuse, which could also have a positive impact on the mental health of workers. This approach emphasizes the importance of providing accessible health resources and services, as well as education and prevention programs that address the specific problems faced by sex workers.

This approach emphasizes the importance of providing accessible health resources and services, as well as education and prevention programs that address the specific problems faced by sex workers.

From abolitionist positions, on the other hand, it is argued that prostitution is a form of exploitation that negatively affects the mental health of women in prostitution. From their perspective, prostitution not only involves physical risks but can also lead to mental health problems such as depression, anxiety, and trauma due to the violence, stigma, and marginalization they face. In this sense, they believe that the real solution to improve the mental health of women in prostitution is to eliminate it as an option and provide an environment that supports their holistic well-being.

In any case, studies carried out in this regard, such as the study "Post-traumatic stress disorder among female street-based sex workers in the greater Sydney area (2006) give us extremely worrying data on the impact of prostitution on mental health.

This study examines the rates of exposure to work-related violence and other traumas, as lifetime and current prevalence of post-traumatic stress disorder (PTSD) among female street sex workers. In his study, it is associated with psychiatric comorbidity, risk behaviors, and trauma history.

About 87% of sex workers reported depressive symptoms, 54% severe depressive symptoms, and 74% suicidal thoughts. In addition, 42% attempted suicide, 40% consulted a health professional in the past 6 months, and 79% of those consultations were for depression.

According to the study "Mental and physical problems of prostitution: a review of the PubMed database," Laura Guillén Javaloyes concludes that "mental and physical health in prostitution shows that conditions such as depression are greater in women in prostitution than in women in general.

Added to this are the consequences of stigma, social isolation, lack of support, drug use, and economic poverty, increasing the causes of anxiety and disorders such as post-traumatic stress disorder, addictions, suicidal thoughts, and, in general, lack of self-esteem.

The study entitled "Health care for people in prostitution Guide of recommendations for socio-health professionals in Primary Care points out that" women in prostitution refer more depression, suicidal thoughts or low quality of life, and that there are studies indicating that the prevalence of depression among these women is 62.4% [15]. There are also studies showing that these women suffer post-traumatic stress disorder (PTSD) as a result of rape sustained over time.

33.8 How Do We Intervene in Askabide?

The diversity of the group, their identities, needs, and experiences inside and outside the activity tells us about a complex group, with dualities, ambivalences, and vulnerabilities, and, at the same time, with strengths and capacity for decision and agency.

Outside the world of debates and proposals on prostitution, we find the day-to-day life of the women who carry out this activity, who live in the most diverse situations, difficult to address with a single proposal for action.

Askabide intervenes considering all the dimensions of the woman's life, including her physical and mental health, economic situation, social and family context, and any other vulnerability she may be facing.

The basic principle that guides our intervention is the recognition of the reality of each woman and the various intersections that cross them, addressing their situation from an individual dimension, respecting and valuing the identities and life experiences of each one of them; and from a socio-community dimension, with the design of flexible strategies that try to respond to all this complexity.

All of these women often face an intersection of challenges that require an approach that is specific and sensitive to their realities in order to effectively address social exclusion.

We firmly believe that it is they, the people who live the reality of prostitution on a daily basis, who must be the protagonists of their growth and destiny, reflecting on issues that affect them, proposing solutions, and making decisions that can transform the scenario in which prostitution takes place.

In this line, Askabide works to generate individual and collective empowerment processes that allow women to be autonomous in accessing different resources, in claiming and developing their rights, and in the search for and creation of their own useful tools to get out of the situation of social exclusion in which they find themselves.

An attitude of conscious respect, acknowledgement, and nonjudgment is our way of combating the stigma that these people endure.

We also take into account the importance of recognizing and respecting cultural and contextual differences that may influence a woman's experience. This includes being aware of linguistic and cultural barriers.

An attitude of conscious respect and recognition, without making value judgments, is the way we have to fight against the stigma that these people endure.

In this way, we have managed to create a meeting place for them, a place free of prejudice, where they can share their concerns with other colleagues, professionals, and volunteers on an equal footing.

With this way of doing things, we have managed to create a meeting place for them, free of prejudice, where they can share their concerns, needs, dreams, in short, their daily lives, with other colleagues, professionals, and volunteers on an equal footing.

33.9 Psychological Support Service at Askabide

Askabide has a psychological care service for women in prostitution.

In 2024, 177 of the 1235 requests we attended to at the Shelter Center were in the area of psychology.

In our intervention in this area, it is important to point out that 163 of these interventions were in what Askabide calls "psychoeducational assistance" and 14 were individual psychological support.

Askabide proposes a psychosocial intervention approach as the most effective way to address the mental problems presented by the women we serve.

Psychosocial intervention is an approach that combines psychological and social aspects to address the problems that affect the well-being of these women.

We believe that we cannot make a "therapeutic" intervention without a parallel social intervention.

We believe that our intervention must be comprehensive, taking into account both psychological factors (emotions, thoughts, and behaviors) and social factors (such as the environment, interpersonal relationships, and socioeconomic conditions) that influence the lives of these women.

This service, in which we offer emotional support, works in coordination with other professionals of the entity that address other services such as legal advice (administrative procedures, protection against exploitation, violence, etc.) and social (access to residential resources, training-labor programs, access to health services, etc.).

We guarantee a safe space where women can express themselves without fear of being judged or having their identity or situation revealed. Obviously, confidentiality is essential to create an environment of trust.

Our work with them tries to be empathetic, nonjudgmental, and non-stigmatizing. Women in prostitution often face a great deal of social stigmatization, so the service is inclusive and respectful, without condemnation.

We also include interventions at the community level, seeking to strengthen support networks and foster social cohesion.

For all these reasons, we work with a variety of techniques and approaches, such as individual or group therapy, empowerment and personal growth workshops, education and awareness programs, and recreational and cultural activities.

The main objective of our intervention is to empower these women by helping them develop skills and resources that allow them to confront their problems and improve their situation.

Finally, we would like to point out that this work methodology involves the collaboration of professionals from various disciplines, such as psychologists, social workers, educators, and physicians, to comprehensively address their needs.

33.10 Mental Health Disorders

33.10.1 Depressed Disorders

Prostitution may be associated with feelings of hopelessness, sadness, and loss of interest in previously pleasurable activities, and these women, throughout their lives, have suffered consecutive painful losses. Whose mourning has never been elaborated in a healthy way.

33.10.2 Anxiety Disorders

Uncertainty, fear of violence, rejection or stigmatization, and the very conditions in which prostitution is practiced generate high levels of anxiety in these women, which can manifest themselves as panic attacks, generalized anxiety disorders, and other related symptoms.

33.10.3 Low Self-Esteem

The experiences of rejection and discrimination affect the self-image and self-esteem of these women, leading them to feel unworthy or belittled.

33.11 Substance Use Disorders

Addiction to different drugs can be generated by the very development of the activity, not only as a personal option to escape from tensions and problems of their activity. To some extent, prostitution facilitates the consumption of substances; women must invite clients to drink and use drugs because the profits from the service are greater or because the owners of the clubs demand it.

Social Isolation Stigmatization and social rejection lead them to isolation. These women develop their lives in a reduced environment that often does not go beyond the people close to them (friends at the club, clients, managers, owners, etc.). The conditions in which prostitution takes place (schedules, lack of rest days, etc.) make it difficult to relate to other people outside this environment. Both circumstances drastically reduce any possibility of integrating into any social network outside this world.

Relationship Problems They present difficulties in interpersonal relationships, whether with partners, family, or friends, affecting their ability to establish healthy connections.

Eating and Sleeping Disorders Some women develop eating disorders as a way of coping with stress or social pressure related to body image.

Feelings of Guilt and Shame Many women experience feelings of guilt or shame about their situation, and also about disappointing their family and environment.

Defeatist Attitudes Some of these women assume that their life is a dead-end option; they recognize their personal defeat, and this causes them to behave in a completely defeatist way.

Difficulties in Emotional Regulation Constant exposure to stressful and traumatic situations hinders their ability to manage their emotions in a healthy way.

33.12 Improving Mental Health for Women in Prostitution at Askabide

- Ensure access to individual and group psychological support services, where MEPs can share experiences and emotional management strategies in a safe and nonjudgmental space.
- Work from a person-centered intervention approach, where, through empathy and unconditional acceptance, women feel valued and understood.
- Many of the achievements in our work have to do with the "bond" we establish with them. These are very damaged women, and it is very difficult for them to establish healthy bonds.
- Creating safe and welcoming environments where women feel comfortable sharing their experiences. Thus, through empowerment, we promote self-esteem, self-confidence, and coping skills of these women.

At Askabide, we continuously develop "workshops" on social skills, leadership, personal development, and empowerment, in which we provide information on mental health, rights, and available resources that empower women and help them make informed decisions about their well-being.

- To develop information, awareness and social denunciation projects about the situation of this group. We believe that combating stigma is key to improving their mental health. We have already mentioned that social rejection and criminalization generate anxiety, depression, and feelings of isolation in these women.
- Ensure that these women have access to health services, both physical and mental, including not only sexual and reproductive health, but also general medical care and disease prevention programs.
- Offer educational and training programs for MEPs who demand them, thus enabling them to improve their employment opportunities. This can give them

more control over their lives and finances, which in turn can reduce stress and anxiety.

- Ensure that they carry out this activity in an environment free of violence and exploitation.
- Encourage the creation of support networks among the MEPs. Encourage the creation of peer support groups that allow them to share coping strategies and reduce feelings of isolation.
- Ensure that MEPs have access to legal support and protection from violence, exploitation, or abuse, both within and outside the prostitution environment.

References

1. Research Study "Gender violence and prostitution", Askabide. Ed. Mensajero; 2006.
2. Research Study "The profile of prostitution clients in Bizkaia", Askabide. Ed. Mensajero; 2008.
3. Elezkano L. (Coord.). Let me tell you: testimonies of women who have suffered violence in the practice of prostitution. Askabide; 2020.
4. Meneses G. (Coord.). Trafficking of women and girls for sexual exploitation in Euskadi: needs and proposals. Emakunde; 2021.
5. Castaños M, Meneses C. Research Study "Labor insertion of women victims of gender violence". Soledad Valle, University of Deusto; 2007. p. 2015.
6. Study "The incidence of human trafficking in the basque autonomous community", Ararteko; 2016.
7. Report "Challenges in advancing towards effective protection of women and girls in situations of trafficking in Euskadi from an international protection approach", CEAR Euskadi; 2019.
8. Research on "The situation of women victims of trafficking in Spain: degree of compliance by authorities in their obligation to detect, identify, and protect potential victims of trafficking, especially among migrant women arriving in Spain", Research and Internal Policy Area of Amnesty International; 2019.
9. Study "Hidden homelessness in the group of people engaged in prostitution and/or in situations of social exclusion", Askabide and University of Deusto; 2019.
10. Study "Prostitution in the digital age: the context of Bizkaia", Askabide and UPV, Social Education; 2022.
11. Association for the Prevention, Reintegration, and Care of Prostituted Women (APRAMP). Prostitution: basic keys to reflect on a problem; 2011.
12. Prostitution situation and mental health: contributions to consider interventions from social work. Margen: J Soc Work Soc Sci. 2018;91:5–11.
13. Roxburgh A, Degenhardt L, Copeland J. Posttraumatic stress disorder among female street-based sex workers in the greater Sydney area, Australia. BMC Psychiatry. 2006;6(1):24.
14. World Health Organization. (2018). World Mental Health Day: Mental health matters.
15. Yuen WW-Y, Tran L, Wong CK-H, Holroyd E, Tang CS, Chai-Wai W. Psychological health and HIV transmission among female sex workers: a systematic review and meta-analysis. AIDS Care. 2016;28(7):816–24.

GPSR Compliance

The European Union's (EU) General Product Safety Regulation (GPSR) is a set of rules that requires consumer products to be safe and our obligations to ensure this.

If you have any concerns about our products, you can contact us on ProductSafety@springernature.com

In case Publisher is established outside the EU, the EU authorized representative is:

Springer Nature Customer Service Center GmbH
Europaplatz 3
69115 Heidelberg, Germany

Batch number: 10726058

Printed by Printforce, the Netherlands